CANCER AND CHEMOTHERAPY

Volume II

CANCER AND CHEMOTHERAPY

Volume I.   Introduction to Neoplasia and
                      Antineoplastic Chemotherapy

Volume II.   Introduction to Clinical Oncology

Volume III.   Antineoplastic Agents

CANCER AND CHEMOTHERAPY

Volume II

Introduction to Clinical Oncology

Edited by

Stanley T. Crooke, M.D., Ph.D.

Research and Development
Smith Kline & French Laboratories
Philadelphia, Pennsylvania
    and
Department of Pharmacology
Baylor College of Medicine
Houston, Texas

Archie W. Prestayko, Ph.D.

Research and Development
Bristol Laboratories
Syracuse, New York
    and
Department of Pharmacology
Baylor College of Medicine
Houston, Texas

Editorial Assistant

Nancy Alder

1981

ACADEMIC PRESS

A Subsidiary of Harcourt Brace Jovanovich, Publishers

New York   London   Toronto   Sydney   San Francisco

ACADEMIC PRESS, INC.
111 Fifth Avenue, New York, New York 10003

United Kingdom Edition published by
ACADEMIC PRESS, INC. (LONDON) LTD.
24/28 Oval Road, London NW1 7DX

Library of Congress Cataloging in Publication Data
Main entry under title:

Cancer and chemotherapy.

   Includes bibliographies and index.
   CONTENTS: v. 1. Introduction to neoplasia and
antineoplastic chemotherapy.--v. 2. Introduction
to clinical oncology.
   1. Cancer--Chemotherapy. 2. Antineoplastic
agents. I. Crooke, Stanley T. II. Prestayko,
Archie W. [DNLM: 1. Neoplasms--Drug therapy.
2. Antineoplastic agents. QZ 267 C214]
RC271.C5C285   616.99'4061   79-8536
ISBN 0-12-197802-8 (v. 2)

PRINTED IN THE UNITED STATES OF AMERICA

81 82 83 84   9 8 7 6 5 4 3 2 1

CONTENTS

List of Contributors   xi

General Preface   xiii

Preface to Volume II   xv

PART I   LEUKEMIAS AND LYMPHOMAS

1   The Acute Leukemias

Arlan J. Gottlieb
     I. Introduction   3
    II. Incidence   4
   III. Classification   4
   IV. Predisposing Factors   8
    V. Presenting Features   9
   VI. Differential Diagnosis   10
  VII. Laboratory Features   11
 VIII. General Therapeutic Considerations   12
   IX. General Clinical Considerations   14
    X. Prognostic Factors   20
   XI. Conclusions   22
      References   22

2   Hairy Cell Leukemia

Frederick R. Davey
     I. Definition   25
    II. Incidence with Age and Sex Ratio   25
   III. Pathology   26
   IV. Pathogenesis   26
    V. Clinical Features   28
   VI. Laboratory Features   29

VII. Treatment	33
VIII. Course of Disease	35
IX. Summary	35
References	36

3 Chronic Lymphocytic Leukemia

Frederick R. Davey

I. Definition	39
II. Epidemiology	40
III. Etiologic Features	40
IV. Pathologic Observations	41
V. Pathogenesis	42
VI. Clinical Features	44
VII. Laboratory Features	45
VIII. Differential Diagnosis	47
IX. Treatment	50
X. Prognostic Factors	51
XI. Course of Disease	53
References	54

4 Chronic Myelocytic Leukemia

Kanti R. Rai and Arthur Sawitsky

I. Special Characteristics	57
II. Clinical Features	59
III. Clinical Course	60
IV. Summary and Conclusions	67
References	68

5 The Lymphomas

John M. Bennett

I. Introduction	69
II. Hodgkin's Disease	71
III. Non-Hodgkin's Lymphomas	82
IV. Conclusion	94
References	94

PART II   SOLID TUMORS

6 Carcinoma of the Breast

James F. Holland

I. Introduction	99
II. Incidence and Causative Factors	100
III. Pathology	101
IV. Clinical Presentation	102
V. Prognostic Features	102
VI. Clinical Course of Metastatic Breast Cancer	103
VII. Surgical Therapy	104

VIII. Radiation Therapy 105
IX. Hormonal Therapy 106
X. Chemotherapy 106
XI. Discussion 109
References 110

7 Clinical Presentations of Gastrointestinal Cancer
Philip Schein
I. Large-Bowel Carcinoma 113
II. Carcinoma of the Pancreas 117
III. Carcinoma of the Stomach 121
References 123

8 Cancers of the Head and Neck
Montague Lane
I. Introduction 125
II. Incidence 127
III. Etiology 127
IV. Histopathology and Spread 129
V. Clinical Manifestations 130
VI. Diagnosis 142
VII. Clinical Staging 142
VIII. Management 143
IX. Conclusions 145
References 146

9 Carcinoma of the Lung
Robert L. Comis
I. Introduction 147
II. Classification 147
III. Evaluation of Lung Cancer 150
IV. Management of Non-Small-Cell Anaplastic Cancer 153
V. Management of Metastatic Non-Small-Cell
Anaplastic Lung Cancer 156
VI. Evaluation and Management of Small-Cell
Anaplastic Carcinoma 158
VII. Conclusion 163
References 163

10 Clinical Characteristics of Cancer in the Brain
and Spinal Cord
Victor A. Levin and Charles B. Wilson
I. Introduction 167
II. Tumors of the Brain 168
III. Meningeal Carcinomatosis 190
IV. Tumors of the Spinal Cord 192
References 197

11 Genitourinary Cancer
    R. Bruce Bracken
        I. Introduction   200
       II. Renal Carcinoma   201
     III. Carcinoma of the Renal Pelvis   206
     IV. Carcinoma of the Ureter   210
      V. Female Urethral Carcinoma   212
     VI. Male Urethral Carcinoma   216
    VII. Penile Carcinoma   218
   VIII. Testicular Tumors   222
     IX. Bladder Cancer   231
      X. Prostate Cancer   237
         References   241

12 Gynecological Cancers
    Laurence H. Baker
        I. Introduction   243
       II. Ovarian Cancer   245
     III. Cancer of the Cervix   250
     IV. Endometrial Carcinoma   254
         References   255

13 Malignant Melanoma
    Frank E. Smith
        I. Introduction   257
       II. Epidemiology   258
     III. Pathology   259
     IV. Clinical Findings   265
      V. Diagnosis   268
     VI. Prognosis   269
    VII. Treatment   270
   VIII. Conclusion   272
         References   272

14 The Sarcomas
    Robert S. Benjamin
        I. Introduction   275
       II. Diagnosis   276
     III. Soft Tissue Sarcomas   277
     IV. Sarcomas of Bone   284
      V. Conclusion   290
         References   290

15 Pediatric Cancer
    Lawrence Helson
        I. Introduction   295
       II. Tumors   296
     III. Conclusions   315

PART III   NUTRITIONAL AND INFECTIOUS DISEASE ASPECTS OF CANCER

16   Infectious Complications in the Cancer Patient
Gerald P. Bodey
      I. Introduction   319
     II. Types of Infection in Cancer Patients   328
    III. Diagnosis of and Therapy for Infection   343
     IV. Therapy for Nonbacterial Infections   353
      V. Granulocyte Transfusion   354
     VI. Prophylaxis of Infection   356
    VII. Conclusions   359
          References   359

17   Nutrition in Cancer Patients
Brian F. Issell
      I. Introduction   363
     II. Cancer–Malnutrition Associations   363
    III. Mechanisms of Cancer-Associated Malnutrition   364
     IV. Advantages of Nutritonal Support   365
      V. Methods of Nutritional Support   368
     VI. Conclusion   369
          References   369

Index   371

LIST OF CONTRIBUTORS

Numbers in parentheses indicate the pages on which the authors' contributions begin.

Laurence H. Baker (243), Harper Hospital, Wayne State University, Detroit, Michigan 48201

Robert S. Benjamin (275), University of Texas System Cancer Center, Texas Medical Center, Houston, Texas 77030

John M. Bennett (69), Cancer Center of the University of Rochester Medical Center, Rochester, New York 14642

Gerald P. Bodey (319), Chemotherapy Branch and Infectious Diseases, M. D. Anderson Hospital and Tumor Institute, University of Texas System Cancer Center, Texas Medical Center, Houston, Texas 77030

R. Bruce Bracken (199), Department of Urology, M. D. Anderson Hospital and Tumor Institute, University of Texas System Cancer Center, Texas Medical Center, Houston, Texas 77030

Robert L. Comis (147), Section of Oncology, State University of New York–Upstate Medical Center, Syracuse, New York 13210

Frederick R. Davey (25, 39), Pathology Department, State University of New York–Upstate Medical Center, Syracuse, New York 13210

Arlan J. Gottlieb (3), Section of Hematology, State University of New York–Upstate Medical Center, Syracuse, New York 13210

Lawrence Helson (295), Pediatric Cancer Research Laboratory, Memorial Sloan-Kettering Cancer Center, New York, New York 10029

James F. Holland (99), Department of Neoplastic Diseases, Mount Sinai Medical Center, New York, New York 10029

Brian F. Issell (363), Clinical Cancer Research, Bristol Laboratories, Syracuse, New York 13201

Montague Lane (125), Department of Pharmacology, Baylor College of Medicine, Houston, Texas 77025

Victor A. Levin (167), Brain Tumor Research Center, University of California School of Medicine, San Francisco, California 94143

Kanti R. Rai (57), Division of Hematology/Oncology, Long Island Jewish–Hillside Medical Center, New Hyde Park, New York 11042, and Health Sciences Center, State University of New York, Stonybrook, New York 11790

Arthur Sawitsky (57), Division of Hematology/Oncology, Long Island Jewish–Hillside Medical Center, New Hyde Park, New York 11042, and Health Sciences Center, State University of New York, Stonybrook, New York 11790

Philip Schein (113), Section of Hematology, Vincent T. Lombardi Cancer Research Center, Georgetown University School of Medicine, Washington, D.C. 20037

Frank E. Smith (257), Department of Pharmacology, Baylor College of Medicine, Houston, Texas 77025

Charles B. Wilson (167), Department of Neurological Surgery, Mount Sinai Medical Center, San Francisco, CA 94143

GENERAL PREFACE

With the rapid development of new chemotherapeutic approaches and new agents used in the treatment of patients with cancer, a basic instructional workbook describing in some detail the drugs currently employed, current therapeutic approaches, and agents in development is essential. However, to understand fully cancer chemotherapeutic agents and their use, one must understand various aspects of anticancer drug development, the molecular and cellular biology of malignant disease, and the clinical characteristics of the most common neoplasms. Only with this information can a detailed discussion of anticancer drugs be presented.

It was with these thoughts in mind that *Cancer and Chemotherapy* was developed; the goal: to provide in a single source the information necessary for a detailed understanding of the major antineoplastic agents. Thus, Volume I is designed to provide the fundamental information concerning the molecular and cellular biology of cancer, carcinogenesis, and the basics of anticancer drug development. Volume II will provide clinical information relative to the most common human malignancies and discusses the use of chemotherapeutics in the treatment of those diseases. In Volume III the antineoplastic agents will be discussed. It contains reviews of all the major anticancer drugs and a review of agents in development. Furthermore, in two sections—the molecular pharmacology of selected antitumor drugs and the clinical pharmacology of selected antitumor drugs—significantly more detailed discussions of certain drugs are provided. These drugs were selected because they have interesting characteristics, and adequate data are available to allow a more detailed discussion. These two sections should be of particular value to individuals who have an interest in certain aspects of particular drugs.

Stanley T. Crooke
Archie W. Prestayko

PREFACE TO VOLUME II

In Volume II, leading oncologists present a review of the clinical features of the major tumor categories. Each chapter discusses the history, etiology, pathology, course of the disease, prognosis, accepted therapies, and the role of chemotherapy in advanced disease. The information presented in this volume is designed to provide a basic framework to allow better understanding of the antineoplastic drugs discussed in Volume III.

Stanley T. Crooke
Archie W. Prestayko

Part I
Leukemias and Lymphomas

1

THE ACUTE LEUKEMIAS
Arlan J. Gottlieb

I.	Introduction	3
II.	Incidence	4
III.	Classification	4
IV.	Predisposing Factors	8
V.	Presenting Features	9
VI.	Differential Diagnosis	10
VII.	Laboratory Features	11
VIII.	General Therapeutic Considerations	12
IX.	General Clinical Considerations	14
	A. Thrombocytopenic Bleeding	14
	B. Infection	15
	C. Central Nervous System Leukemia	18
	D. Leukostasis	20
X.	Prognostic Factors	20
XI.	Conclusions	22
	References	22

I. INTRODUCTION

The acute leukemias are primary malignant proliferations of the precursors of the formed blood elements. Characteristically, there is a progressive infiltration of the bone marrow, lymph nodes, and other organs by the immature neoplastic cells. As a consequence of the proliferation and accumulation of the leukemic cells in the bone marrow, the clinical course of leukemia is associated with a depletion of the normal cellular constituents of the blood. Thus, anemia, granulocytopenia, and thrombocytopenia—with resultant weakness, increased susceptibility to infection, and bleeding—become part of the clinical picture of acute leukemia. In the vast majority of cases, acute leukemia involves either the lymphocytic cell line (acute lymphocytic leukemia) or the granulocyte-erythroid–megakaryocytic cell line (acute non-lymphocytic leukemia).

CANCER AND CHEMOTHERAPY, VOL. II
3

II. INCIDENCE

The incidence of acute leukemia is between 3.5 and 5 cases per 100,000 population. Acute lymphocytic leukemia (ALL) is the most common malignancy of childhood and accounts for approximately 80–90% of the acute leukemia in the pediatric population. Ninety percent of patients with acute non-lymphocytic leukemia (ANLL) are adults. One-third of these patients are over 60 years old (Fraumeni, 1967). Acute leukemia has been thought to be rare in blacks. However, perhaps as a result of the increased entry of black patients into the health care delivery system, a rising incidence of acute leukemia in blacks has been recently noted.

III. CLASSIFICATION

The classification of, and distinction between, the acute leukemias has in the past been made on the basis of cell morphology. The morphologic features used to distinguish ANLL from ALL are given in Table I. The hematopathologist considers both the morphology of the individual neoplastic cell and the features of the cellular environment. Thus, morphologic similarity between a neoplastic blast and a cell that clearly contains promyelocytic granulation helps establish the myeloid nature of the blast.

The granulocyte, erythrocyte, and megakaryocyte—but not the lymphocyte—share a common cell of origin (committed stem cell), which normally undergoes differentiation and proliferation when appropriately stimulated *in vivo*. In acute leukemia, differentiation is aborted and proliferative capacity retained and the effects of neoplastic transformation are frequently shared by all the progeny of the transformed stem cell. For these reasons, disturbances in the morphology and maturation of the erythroid series and of the megakaryocyte are often observed in the ANLLs. A delay in nuclear, as compared to cytoplasmic, maturation (as might be expected with a disorder involving DNA) and morphologic abnormalities of the nuclear chromatin are seen. These changes are categorized as "cytonuclear dissociation" and "megaloblastic changes." The presence of these disturbances of morphology, which are similar to those observed in nutritional deficiencies of B_{12} or folic acid, weigh in favor of a diagnosis of ANLL as opposed to ALL.

The distinction between ANLL and ALL on the basis of morphology alone is not always accurate. Increased reliance has now been placed upon a series of cytochemical reactions that apparently allow a more objective evaluation and characterization of the neoplastic (blast) form. As compiled by a French–American–British (FAB) cooperative group, these cytochemical reactions have been employed in an alternative classification of the acute leukemias which

TABLE I

Morphologic and Immunologic Distinction of Acute Lymphocytic Leukemia (ALL) from Acute Non-lymphocytic Leukemia (ANLL)[a]

Morphology	
ALL	ANLL
High nuclear/cytoplasmic ratio	More cytoplasm
One or two nucleoli	Two or more nucleoli
Clumped chromatin	Fine lacelike chromatin
Homogenous cell population	More heterogeneous cell population with microblasts
Round nuclei	Auer rods
	Granules in primitive cells
	Nuclear detail similar in blast and promyelocyte
	Megaloblastosis and red cell dysplasia
	Folded, indented nuclei (myelo-monocytic)

Immunology

Surface membrane immunoglobulin
Intracytoplasmic immunoglobulin
Immune or nonimmune rosette
  formation (monocyte Fc receptor
  must be excluded)

[a] Adapted from Keating et al. (1977).

appears logical, useful, and reproducible (Table II) (Gralnick et al., 1977; Bennett et al., 1976).

Histochemistry also serves as an aid in distinguishing the malignant cell of ANLL from that of ALL (Table II). Additionally, identification of lymphoid cells by the presence of cell surface characteristics such as surface-membrane immunoglobulin, complement, and the Fc receptor, or the capacity of the cell to form rosettes with sheep erythrocytes, may also be of diagnostic value. Unfortunately for the nosologist, the malignant lymphocytes of approximately three-fourths of the cases of ALL lack the distinct surface membrane characteristics that are presently identifiable. Consequently they are classed as "null" or non-T, non-B lymphoblasts (Davey and Gottlieb, 1974; Belpomme et al., 1977; Brouet and Seligmann, 1978). The null cell may, perhaps, be distinguished by specific antisera (Greaves et al., 1975). At times, the presence of intracytoplasmic immunoglobulin may be demonstrated ("pre-B cell") (Vogler et al., 1978).

TABLE II

Cytochemical Reactions in the Acute Leukemias[a,b]

| FAB classification | Myelocytic | | Promy-elocytic | Myelomono-cytic | Monocytic | Lympho-cytic |
	M_1	M_2	M_3	M_4	M_5	$L_{1,2,3}$
Histochemical stain						
Peroxidase	1+	3+	3+	2+	+/−	−
Sudan black B	1+	3+	3+	2+	+/−	−
NASDA	1+	2+	2+	3+	3+	+/−
NASDA-fluoride	1+	2+	2+	2+/1+	+/−	+/−
PAS	+/−	1+	1+	2+/1+	2+/1+	3+/−

[a] Cellular reactivity is classed as follows: 1+ indicates greater than 3% of blast forms are reactive; 2+, greater than 25% of blast forms are reactive; and 3+ indicates greater than 50% of the malignant cells are reactive with the cytochemical stains. Naphthol chloroacetate (NASDA) was used as a substrate to determine cellular esterase activity.

[b] Adapted from Gralnick et al. (1977).

The various nomenclatures applied to the morphologic subgroups of the ANLLs appear to have had a rather constant and rapid growth rate. Included are the myelocytic, myelomonocytic, promyelocytic, monocytic, and erythroid leukemic variants of acute non-lymphocytic leukemias. To some extent, these morphologic groupings are associated with characteristic clinical signs. For example, numerous Auer rods and disseminated intravascular coagulation have been associated with promyelocytic leukemia, whereas gingival hypertrophy and heavy lysozyminuria is most commonly observed with acute monocytic and myelomonocytic leukemia. Nonetheless, a distinct pattern of therapeutic response has not emerged from the older nosology of ANLL. The newer proposed classification appears to offer greater coherency and reproducibility than those previously employed.

According to the French–American–British (FAB) classification, the acute non-lymphocytic leukemias would now be grouped as follows (Table II):

M_1 Those cases of acute myelocytic leukemia showing minimal evidence of differentiation along the granulocytic pathway

M_2 Acute myelocytic leukemia. Some granulocytic maturation to the promyelocyte and beyond is evident

M_3 Acute hypergranular promyelocytic leukemia

M_4 Acute myelomonocytic leukemia; usually characterized by monocytoid cells in the peripheral blood and a more myeloblastic component in the marrow

M_5 "Pure" monocytic leukemia

M_6 Acute erythroleukemia

The degree to which this newer classification will replace the multitude of terms now in common parlance and whether prognostic significance may be assigned the subclasses of ANLL must, however, await the test of time.

The diagnostic criteria for ANLL have also been addressed (Gralnick *et al.*, 1977; Bennett *et al.*, 1976). It has been suggested that the minimum number of marrow blasts and promyelocytes required for a diagnosis of acute leukemia be set liberally high (greater than 50% blasts plus promyelocytes). Generally, greater than 30% blasts plus promyelocytes in a bone marrow in which dysmyelopoiesis and dyserythropoiesis are also evident, has been previously accepted. The newer classification would thus tend to minimize the number of cases of subacute leukemia, "preleukemia," and other dysmyelopoietic states that would be diagnosed as acute leukemia, but would exclude some cases of acute leukemia.

The FAB classification of acute lymphocytic leukemia is summarized below (Bennett *et al.*, 1976):

L_1 There is a homogenous cell population. Nucleoli are sparse and nuclear chromatin is dense. Approximately three-fourths of the cases are of the null cell type. The L_1 type represents three-fourths of the cases of ALL encountered in children and one-half those seen in adults.

L_2 The cell population is more heterogeneous, with large and small lymphoblasts with prominent nucleoli. At times the nuclei are distinctly clefted. Surface markers are null in two-thirds of the cases. Histochemical reactions for acid phosphatase and terminal transferase activity are often present in the T cell form (Gralnick *et al.*, 1977).

L_3 This designation is reserved for leukemia characterized by a large, highly malignant-appearing cell with prominent nucleoli and intensely basophilic cytoplasm. The neoplastic cell closely resembles the malignant lymphocyte found in Burkitt's lymphoma. There are often cytoplasmic vacuoles, which stain brightly with Oil Red. These cells usually display surface membrane immunoglobulin and are of the "B" cell type.

It must be noteu that the presence of distinctive surface markers on the leukemic lymphocyte appears to affect adversely the response to therapy and thus prognosis (Belpomme *et al.*, 1977). Prognostic differences may also be emerging between the L_1 and L_2 types of childhood ALL (Keleti *et al.*, 1978). The poor prognosis of the Burkitt's cell line (L_3) has been evident for a number of years. It is clear that the implications of the newer immunologic and morphologic subdivision of the acute lymphocytic leukemias will continue to develop rapidly over the next several years.

The varieties of "preleukemic" or "dysmyelopoietic" syndromes that have a high frequency of developing into acute myeloid leukemia have also been codified.

Although beyond the scope of the current discussion, excellent reviews are available (Linman and Saarni, 1974; Linman and Bagby, 1978; Gralnick *et al.*, 1977).

IV. PREDISPOSING FACTORS

There appears to be a four- to sevenfold increase in the incidence of acute leukemia in first-degree relatives of patients with acute leukemia. The likelihood that the monozygotic twin of a patient with acute leukemia will also develop acute leukemia is almost 25% when the leukemia is acquired before the age of 10 (Miller, 1971). The incidence of acute leukemia has been reported to be increased in Down's symdrome and in several other developmental disorders (Bloomfield and Brunning, 1976). A clear distinction should be made, however, between the increased incidence of acute lymphocytic leukemia and the benign, spontaneously reversible, inappropriate granulopoiesis that is observed in newborns with Down's syndrome.

Exposure to ionizing radiation is a clear predisposing factor in the development of acute non-lymphocytic leukemia. An increased incidence has been found in the survivors of atomic catastrophies and in patients treated with irradiation for ankylosing spondylitis and other disorders (Cronkite *et al.*, 1960). X-Ray pelvimetry of pregnant women has been shown to increase the risk of leukemia in the offspring by almost 40% (MacMahon, 1962).

Bone marrow or chromosomal injury after exposure to a variety of chemicals has been associated with the development of ANLL. Nonetheless, the most reliable current data incriminate only extensive benzene exposure (Bloomfield and Brunning, 1976). Most notable is the incidence of acute leukemia in shoe workers in Istanbul, which was 2–3 times greater than anticipated (Askoy *et al.*, 1974).

The increased incidence of acute non-lymphocytic leukemia observed in patients treated for a variety of malignant and premalignant disorders is distressing. Some diseases such as polycythemia vera and multiple myeloma carry a clear predisposition to the development of acute non-lymphocytic leukemia. In some cases (Landaw, 1976; Rosner and Grunwald, 1974, 1975; Rosner, 1976), ANLL has been found in the patient at presentation (Rosner and Grunwald, 1974). The therapeutic use of alkylating agents in particular, such as phenylalanine mustard, appears to impose an additional risk factor. A report by Bergsagel *et al.*, (1979) has indicated that the actuarial risk of developing acute leukemia in patients treated for multiple myeloma is 17.4% of survivors at 50 months.

Leukemia has also been observed in several other disorders wherein acute non-lymphocytic leukemia is not otherwise part of the natural history. Included in this latter group are Hodgkin's disease, non-Hodgkin's lymphoma, and ovarian carcinoma (Canellos *et al.*, 1975; Coleman *et al.*, 1977; Reimer *et al.*, 1978; Pajak *et al.*, 1978). It has been estimated that the incidence of ANLL in patients treated for Hodgkin's disease with chemotherapy and/or radiotherapy may approach 5% in the group at long-term risk. In an ongoing study of Cancer and Leukemia Group B (CALGB) (Pajak *et al.*, 1978), the incidence of ANLL in 1850 patients treated for Hodgkin's disease in studies commencing in 1966 is 1%. The median time to development of ANLL was over 6 years. The incidence of ANLL seems highest in the group treated with both chemotherapy and radiotherapy (Cannellos *et al.*, 1975; Pajak *et al.*, 1978). The development of ALL other lymphatic malignancies appears to be prevalent in the immunodeficiency diseases and as an apparent consequence of medication that is immunosuppressive (Gatti and Good, 1971; Louie and Schwartz, 1978).

Although chromosomal analysis has failed to reveal any specific chromosomal abnormalities in acute leukemia, to date, some 50% of patients with ANLL display a variety of chromosomal translocations, breaks, or chromosomal loss. Several repetitive patterns have now been identified (Rowley, 1978). The role of X-ray exposure and alkylating agents in inducing chromosomal damage has drawn extensive comment. Almost 90% of cases of chronic granulocytic leukemia display a consistent chromosomal translocation (the Philadelphia chromosome). The incidence of termination of this disorder in acute leukemia (blastic crisis) is striking. It is worthy of note that the appearance of blast crisis is usually preceded or accompanied by the appearance of additional chromosomal aberrations (Lilleyman *et al.*, 1978).

V. PRESENTING FEATURES

The clinical signs and symptoms of acute leukemia arise from the compromise of normal function consequent to the progressive infiltration of the bone marrow and other organs by malignant cells. Included are common nonspecific signs and symptoms such as fatigue, malaise, weight loss, anemia, and fever. Other signs and symptoms are more specific and may often be related to leukemia or its consequences. Thus, granulocytopenia may result in acute or refractory recurrent infection and may be represented by a spectrum of illnesses ranging from pneumonitis to ulcerative stomatitis, gingivitis, and perianal abscesses.

Clinical problems related to thrombocytopenia, such as purpura, hematomata, and retinal and central nervous system hemorrhage, occur frequently. Pain may result from organ enlargement. Notable is the periarticular and sternal pain resulting from bone marrow, periosteal, and synovial involvement. Cranial nerve palsies, headache, or an altered state of consciousness may appear, because of central nervous system involvement by the leukemic process. A stiff neck or papilledema may also be present.

VI. DIFFERENTIAL DIAGNOSIS

The presence of acute leukemia is almost invariably suggested by analysis of the peripheral blood counts and blood film. In a review of the experience at M.D. Anderson Hospital, an initial hemoglobin of less than 10 gm% was observed in 60% of patients presenting with acute leukemia (Keating *et al.*, 1977). The white blood count was less than 5000/mm³ in 30% of the patients; between 5000 and 10,000/mm³ in 15%; between 10,000 and 50,000/mm³ in 30%; and greater than 50,000/mm³ in 25% of the patients. The platelet count was less than 150,000/mm³ in 85% of the patients and less than 50,000 in 40%. Blast cells could be demonstrated in a peripheral blood flim of 90% of patients with appropriate examination.

A diagnosis of acute leukemia may often be strongly suggested by examination of the blood smear, particularly when the rodlike inclusions (Auer bodies) diagnostic of ANLL are found within the abnormal granulocyte precursor. Nonetheless, the serious nature and implications of the diagnosis require complete documentation. For this purpose, an adequate bone marrow aspirate and biopsy should be obtained. Examination of the bone marrow will almost invariably show hypercellularity with a preponderance of immature cellular forms. As previously noted, morphologic abnormalities of the megakaryocyte and erythrocyte series are usually seen in the bone marrow of patients with acute non-lymphocytic leukemia.

Differentiation between acute non-lymphocytic leukemia and a leukemoid reaction, or overwhelming sepsis with marked granulocytic hyperplasia and a shift to less mature granulocyte precursors, is usually not diffucult. A diagnostic, or at least a nosologic, problem may arise when one of the various dysmyelopoetic or dyserythropoetic syndromes is encountered (Gralnick *et al.*, 1977; Linman and Saarni, 1974; Linman and Bagby, 1978). At times these syndromes may prove to be clearly and rapidly preleukemic in nature, whereas on other occasions they may run a more stable, protracted course. The slow evolution of subacute leukemia, wherein some granulocyte maturation is retained in association with 10–30% abnormal blast forms, may present a problem regarding the timing of therapeutic intervention.

The erythroleukemic variant (M_6) of acute non-lymphocytic leukemia deserves particular mention (Hetzel and Gee, 1978). The disorder is characterized by a bone marrow that displays abnormal erythropoesis with erythroid hyperplasia, severe nuclear fragmentation, and "budding." The bizarre megaloblastic changes that are observed are usually most marked in the erythroid series. The abnormal red cell precursors may be strongly positive to periodic acid–schiff (PAS) stain. Ringed sideroblasts and an increased number of myeloblasts are often present. The morphology of the marrow erythrocytic, granulocytic, and megakaryocytic series and the immaturity of the granulocytic series in the peripheral blood film are usually sufficient to suggest the presence of a leukemic process on a single examination, and the rapid progression to a more typical picture of an acute myeloid leukemia makes serial diagnostic evaluation moot.

However, the evolution of this disorder may be more protracted (chronic erythemic meylosis). In these circumstances the diagnostic distinctions between the nutritional megaloblastic anemias, the untoward effects of drugs or environmental toxins, and the refractory anemias and leukemia may require successive evaluation. The elevation of serum lactic dehydrogenase (isoenzymes 1 and 2) found in the majority of patients with nutritional megaloblastic anemia helps to distinguish these patients. Most clinicians will attempt to document the presence of a nutritional deficiency and institute a therapeutic trial of vitamin B_{12} and folic acid and perhaps pyridoxine.

The differential diagnosis of acute lymphocytic leukemia includes the various causes of marked atypical lymphocytosis (e.g., infectious mononucleosis, cytomegalovirus infection, pertussis, or toxoplasmosis). In these cases the bone marrow biopsy and aspiration fails to show infiltration by immature lymphocytes. At times, only lymphocytes may be obtained on bone marrow aspiration of a patient with aplastic anemia. An adequate bone marrow biopsy will usually clarify this apparent dilemma.

Blood and bone marrow involvement with lymphoblasts is commonly seen in the poorly differentiated lymphosarcomas. A more focal, rather than diffuse, pattern is often seen on marrow biopsy in these disorders. The clinical presentation and history of the patient will often provide additional information regarding classification. For most, if not all, of the poorly differentiated lymphomas, bone marrow involvement represents a poor prognostic finding. Thus, as therapy for many of these latter disorders becomes more aggressive, the distinction between them and ALL may become less important than it has seemed to be in the past.

VII. LABORATORY FEATURES

Hyperuricemia arising as a consequence of an increased metabolic turnover of nuclear protein is commonly observed. This feature of the disease should be treated by blocking the *de novo* synthesis of uric acid from xanthine and hypoxanthine with allopurinol and, where appropriate, urinary alkalinization. A consequence of hyperuricemia, which may be exaggerated by cell lysis during therapy, is the syndrome of renal insufficiency secondary to the deposition of uric acid crystals in the renal tubule. Doses of 600 mg or greater of allopurinol and generous hydration are commonly employed to lower abruptly the uric acid when renal compromise is threatened or when the prompt institution of therapy is mandated despite marked hyperuricemia.

Hypercalcemia—with its metabolic consequences of polyuria, polydipsia, dehydration, and disturbances of consciousness—is uncommonly encountered. With rapid cell lysis following therapy, hypocalcemia and hypomagnesemia may supervene as a result of the release of intracellular phosphates into the plasma. Although more common in ALL, particularly the L_3 form, the "tumor lysis" syndrome may also be seen when ANLL is associated with markedly elevated peripheral white blood counts.

A variety of renal tubular defects may also be observed in ANLL. Most commonly, hypokalemia, which requires potassium supplementation, presents problems in clinical care of the patient (O'Regan et al., 1977).

Disturbances in the fluid phase of blood coagulation (as distinct from those changes related to thrombocytopenia) are not uncommon. Prolongation of the prothrombin time, partial thromboplastin time, and thrombin time, in association with hypofibrinogenemia and an elevation of fibrin split products, may be seen as a consequence of disseminated intravascular coagulation. This syndrome is frequently encountered in the hypergranular promyelocytic variant (M_3) of ANLL, and may relate to the clot-promoting activity of the blast cell itself (Gralnick and Sultan, 1975). This complication appears to be best treated by rapid and aggressive cytolytic therapy of the acute leukemia. The supplemental use of heparin in addition to the replacement of coagulation factors and platelets in the treatment of the syndrome of paracoagulation has been advocated (Gralnick and Sultan, 1975; Collins et al., 1978).

VIII. GENERAL THERAPEUTIC CONSIDERATIONS

The survival of the patient with acute leukemia is most influenced by the attainment of a complete clinical and hematologic remission. Although some prolongation of survival is observed in patients who achieve partial remission, long-term survival is seen almost exclusively in patients achieving and maintaining a complete therapeutic response.

Contemporary therapy for acute leukemia consists of an induction and a maintenance phase. These phases of therapy are considered from the standpoint of cell kinetics and leukemic cell kill elsewhere in this volume. The general therapeutic strategy is to employ combinations of agents for remission induction followed by cyclic drug combinations in order to maintain the remission.

The goal of induction therapy is the rapid and complete obliteration of all clinically evident disease. Complete remission is indicated by (1) a bone marrow of normal or near-normal cellularity, containing no more than 10% blast forms, and at least 25% normal granulocytic elements and 15% erythroid precursors; (2) the absence of any distinctly leukemic cells (M_1 marrow); and (3) a disappearance of all clinical and laboratory signs of acute leukemia. Confirmation of the status of the marrow as assessed by marrow biopsy and an analysis of individual cell morphology on the aspirate provide the most reliable confirmation of marrow remission. It is estimated that at least a 2-log reduction (or 99%) in the leukemic cell population is required for this goal to be achieved.

In the past 15 years the remission frequency in ANLL has risen from 10–20% to 50–70% as a result of increasingly aggressive multiagent chemotherapeutic programs. Generally, these therapies consist of continuous intravenous infusion of cytosine arabinoside and pulsed doses of anthracycline. The evolution and current status of these programs have recently been reviewed (Gale, 1979).

Unfortunately, the lack of a high degree of specificity of the chemotherapeutic agent for the leukemic cell population as compared to the normal cell population produces significant morbidity in the patient. The relationship between leukemic cell kill and the drug dose administered requires the administration of the therapeutic agents at hand at rather toxic levels. A complete obliteration of the normal as well as the abnormal bone marrow elements is the usual result of adequate therapy. Infection and bleeding commonly appear as a consequence, and increasingly sophisticated systems for support of the patient during periods of marrow hypoplasia are mandated.

Induction therapy for childhood ALL is usually less toxic than that employed in ANLL. Nonetheless, the relationship between cell kill, drug dose, and maximally effective therapy remains critical. In adults with ALL, conventional induction programs with vincristine, prednisone, and asparaginase are less effective than in children. In patients older than 16 years, the addition of an anthracycline to vincristine and prednisone increases the frequency of complete remission from approximately 50 to 75% of patients (Gottlieb and Weinberg, 1979). Given the added myelotoxicity of the anthracyclines, the problems in patient support that arise are similar to those encountered in the therapy of acute non-lymphocytic leukemia.

Maintenance therapy is the treatment of the patient in remission. Its goal is continued reduction of the leukemic cell population with the ultimate obliteration of the entire population of neoplastic cells. Maintenance programs must be sufficiently aggressive to provide continued cell kill and sufficiently varied in the metabolic attack upon the neoplastic cell to prevent the emergence of drug-resistant clones. At the same time these programs must permit sufficient recovery of the host to avoid inordinate morbidity and mortality (Pinkel et al., 1971). Intensification or consolidation therapy has been shown of value during maintenance therapy. These programs usually employ periodic use of the drugs employed during induction at relatively high doses. The value of maintenance therapy is best seen then in the early studies of ALL wherein the median duration of unmaintained remission after induction with vincristine and prednisone was less than 6 months! For reasons previously stated, current maintenance programs are of necessity toxic. For example, the mortality rate in children in complete remission consequent to the initial curative programs employed by St. Jude

Hospital was 16%. The most frequent cause of mortality was infection (Simone *et al.*, 1972).

In ALL, prophylactic therapy aimed at prevention of meningeal leukemia and reintensification or consolidation therapy during maintenance (Fernbach *et al.*, 1975) for patients attaining complete remission result in distinct benefits in the overall duration of the complete remission, and an increased incidence of un-maintained long-term survival.

In ANLL, the incidence of central nervous system (CNS) leukemia, both at presentation and during the course of complete remission, appears to be lower than in ALL. The benefits of conventional maintenance therapy are similarly less clear (Embury *et al.*, 1977). Thus, in ANLL, the value of CNS prophylaxis, more aggressive programs of maintenance, early and late intensification of therapy, and reinduction therapy are currently under study. Early results from these more aggressive maintenance programs are encouraging, with prolongation of the duration of the initial remission (Freireich *et al.*, 1978). The climate established by the increasing incidence of long-term survivorship and the success of noncomparative programs employing intensification during remission make a contemporary randomized comparative trial of maintained versus unmaintained remission in ANLL unlikely.

IX. GENERAL CLINICAL CONSIDERATIONS

The patient with acute leukemia often presents with granulocytopenia and thrombocytopenia. Additionally, there appears to be a degree of immune sup-pression associated with ANLL as well as ALL. As a consequence, a markedly increased susceptibility to both infection and bleeding exists prior to the initiation of therapy. Moreover, as noted above, granulocytopenia and thrombocytopenia supervene as a consequence of chemotherapy.

A. Thrombocytopenic Bleeding

The prevention of and therapy for thrombocytopenic bleeding represent a primary consideration during the therapeutic management of a patient with acute leukemia. Of particular importance in patient mortality is CNS bleeding. The increased availability and use of platelet transfusions have dramatically de-creased the incidence of thrombocytopenic bleeding as a cause of patient demise during induction therapy for acute leukemia (Hersh *et al.*, 1965; Ketchel and Rodriguez, 1978). Since the frequency and seriousness of bleeding episodes increase markedly in patients with platelet counts below 20,000/mm^3, prophylac-tic platelet transfusions are employed to maintain the platelet count above this level (Gaydos *et al.*, 1962).

The continued efficacy of these platelet transfusions is limited mainly by histocompatibility antigen (HLA) sensitization. For this reason, it appears best to employ, where possible, single-donor platelet transfusions obtained by plateletphoresis. When HLA sensitization occurs, as manifested by a failure of the platelet count to increase appropriately following platelet transfusion, a new donor with unshared HLA determinants is selected. HLA typing should be routinely performed at patient presentation. Since contemporary therapy of adult leukemia is by necessity ablative to the bone marrow, the availability and use of platelet transfusions is mandatory. Similar considerations exist in the therapy of childhood leukemia.

B. Infection

Infection has become the leading cause of death of patients with acute leukemia (Hersh et al., 1965; Chang et al., 1976; Ketchel and Rodriguez, 1978). Approximately 75% of treated patients die of infection. The fatal infection proves to be bacterial in origin in three-fourths of the patients (Ketchel and Rodriguez, 1978). The prime factor predisposing to infection is absolute granulocytopenia. During therapy for acute leukemia, blood granulocytes are almost invariably low and the activity of the proliferative marrow pool is suspended. Bodey et al. (1966) first established that the number of febrile episodes endured by the patient with acute leukemia could be related to the degree of granulocytopenia. There were 43 episodes per 1000 hospital days encountered in patients with fewer than 100 granulocytes per mm^3, as compared to 19 episodes per 1000 days when granulocytes were 100–500/mm^3. Patients with more than 500 granulocytes per mm^3 were at a comparatively reduced risk. A favorable response to infection, moreover, can be related to the imminence of marrow recovery (Bodey et al., 1971). Overall, patients were febrile for one quarter of their hospital days.

Similar data regarding the association of infectious febrile episodes and the absolute granulocyte count are provided in the representative studies of Sickles et al. (1975) and Gurwith and co-workers (1978). In the former study, fever was present for 44% of the hospital days of patients with granulocytes below 1000/mm^3 as compared to 69% of days for patients with fewer than 10 granulocytes per mm^3.

Except for fever, the clinical signs and symptoms characteristic of infection may not be present, at least initially, in the granulocytopenic host (Sickles et al., 1975). Thus, all too frequently the physician is faced with a febrile and granulocytopenic patient who lacks a specific site and/or organism as the source of infection. Nonetheless, more than two-thirds of these febrile episodes can be shown to be infective (Bodey and Rodriguez, 1978). Disseminated infection and pneumonia were found in 60% of 1209 infections in 494 patients with acute leukemia. In one-third of the febrile episodes the cause of the fever could not be identified. In only 1% could the febrile response be shown to be noninfectious. In 192 febrile episodes in 126 granulocytopenic patients (Gurwith *et al.*, 1978), infection was identified in 86 of 128 episodes in adults and 19 of 64 occasions in children. Moreover, 44 bacteremic episodes were observed.

The high frequency with which fever is coupled with bacteremia and its relationship to the total granulocyte count are shown in the data drawn from the study of Sickles *et al.* (1975) (Table III). It should be underscored that the cause of the febrile episodes in most reports was established by rigorous and aggressive use of surveillance cultures, serologic techniques, interventive diagnostic procedures, and necropsy. In most institutions, the cause of a febrile episode cannot be documented with the same high frequency.

The most common offending organisms are gram-negative bacilli and include *Klebsiella penumoniae, Escherichia coli, Pseudomonas aeruginosa,* and the Enterobacter group. These pathogens appear to account for up to 80% of all proven infections and approximately half of those with a fatal outcome (Ketchel and Rodriguez, 1978). The relative frequency and pattern of antimicrobial resistance for each organism varies among treatment centers.

There is a rising incidence of infections due to resistant organisms such as *Serratia marcescens* and previously unusual gram-positive bacilli such as *Bacillus cereus*. Similarly, the frequency of fungal infection is rising, undoubtedly because of the frequent and prolonged use of multi-agent antibiotic therapy. *Candida* is the most common fungus encountered. Systemic and local infection with *Aspergillus* and the Phycomycetes group are also seen. The diagnosis of fungal infection is infrequently made antemortem since the fungi have proved

TABLE III

Bacteremic Episodes in Granulocytopenic Patients Undergoing Cancer Therapy as a Function of the Absolute Granulocyte Count.[a]

Site of infection	Absolute granulocyte count					
	0–100 mm^3		101–1000 mm^3		>1000 mm^3	
Pharynx	5/15[b]	(33%)[c]	1/10	(10%)	0/6	(0%)
Skin	4/19	(19%)	1/8	(13%)	2/24	(8%)
Anorectal	6/13	(46%)	1/5	(20%)	0/3	(0%)
Urinary tract	5/9	(56%)	2/7	(29%)	5/38	(13%)
Lung	23/42	(55%)	7/34	(21%)	10/58	(17%)
Total	43/100	(43%)	12/64	(19%)	17/129	(13%)

[a] Data from Sickles *et al.* (1975).
[b] Bacteremic episodes per patients undergoing therapy.
[c] Frequency with which fever is coupled with bacteremia.

difficult to culture from the bloodstream, even in the patient with disseminated candidiasis. The presence of a disseminated fungal infection should be suspected in the febrile antibiotic-unresponsive patient. Biopsy is often the only way to confirm a clinical suspicion of invasive, disseminated mycotic infection. In the M.D. Anderson Hospital experience, fungal infections have been found in the necropsies of up to 30% of patients (Ketchel and Rodriguez, 1978). Eleven fungal infections were found in 192 febrile episodes observed in 126 hospitalized granulocytopenic patients (Gurwith *et al.*, 1978).

Pneumocystis carinii and *Toxoplasma* are protozoal pathogens. The wide variation in the frequency of infection with these organisms among various institutions probably represents true differences in epidemiology. The diagnosis of, and consequently specific therapy for, intercurrent infection in patients with acute leukemia are further complicated by the increased susceptibility of these patients to viral infection.

A mortality rate of 20–40% from untreated bacterial sepsis may be anticipated in the first 48 hours of infection in the compromised granulocytopenic host (Ketchel and Rodriguez, 1978). Close surveillance of temperatures is thus mandatory in this group at risk.

Given the high frequency of bacterial sepsis associated with febrile episodes, its rapid and high mortality, and the paucity of associated signs of infection, sustained (two or more consecutive) temperatures of greater than 101°F that are not otherwise explicable are an urgent indication for the antimicrobial therapy even in the compromised, site-negative, organism-negative individual. After appropriate cultures have been obtained and clinical evaluation performed, broad-spectrum antibiotic coverage for both gram-negative and gram-positive organisms is mandatory. An aminoglycoside plus a cephalosporin or carbenicillin, or a combination of all three drugs, is the most commonly employed combination. When a specific organism or site of infection is clarified, therapy may be tailored to more specific agents. For infections with *Pneumocystis* or *Toxoplasma,* a combination of trimethoprim and sulfamethoxazole may be employed. Although systemic fungal infection is often successfully treated with amphotericin in the noncompromised host, such an infection is usually fatal in the patient with acute leukemia, unless the patient rapidly enters a complete remission.

In patients in whom a specific site of infection or organism is identified, the duration of therapy presents less of a dilemma than in the continuingly febrile patient who remains febrile despite persistently negative cultures and examinations. Since more than three-fourths of this latter group will prove to be *apparently* antibiotic responsive, and since recrudescence of an underlying infection following premature termination of antibiotics has a poor prognosis, antibiotics are generally continued for a minimum of 7–10 days (Rodriguez *et al.,* 1973).

The patient who fails to respond to antibiotic therapy represents a difficult therapeutic dilemma. The length of time before antibiotics are stopped, the timing of the reassessment of the patient by culture, and the level of diagnostic intervention that should be employed must remain a function of the individual clinical circumstance. The combination of trimethoprim and sulfamethoxazole has been used to some advantage in this setting (Grose *et al.*, 1977). Clearly it is just such a patient in whom a generalized fungal infection should be considered.

The use of white blood cell transfusions has recently been shown to be efficacious in the support of patients during periods of granulocytopenia and infection, and will play an increasing role in supportive care in the next decade (Freireich *et al.*, 1978). Stringent patient isolation employing ''life islands'' and prophylactic antibiotics directed against enteric pathogens have their advocates but have not seen widespread use (Preisler and Bjornsson, 1975; Levine and Deisseroth, 1978).

Levine *et al.* (1974) underscored the measures that may be routinely employed in the prevention of infection. Given the magnitude and seriousness of the problem, these procedures, which are within the scope of every treatment facility, should be rigorously advocated (Table IV).

C. Central Nervous System Leukemia

Central nervous system leukemia frequently develops in the absence of therapy directed toward eradication of the leukemic cell from the CNS. The prolonged survival of the patient attaining complete hematologic remission without prophylatic therapy of the CNS places such a patient at highest risk for CNS leukemia. It results from the seeding and proliferation of leukemic cells in a ''sanctuary'' area. In this case the CNS is excluded from the effects of conventional systemic chemotherapy because these agents do not penetrate the blood–brain barrier.

Pinkel *et al.* (1971) have indicated that clinical or necropsy evidence of CNS leukemia was found in 83% of 42 chemotherapeutically responsive children with ALL who were not treated prophylactically for CNS disease. In adults with hematologically responsive ALL, the attack rate for CNS disease in the absence of specific CNS prophylaxis appears similar (Wolk *et al.*, 1974). When CNS prophylaxis is not given to adults, clinical signs of CNS involvement were found in 40% of patients with ALL and 6.5% of patients with ANLL. The incidence of necropsy was 40% for ALL and 19% for ANLL (Wolk *et al.*, 1974). It is uncertain whether the differences in incidence of CNS leukemia between ALL and ANLL relate only to increased survivorship, and thus time at risk, for children with ALL. However, CNS involvement appears to be more common at presentation in ALL than in ANLL. Excellent descriptions of the clinical and pathologic findings of CNS leukemia are avialable (Shaw *et al.*, 1960).

Typically, CNS leukemia is marked by the signs and symptoms of diffuse

TABLE IV

General Principles of the Prevention of Infection in the Granulocytopenic Host[a]

Reduce acquisition of organisms from the hospital environment
Avoid hospitalization when ambulatory care will suffice. Avoid crowding in treatment facilities.
Enforce strict hygiene among physicians, nurses, aides, and other contacts.
Decrease contacts with nonessential personnel.
Remove the patient from the general hospital environment at periods of greatest risk. (Mask and gown isolation, laminar air flow rooms.)

Avoid invasive procedures where possible
Indwelling intravenous or arterial lines or indwelling catheters should not be employed except when absolutely necessary.
Change "butterfly" needles, tubing, and intravenous bottles daily.
Take scrupulous care of intravenous sites.
Use oral temperatures whenever possible; avoid rectal administration of medications.
Use blood and blood products screened for hepatitis-associated antigens.

Reduce numbers of colonizing organisms and sites of colonization
Remove or reduce the number of catheters and episodes of venipuncture.

Bolster the host defense mechanisms
Support good personal hygiene and employ preventive medicine in the intervals between therapy (good dental hygiene, remove carious teeth).
Promptly treat intracurrent infections.
Use active anti-bacterial immunization (pneumococcal vaccine).
Employ passive immunization where appropriate.
Encourage adequate nutrition and exercise.
Improve respiratory toilet.
Treat comorbid disease (e.g., heart failure).

Decrease the patient's time at risk
Appropriately and aggressively treat the primary disease in such a manner as to avoid the untoward effects of multiple courses of suboptimal therapy.

---

[a] Adapted from Levine *et al.* (1974).

cerebritis, cranial nerve palsy, or visual difficulties secondary to papilledema. CNS leukemia may occasionally be observed in the otherwise asymptomatic patient. Blast forms are usually present in the cerebral spinal fluid. Serial examinations may be necessary for cytologic documentation. Cerebrospinal fluid is best examined following staining of a cytocentrifuged preparation. The CSF protein may be elevated.

Therapy of established, clinically evident CNS leukemia is poor and few patients are alive 2–3 years after its onset. The pioneering experiments at St. Jude Hospital have established the value of prophylactic CNS therapy directed at the irradication of microscopic foci of CNS leukemia. Such therapy, rendered soon after the induction of complete remission, is mandatory in ALL. At present, prophylactic therapy consists of either intrathecal medication (methotrexate or cytosine arabinoside) or cranial irradiation, or both. The ability of systemic therapy (e.g., methotrexate) in sufficient dosage to provide effective concentration of drug within the CNS is currently being evaluated. If successful, this approach will help obviate the leukoencephalopathy, cerebral atrophy, growth and hormonal disturbances, and risk of second malignancies in areas of irradiation produced in children by cranial irradiation (D'Angio, 1978), or the arachnoiditis produced by multiple intrathecal instillations of methotrexate. Data obtained in ALL of childhood have indicated that with adequate CNS prophylaxis, the CNS is an extremely uncommon site of initial relapse (George *et al.*, 1979).

D. Leukostasis

Infiltrative white cell aggregates that injure the endothelium of small arteries and veins are commonly seen in patients with large numbers of circulating blast cells (McKee and Collins, 1974). These lesions are uncommon when the blast count is less than 150,000, but become progressively more common in patients in whom the blast count is higher. These white cell aggregates predispose to hemorrhage presumably due to endothelial damage. The best therapy for this condition is effective and rapidly cytolytic drug therapy or leukophoresis. The CNS and lung are the sites where this phenomenon is most evident clinically.

X. PROGNOSTIC FACTORS

A number of clinical and laboratory features of acute leukemia have been identified that influence the frequency with which the patient will attain complete remission and, to an extent, the duration of the remission attained. The factors most consistently reported are summarized in Table V. In addition, black patients have been reported to do more poorly than those of other races. Identification of these prognostic factors has important clinical significance in the individual patient and allows for more appropriate study design. Stratification for risk factors may be employed, in study design which, in turn, allows alternative and more effective therapies to be employed for various groupings. Additionally, the results of therapy may be compared between more comparable groups (Gehan *et al.*, 1976). Those factors that will definitively distinguish which patients will relapse on a particular therapeutic program are not, as yet, known.

In both the pediatric and adult population, age is the most consistent prognostic factor. Between the ages of 2 and 10 some 90% of children with ALL enter complete remission following therapy with vincristine, prednisone, and asparaginase. Below age 2 and above the ages of 8–10, a significant decrement in the frequency of complete remission is observed; no more than 50% of patients

TABLE V

Favorable Prognostic Factors in Acute Leukemia

ALL	ANLL
Age (2–10 yr)	Age (<40 yr)
Normal or near-normal white blood count (lower level of circulating "blasts")	Normal or near-normal white blood count (lower level of circulating "blasts")
Absence of CNS leukemia	Absence of CNS leukemia
Absence of other major illness	Absence of other major illness
Good performance status	Good performance status
Presence of null type rather than B or T cell type	—
Absence of hepatosplenomegaly	Absence of hepatosplenomegaly?
—	Absence of previously treated malignancy (i.e., Hodgkin's disease, polycythemia vera, ovarian carcinoma, chronic granulocytic leukemia, myeloma)
L_1 rather than L_2 type? (FAB)	—

over age 20 enter complete remission with similar therapy [Cancer and Leukemia Group B (CALGB) studies 7113 and 7612, Gottlieb and Weinberg, 1979]. Moreover, regression analysis clearly indicates a poorer outlook for the attainment of complete remission as the age decade increases. Between 25 and 45% of children with ALL who attain complete remission now represent long-term unmaintained survivors, and are potentially cured of their disease.

No such clear tendency toward long-term survival has as yet emerged in adult ALL, and a continuous pattern of relapse on maintenance therapy is observed. The appearance of CNS leukemia represents a poor prognostic finding for long-term survival. When CNS relapse occurs it appears to presage marrow relapse, and reinduction therapy at the time of CNS relapse may be advisable. In children induced and maintained on the programs of St. Jude Hospital, the adverse effects of poor prognostic factors on survival and "cure" are no longer applicable should the patient remain in complete remission after 2 1/2 years of maintenance therapy (George et al., 1979).

Between 50 and 75% of all adults treated for ANLL now regularly attain complete remission following chemotherapy (Keating et al., 1977; Ellison and Glidewell, 1979). The median duration of remission is in excess of 1 year. A significant trend toward longer initial remissions is now observed. Recent studies indicate that approximately 25% of adults attaining complete remission will remain continuously disease-free for at least 3 years (Keating et al., 1977; Ellison and Glidewell, 1979). In the younger adult (under age 40), the remission induction frequency increases to 70–80% of patients. In all groups of higher frequency of remission induction is observed in the absence of other significant co-morbid disease and in patients with the best initial performance status.

There have been major advances in the understanding and therapy of the acute leukemias over the past decade. Childhood acute lymphocytic leukemia is now curable in a significant percentage of patients, and the frequency of complete remission following induction in adult lymphocytic leukemia has climbed from 50 to 75% of patients currently beginning therapy. Ten years ago the attainment of therapeutically induced complete remission in 25% of patients with ANLL was considered exceptional. The efficacy of current programs of induction has already been noted. In addition, the duration of complete response in ANLL is lengthening, and new approaches to the maintenance of patients are under evaluation. Most important, an enlarging fraction of patients with ANLL remains in complete and continuous remission for 3, 4, and 5 years following induction, and a group of unmaintained long-term survivors of ANLL is now increasingly identifiable (Bloomfield, 1978; Ellison and Glidewell, 1979; Keating et al., 1977).

XI. CONCLUSIONS

Significant progress in the therapy of acute leukemia has resulted from the research activities of multi-institutional cooperative groups and selected single institutions. The facilities of these organizations combine patient access, clinical expertise, and basic research and development. Contemporary therapy of acute leukemia requires the clinical skill and commitment of the professional staff, the designation of institutional facilities, and the forebearance of the patient. In view of the progress to date these continued efforts are clearly justified.

ACKNOWLEDGMENTS

These studies were supported in part by a grant (R10CA21060) from the National Institutes of Health, National Cancer Institute, DHEW.

Tables I, III, IV, and V were prepared for this discussion. They have been presented together with a discussion of infection in the *Whole Internist Catalog* by Gottlieb, A. J., Zamkoff, K. W., Jastremski, M. S., Scalzo, A., and Imboden, K. J. (1980), published by W. B. Saunders Co., Philadelphia, and are reproduced with permission. Original source references for these data are provided in text.

REFERENCES

Askoy, M., Erdem, S., and Dincol. G. (1974). *Blood* **44,** 837–841.
Belpomme, D., Mathé, G., and Davies, A. J. S. (1977). *Lancet* **1,** 555–558.

Bennett, J. M., Catovsky, D., Daniel, M., Flandrin, G., Galton, D. A. G., Gralnick, H. R., and Sulton, C. (1976). *Br. J. Haematol.* **33**, 451-458.

Bergsagel, D. E., Bailey, A. J., Langley, G. R., MacDonald, R. N., White, D. F., and Miller, A. B. (1979). *N. Engl. J. Med.* **301**, 743-748.

Bloomfield, C. D. (1978). *Arch. Intern. Med.* **138**, 1333-1334.

Bloomfield, C. D., and Brunning, R. D. (1976). *Semin. Oncol.* **3**, 297-317.

Bodey, G. P., and Rodriguez, V. (1978). *Semin. Hematol.* **15**, 221-261.

Bodey, G. P., Buckley, M., Sathe, Y. S., and Freireich, E. J. (1966). *Ann. Intern. Med.* **64**, 328-340.

Bodey, G. P., Whitecar, J. P., Jr., and Middleman, E. (1971). *J. Am. Med. Assoc.* **218**, 62-66.

Brouet, J. C., and Seligmann, M. (1978). *Cancer* **42**, 817-827.

Canellos, G., DeVita, V. T., Whang-Peng, J., Johnson, R. C., and Arseneau, J. C. (1975). *Lancet* **1**, 947-949.

Chang, H. Y., Rodriguez, V., Narboni, G., Bodey, G. P., Luna, M. A., and Freireich, E. J. (1976). *Medicine (Baltimore)* **55**, 259-268.

Coleman, C. N., Williams, C. J., Flint, A., Glatstein, E. J., Rosenberg, S. A., and Kaplan, H. S. (1977). *N. Engl. J. Med.* **297**, 1249-1252.

Collins, A. J., Bloomfield, C. D., Peterson, B. A., McKenna, R. W., and Edson, J. R. (1978). *Arch. Intern. Med.* **138**, 1177-1178.

Cronkite, E. P., Moloney, W., and Bond, V. P. (1960). *Am. J. Med.* **28**, 673-682.

D'Angio, G. J. (1978). *Cancer* **42**, 1015-1022.

Davey, F. R., and Gottlieb, A. J. (1974). *Am. J. Clin. Pathol.* **6**, 818-822.

Ellison, R. R., and Glidewell, O. (1979). *Proc. Am. Assoc. Cancer Res.* **20**, 161a.

Embury, S. H., Elias, L., Heller, P. H., *et al.* (1977). *West. J. Med.* **126**, 267-272.

Fernbach, D. J., George, S. L., Sutow, W. W., Ragab, A. H., Lane, D. M., Haggard, M. E., and Lonsdale, D. (1975). *Cancer* **36**, 1552-1559.

Fraumeni, J. F. (1967). *J. Natl. Cancer Inst.* **38**, 593-605.

Freireich, E. J. (1966). *Transfusion* **6**, 50-54.

Freireich, E. J., Keating, M. J., Gehan, E. A., McCredie, K. B., Bodey, G. P., and Smith, T. (1978). *Cancer* **42**, 874-882.

Gale, R. P. (1979). *N. Engl. J. Med.* **300**, 1189-1199.

Gatti, R. A., and Good, R. A. (1971). *Cancer* **28**, 89-98.

Gaydos, L. A., Freireich, E. J., and Mantel, N. (1962). *N. Engl. J. Med.* **266**, 905-909.

Gehan, E. A., Smith, T. L., Freireich, E. J., Bodey, G. P., Rodriguez, V., Speer, J., and McCredie, K. (1976). *Semin. Oncol.* **3**, 271-282.

George, S. L., Aur, R. J. A., Mauer, A. M., and Simone, J. V. (1979). *N. Engl. J. Med.* **300**, 269-273.

Gottlieb, A. J., and Weinberg, V. (1979). *Blood* **54**, 189a (Suppl. 1).

Gralnick, H. R., and Sultan, C. (1975). *Br. J. Haematol.* **29**, 373-376.

Gralnick, H. R., Galton, D. A. G., Catovsky, D., Sultan, C., and Bennett, J. M. (1977). *Ann. Intern. Med.* **87**, 740-753.

Greaves, M. F., Brown, G., Rapson, N. T., and Lister, T. A. (1975). *Clin. Immunol. Immunopathol.* **4**, 67-84.

Grose, W. E., Bodey, G. P., and Rodriguez, V. (1977). *J. Am. Med. Assoc.* **237**, 352-354.

Gurwith, M. J., Brunton, J. L., Lank, B. A., Ronald, A. R., and Harding, G. K. M. (1978). *Am. J. Med.* **64**, 121-126.

Hersh, E. M., Bodey, G. P., Nies, B. A., and Freireich, E. J. (1965). *J. Am. Med. Assoc.* **193**, 105-109.

Hetzel, P., and Gee, T. S. (1978). *Am. J. Med.* **64**, 765-772.

Keating, M. J., Freireich, E. J., McCredie, K. B., Bodey, G. P., Hersh, E., Hester, J. P., Rodriguez, V., and Hart, J. (1977). *Ca* **27**, 1-25.

Keleti, J., Revesz, T., and Schuler, D. (1978). *Br. J. Haematol.* **40**, 501–502.
Ketchel, S. J., and Rodriguez, V. (1978). *Semin. Oncol.* **5**, 167–179.
Landaw, S. A. (1976). *Semin. Hematol.* **13**, 33–48.
Levine, A. S., and Deisseroth, A. B. (1978). *Cancer* **42**, 883–894.
Levine, A. S., Schimpff, S. C., Graw, R. G., Jr., and Young, R. C. (1974). *Semin. Hematol.* **11**, 141–202.
Lilleyman, J. S., Potter, A. M., Watmore, A. E., Cooke, P., Sokol, R. J., and Wood, J. K. (1978). *Br. J. Haematol.* **39**, 317–323.
Linman, J. W., and Bagby, G. C., Jr. (1978). *Cancer* **42**, 854–864.
Linman, J. W., and Saarni, M. I. (1974). *Semin. Hematol.* **11**, 93–100.
Louie, S., and Schwartz, R. S. (1978). *Semin. Hematol.* **15**, 117–138.
McKee, L. C., and Collins, R. D. (1974). *Medicine (Baltimore)* **53**, 463–478.
MacMahon, B. (1962). *J. Natl. Cancer Inst.* **28**, 1173–1191.
Miller, R. W. (1971). *J. Natl. Cancer Inst.* **46**, 203–209.
O'Regan, S., Carson, S., Chesney, R. W., and Drummond, K. N. (1977). *Blood* **49**, 345–353.
Pajak, T., Gottlieb, A. J., and Bloomfield, C. D. (1978). *Blood* **52**, 268, Suppl. 1.
Pinkel, D., Hernandez, K., Borella, L., Holton, C., Aur, R., Samoy, G., and Pratt, C. (1971). *Cancer* **27**, 247–256.
Preisler, H., and Bjornsson, S. (1975). *Semin. Oncol.* **2**, 369–377.
Reimer, R. R., Hoover, R., Fraumeni, J. F., and Young, R. C. (1978). *N. Engl. J. Med.* **297**, 177–181.
Rodriguez, V., Burgess, M. A., and Bodey, G. B. (1973). *Cancer* **32**, 1007–1012.
Rosner, F. (1976). *Cancer* **37**, 1033–1042.
Rosner, F., and Grunwald, H. (1974). *Am. J. Med.* **57**, 927–939.
Rosner, F., and Grunwald, H. (1975). *Am. J. Med.* **58**, 339–353.
Rowley, J. D. (1978). *Semin. Hematol.* **15**, 301–319.
Shaw, R. K., Moore, E. W., Freireich, E. J., and Thomas, L. B. (1960). *Neurology* **10**, 823–833.
Sickles, E. A., Greene, W. H., and Wiernik, P. H. (1975). *Arch. Intern. Med.* **135**, 715–719.
Simone, J. V., Holland, E., and Johnson, W. (1972). *Blood* **39**, 759–770.
Vogler, L. B., Crist, W. M., Bockman, D. E., Pearl, E. R., Lawton, A. R., and Cooper, M. D. (1978). *N. Engl. J. Med.* **298**, 872–878.
Wolk, R. W., Masse, S. R., Conklin, R., and Freireich, E. J. (1974). *Cancer* **33**, 863–869.

2

HAIRY CELL LEUKEMIA
Frederick R. Davey

I.	Definition	25
II.	Incidence with Age and Sex Ratio	25
III.	Pathology	26
IV.	Pathogenesis	26
V.	Clinical Features	28
VI.	Laboratory Features	29
VII.	Treatment	33
VIII.	Course of Disease	35
IX.	Summary	35
	References	36

I. DEFINITION

In 1958, hairy cell leukemia (HCL) was first described as an independent clinical–pathological entity under the term leukemic reticuloendotheliosis by Bouroncle and co-workers. The disease is characterized clinically by splenomegaly and pancytopenia. HCL can be differentiated from other lymphoproliferative disorders by the presence of abnormal mononuclear cells containing long protoplasmic projections in the peripheral blood and bone marrow.

II. INCIDENCE WITH AGE AND SEX RATIO

Hairy cell leukemia is a rare disorder that represents approximately 2% of all leukemias (Bouroncle, 1979). It occurs most frequently in middle-aged persons. The average and median age range is from 50 to 55 years (Bouroncle, 1979; Burke *et al.*, 1974; Golomb *et al.*, 1978). However, patients in their twenties as well as patients in the eighties are afflicted with HCL. The approximate male-to-female ratio is 4:1 (Bouroncle, 1979; Golomb *et al.*, 1978; Katayama and Finkel, 1974; Burke *et al.*, 1974; Catovsky, 1977).

III. PATHOLOGY

Bone marrow biopsies reveal collections of small mononuclear cells. In early stages, the infiltrates are focal but later the marrow is diffusely involved. Mitoses are rare. Megakaryocytes, granulocytes, and erythroid precursors are usually decreased. Reticulum fibers are increased and probably account for difficulties in obtaining an adequate marrow aspirate.

Spleens from patients with HCL are characteristically enlarged and weigh between 350–6000 gm. Grossly, the spleens are firm. The cut surface is homogeneously dark red and is firm in consistency. Microscopically, the red pulp sinusoids and cords contain numerous abnormal mononuclear cells. This infiltrate encroaches upon the white pulp, reducing the size of the Malpighian corpuscles. Pseudosinuses lined by "hairy" cells and containing erythrocytes are characteristic findings (Nanba et al., 1977).

The liver is usually enlarged at postmortem examination. Small nodular areas of leukemic infiltrates may be present (Katayama and Finkel, 1974). Histopathologic sections demonstrate a collection of mononuclear cells throughout the hepatic sinuses. The infiltrates are usually diffuse but may be focal. Mononuclear cells also occur in periportal areas. Angiomatous lesions consisting of numerous dilated spaces resembling blood vessels filled with erythrocytes have been observed in the livers of patients with HCL (Nanba et al., 1977).

Lymph nodes are less frequently involved than the spleen or liver. When infiltrated, the histology of the nodes is altered by a collection of abnormal mononuclear cells in the subcapsular and interfollicular sinuses and medullary cords. Lymphoid follicles are frequently preserved.

Leukemic infiltrates of the skin may occur in approximately 5% of the cases (Katayama and Finkel, 1974). Other organs involved at postmortem include kidneys, pancreas, and adrenal glands (Bouroncle, 1979).

IV. PATHOGENESIS

The lack of mitoses in tissue sections suggests that "hairy" cells have a low proliferative capacity. A decreased uptake of tritiated thymidine in in vitro cultures of hairy cells using liquid scintillation techniques (Davey et al., 1980) and autoradiographic methods (Braylan et al., 1978) also indicates a low proliferative rate. In addition, Braylan et al. (1978), using a flow microfluorometer, determined that enriched populations of hairy cells contained few cells in S phase. Since hairy cells appear to multiply slowly, their accumulation in the lymphoreticular tissues, bone marrow, and blood may be the result of a prolonged survival. However, the determination of the life span of neoplastic cells in HCL has not been adequately studied.

Debusscher and co-workers (1975) labeled hairy cells with tritiated cytidine and then infused them into a patient. After a rapid disappearance of 67% of the labeled cells, a slow exponential decrease with a intravascular half-time of 150 hr was observed. The rapid decrease in labeled cells was thought to be the result of the redistribution of labeled cells between vascular and extravascular pools.

Numerous studies have been performed to determine the lineage of hairy cells. Some investigators believe that these neoplastic cells are a subtype of B lymphocytes (Catovsky *et al.*, 1974; Debusscher *et al.*, 1975; Golde *et al.*, 1977; Haak *et al.*, 1974; Jansen *et al.*, 1979). Other studies indicate that hairy cells have monocyte-like characteristics (Jaffe *et al.*, 1974; King *et al.*, 1975; Seshadri *et al.*, 1976; Trubowitz *et al.*, 1971). In addition, several studies indicate that the hairy cell may be a hybrid containing characteristics of B lymphocytes and monocytes/histiocytes (Boldt *et al.*, 1977; Braylan *et al.*, 1978; Fu *et al.*, 1974; Utsinger *et al.*, 1977; Davey *et al.*, 1979; Golomb, 1978).

Neoplastic cells from most cases of HCL have surface-membrane immunoglobulin (Boldt *et al.*, 1977; Braylan *et al.*, 1978; Catovsky *et al.*, 1974; Fu *et al.*, 1974; Davey *et al.*, 1979). In addition, several studies indicate that hairy cells can synthesize immunoglobulin (Debusscher *et al.*, 1975; Leech *et al.*, 1975; Golomb, 1978; Davey *et al.*, 1979). The presence of surface-membrane immunoglobulin and the ability to synthesize immunoglobulin are major characteristics of B lymphocytes.

In most cases of HCL, intracytoplasmic immunoglobulin is not present in the neoplastic cells (Braylan *et al.*, 1978; Davey *et al.*, 1979). However, one case has been reported in which a variable portion of the cells contained intracytoplasmic IgM immunoglobulin, and a second case with cytoplasmic IgG immunoglobulin (Golde *et al.*, 1977). In both cases the patient's serum contained the corresponding monoclonal immunoglobulin.

Most investigators agree that hairy cells contain receptors for the Fc portion of IgG immunoglobulin (Haegert *et al.*, 1974; Jaffe *et al.*, 1974; King *et al.*, 1975; Fu *et al.*, 1974). Fc receptors have been described on B and T lymphocytes as well as monocytes.

Ia-like or HLA-D histocompatibity antigens have been described on the membranes of hairy cells (Cawley *et al.*, 1978; Naeim *et al.*, 1978; Salsano *et al.*, 1979). HLA-D antigens are present on B lymphocytes, monocytes, and activated T lymphocytes.

The demonstration of a complement receptor has not been resolved. When the presence of the complement receptor was tested by incubating the mononuclear cell suspensions with sensitized sheep erythrocytes coated with mouse complement (EAC rosettes), negative results were usually obtained (Jaffe *et al.*, 1974; King *et al.*, 1975; Huber *et al.*, 1976; Davey *et al.*, 1979). However, complement receptors have been demonstrated on hairy cells using human red blood cells and mouse complement (Catovsky, 1977) and ox erythrocytes coated with

IgM and complement. Since the latter two assays measure the presence of the C_3d receptor, it is possible that hairy cells contain only this receptor. B lymphocytes contain both C_3b and C_3d receptors, whereas monocytes have predominantly the C_3b receptor (Catovsky, 1977).

Several studies have indicated that hairy cells phagocytize latex (Boldt et al., 1977; Braylan et al., 1978; Fu et al., 1974; Davey et al., 1979; Utsinger et al., 1977) and zymosan particles (Golomb, 1978). Hairy cells tend not to phagocytize bacteria or fungi (Catovsky et al., 1974; Haak et al., 1974; Jansen et al., 1979). However, Daniel and Flandrin (1974) demonstrated by ultrastructural techniques the ingestion of bacteria by hairy cells. Experiments using other particles or organisms have yielded conflicting results (Catovsky et al., 1974; King et al., 1975; Baker et al., 1976; Schmalzl et al., 1975). Phagocytosis is a major characteristic of monocytes and macrophages. However, there is evidence indicating that a small percentage of lymphocytes may have a phagocytic function (Zucker-Franklin et al., 1966).

In most cases of HCL, the neoplastic cells fail to form spontaneous rosettes with sheep erythrocytes, suggesting that in these cases the tumor cells are not of a T-cell lineage (Braylan et al., 1978; Davey et al., 1979). However, several investigators (Saxon et al., 1978; Cawley et al., 1978) have reported few cases of HCL in which the neoplastic cells possessed only T-cell properties.

In summary data regarding the lineage of hairy cell leukemia suggest that the hairy cell is a distinctive cell possessing both B-lymphocyte and macrophage functions. HCL could be the result of a proliferation of cells that are normally present in small quantities at some early stage of lymphocyte–monocyte differentiation. Hairy cells could also be B lymphocytes that have acquired phagocytic ability. However, the studies of Saxon et al. (1978) and Golde et al. (1977) suggest that HCL may be a heterogeneous disorder in which neoplastic T cells, B cells, macrophages, and perhaps hybrid cells would develop the morphologic appearance and cytochemical characteristics of hairy cells.

V. CLINICAL FEATURES

Hairy cell leukemia is insidious in onset. Nonspecific complaints such as weakness and fatigue are the most common presenting symptoms. Weight loss, easy bruising, abdominal fullness, and splenic pain are less frequent complaints. Occasionally patients present with infection. Sometimes the patients have no symptoms, and the diagnosis of HCL is made as a result of a routine physical examination (Bouroncle, 1979; Golomb et al., 1978).

Splenomegaly occurs in 83–93% of patients, with moderate to marked enlargement observed in 30–50%. Hepatomegaly is observed in 13–40%, and is of moderate degree. Lymphadenopathy has been described in 11–23% and is usually present in only one site. Skin infiltrates are observed in 6–15% of cases (Bouron-cle, 1979; Golomb *et al.*, 1978).

VI. LABORATORY FEATURES

The presence of abnormal mononuclear cells with prominent cytoplasmic projections in the peripheral smear and bone marrow aspirate or bone marrow biopsy touch preparation is a characteristic feature of HCL. In Wright–Giemsa-stained films, the abnormal cells measure 10–15 μm in diameter (Fig. 1). The cytoplasm is abundant and stains light blue or gray. The nucleus is round to oval and is frequently indented. The nuclear chromatin is usually reticular and nucleoli are small and inconspicuous. The examination of a suspension of hairy cells with phase-contrast microscopy helps to identify the hairy-like cytoplasmic projections that cover the surface of the cell.

Studies of hairy cells using scanning electron microscopy show numerous well-developed, undulating ruffles with broad bases (Braylan *et al.*, 1978; Katayama and Schneider, 1977). These surface characteristics can be used to distinguish hairy cells from lymphocytes of patients with chronic lymphocytic leukemia and from normal individuals. However, it is necessary to fix cell

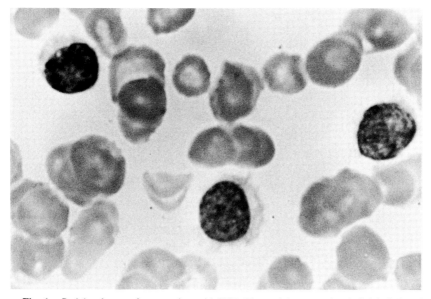

Fig. 1. Peripheral smear from a patient with HCL. The nuclei are round and slightly indented. The cytoplasm contains numerous protoplasmic projections (Wright-Giemsa stain, ×1000).

suspensions immediately at room temperature to avoid artifactitious surface changes (Katayama and Schneider, 1977).

Transmission electron microscopy reveals that the nuclear configuration of hairy cells is markedly variable. Nuclei may be oval or contain multiple lobes as a result of deep indentations. Nuclear pockets, a feature of lymphocytes of other hematologic disorders, are rare. Nucleoli are occasionally seen if the appropriate cross section is examined. The cytoplasm contains ribosome–lamella complexes in almost 50% of the cases (Katayama and Schneider, 1977). In addition, ribosomes and polyribosomes, pinocytotoxic vesicles, mitochondria, and Golgi apparatuses are present. A distinctive feature is the presence of pseudopodia and long cytoplasmic microvilli (Katayama and Schneider, 1977; Haegert et al., 1974; Schnitzer and Kass, 1974) (Figs. 2 and 3).

The use of the tartrate-resistant acid phosphatase reaction (isoenzyme 5) is a helpful cytochemical technique in the diagnosis of HCL (Yam et al., 1971). The acid phosphatase activity is present diffusely throughout the cytoplasm in a variable number of cells (Fig. 4). In rare cases of HCL, tartrate-resistant acid phosphatase has not been demonstrated (Katayama and Yang, 1977).

The presence of α-naphthyl acetate esterase and α-naphthyl butyrate esterase

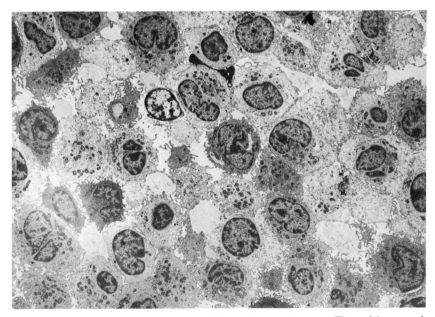

Fig. 2. Suspension of hairy cells viewed with an electron microscope. The nuclei are round, oval, and indented. Most of the cells demonstrate slender protoplasmic projections ($\times$3000). (Courtesy of Gerald B. Gordon, M.D.).

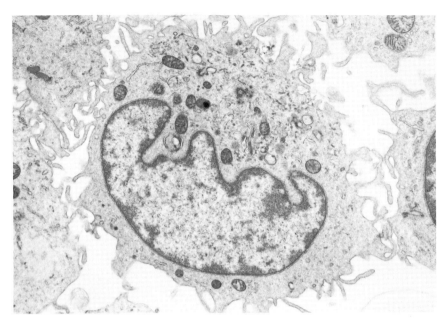

Fig. 3. Electron micrograph of a typical hairy cell showing the long cytoplasmic processes. The cytoplasm contains mitochondria, vesicles, and ribosomes. The nucleus is slightly indented and has heterochromatin along the nuclear membrane ($\times 13,000$). (Courtesy of Gerald B. Gordon, M.D.).

has been described in a variable number of cases (Davey *et al.*, 1979; Braylan *et al.*, 1978; Higgy *et al.*, 1978). It is not clear why there is a variation in the intensity of this reaction product observed in hairy cells within the same preparation and among different cases. Perhaps the variation in intensity of the reaction product reflects different states of activation of the hairy cells. Napthol AS-D chloracetate esterase, peroxidase, and Sudan black B stains are usually negative. The periodic acid–Schiff reactions show weakly positive cytoplasmic granules (Golomb, 1978).

Approximately 70% of patients with HCL are pancytopenic at the time of initial study. The hemoglobin ranges from 5 to 12 gm/dl and the hematocrit from 20–35% in three-fourths of the patients (Bouroncle, 1979). The anemia is usually normocytic–normochromic. In most cases the anemia is the result of a decreased production of erythroid cells, a shorter red cell survival secondary to splenomegaly, or a combination of both processes.

Leukopenia is a frequent finding, with approximately 50% of patients presenting with leukocyte counts of less than $3000/\mu l$. Only 20% of patients exhibit leukocytosis (Golomb *et al.*, 1978).

Abnormal mononuclear cells are present in the peripheral smear in 90–97% of

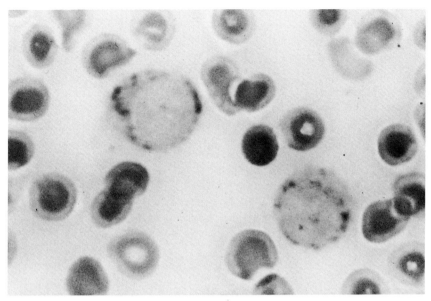

Fig. 4. Peripheral blood smear stained for tartrate-resistant acid phosphatase. The reaction product is seen as small to large cytoplasmic granules (×1000).

patients. However, hairy cells may represent from 1 to over 80% of the leukocyte differential count (Golomb, 1978; Bouroncle, 1979).

Approximately 80% of patients have a platelet count of less than 150,000/μl. Marked thrombocytopenia (less than 20,000/μl) is noted in 10% of patients.

Platelet aggregation studies in 7 of 14 patients with HCL demonstrated a markedly reduced response to epinephrine. No abnormalities were seen in secondary release and aggregation with adenosine diphosphate (ADP) or collagen. None of the patients with abnormal epinephrine aggregation had a clinically significant bleeding problem (Golomb, 1978).

Serum protein electrophoresis and immunoelectrophoresis are frequently normal. However, nondiagnositc alterations may be observed in 30% of cases. A monoclonal IgG immunoglobulin has been reported in one case, and an IgM immunoglobulin in another (Golde et al., 1977).

Numerous studies have been performed on the proliferative activity of hairy cells. Mononuclear cells from patients with HCL respond poorly to phytohemagglutinin (PHA) (Catovsky et al., 1974; Debusscher et al., 1975; Haak et al., 1974; Haegert et al., 1974; King et al., 1975; Naeim et al., 1978; Rieber et al., 1976; Yam et al., 1968). When an enriched population of T lymphocytes is incubated with PHA, a normal proliferative response occurs (Utsinger et al., 1977; Davey et al., 1980). In addition, T-lymphocyte enriched suspensions from spleens of HCL patients respond normally in mixed lymphocyte reactions to allogeneic antigens (Davey *et al.*, 1980). These findings suggest that T-cell function is normal in patients with HCL.

Hairy cells respond poorly to pokeweed mitogen (King *et al.*, 1975; Rieber *et al.*, 1976). When hairy cells are used as timulating cells in an allogeneic mixed lymphocyte reaction, a diminished proliferative response follows (Davey *et al.*, 1980). It is possible that hairy cells either suppress the proliferative response or fail to function normally in *in vitro* cultures.

Golomb (1978) described a chromosomal abnormality in 2 of 19 patients. The karyotype of these two patients revealed a deletion of Y chromosome and a probably extra chromosome number 12. These abnormalities were associated with a rapidly progressive course.

VII. TREATMENT

Assessing the results of therapy of HCL is difficult because of variability in the clinical course. At least one spontaneous remission has been described (Bouroncle, 1979). In addition, some patients have a prolonged chronic disorder with few, if any, symptoms, whereas others have an aggressive disease with numerous systemic difficulties (Golomb *et al.*, 1978).

A major therapeutic goal is to relieve the pancytopenia which is often severe, causing symptoms of excessive bleeding, severe infections, and anemia. The pancytopenia may be the result of hypersplenism secondary to hairy cell involvement of the spleen (Catovsky, 1977; Lewis *et al.*, 1977) or to bone marrow hypofunction due to marrow infiltration (Yam *et al.*, 1977).

Since approximately 20% of patients may require very little or no therapy, it is helpful to observe the patient for a period of time to determine the pace of the disease. Patients who require little or no therapy are older than the average person with HCL. Most of the patients requiring little therapy do not have significant splenomegaly, and although pancytopenia may exist, the median absolute granulocyte count is above $1000/\mu l$ (Golomb *et al.*, 1978).

Symptomatic patients with splenomegaly frequently benefit from splenectomy (Bouroncle, 1979; Golomb *et al.*, 1978). Surgical removal of the spleen should be performed in cases of hemorrhage secondary to thrombocytopenia, infections as a result of leukopenia, increasing transfusion requirements, splenic infarction, or abdominal pain secondary to splenomegaly (Golomb and Vardiman, 1978; Bouroncle, 1979). The examination of platelet and leukocyte counts before and after splenectomy indicates a rise in counts in the majority of patients following surgery (Golomb *et al.*, 1978; Catovsky, 1977).

In one study, 60% of patients achieved complete remission (hemoglobin increase above 11 gm/dl, neutrophils above 1×10^9/liter, and platelets above 100

$\times$ 10^9/liter) 2 weeks following splenectomy(Catovsky, 1977). A partial response (improvement in only one or two blood elements or improvement below the stated levels in three cell lines) was observed in 32%. No evident response was noted in 8% of patients. In the long term, all partial responders and one-half of the complete responders relapsed with pancytopenia. Thus, sustained improvement was observed in one-third of all cases. The interval to relapse is longer in the complete responder than in the partial-responder groups. Patients with the leukemic phase of HCL may benefit from splenectomy because of the increase in platelet count and the lower transfusion requirement that result from splenectomy (Golomb, 1978). Bouroncle (1979) demonstrated that the mean survival time of splenectomized patients was 6.9 years, whereas that of nonsplenectomized individuals was 4.6 years.

Single-drug or combination-drug therapy has not been beneficial as the initial treatment. Drugs that have provided only transient improvement include vinca alkaloids, alkylating agents, androgens, 6-mercaptopurine and procarbazine, and radioactive phosphorus (Katayama and Finkel, 1974; Burke *et al.*, 1974; Bouroncle, 1979; Catovsky, 1977; Plenderleith, 1970).

The use of corticosteroids has produced varied results. Although some successes have been recorded using prednisolone at daily doses of 40–80 mg for 2 to 3 weeks (Catovsky, 1977), remissions have been of short duration. Survival time of patients treated only with corticosteroids is less than patients treated only with splenectomy (Golomb *et al.*, 1978). In addition, the use of corticosteroids may enhance the risk of infections with opportunistic organisms (Bouza *et al.*, 1978).

In one study, splenic irradiation induced a partial response in 16 of 24 patients with HCL. In these individuals there was a decrease in splenic size and improvement in hematologic parameters which lasted from 3–12 months (Bouroncle, 1979).

Additional treatment is required for patients who relapse or fail to respond to splenectomy. Golomb and Mintz (1979) have noted that the daily treatment with an alkylating agent (chlorambucil, 4 mg) provided improvement in blood counts and bone marrow involvement in four patients within 6 months of therapy. Cyclophosphamide at low a dosage, twice weekly, has also proved helpful (Catovsky, 1977).

There is limited experience in treating patients with HCL with anthracyclines. Stewart *et al.* (1979) indicated that one patient with aggressive disease obtained a complete remission, and a second received a partial remission with the use of rubidazone (450 mg/m^2). However, the morbidity of marrow aplasia caused by this agent and the relative youth of the two patients (under 40 years) should caution therapists in the use of this drug in elderly patients and in centers lacking supportive-care programs (Bertino, 1979).

In addition, improvement has been described in a few refractory patients treated with androgens (Lusch *et al.*, 1978) and with leukophoresis (Moore *et al.*, 1977).

In summary, symptomatic patients benefit from splenectomy. Additional drug therapy (usually with an alkylating agent) will be required at a later date in patients whose disease relapses or fails to respond to splenectomy.

VIII. COURSE OF DISEASE

Hairy cell leukemia is, in general, a chronic disease. It varies from a mild disease requiring minimal or no therapy to a steadily progressive illness, necessitating treatment for hemorrhage, infection, or anemia. In one study of 71 patients with HCL, the actuarial survival was 51% at 4 years (Golomb *et al.*, 1978). In a second study involving 82 patients, the average survival was 5 years 9 months. Twelve patients had survived longer than 10 years, and two patients longer than 20 years.

The most common cause of death is infection (Bouroncle, 1979; Golomb *et al.*, 1978). The overall incidence of serious infection in patients with HCL is approximately 40% (Bouza *et al.*, 1978). The incidence of infections is correlated to a neutropenia of less than $500/\mu l$ (Golomb *et al.*, 1978) and to the use of corticosteroid treatment (Bouza *et al.*, 1978). The most common types of infections are pneumonia and septicemia. Urinary tract infections, cellulitis, and abscesses are less frequent (Bouroncle, 1979). The most common offending organisms are *Pseudomonas aeruginosa, Escherichia coli,* and *Staphylococcus aureus.* Other common pathogens are *Klebsiella pneumoniae, Proteus vulgaris,* and salmonella organisms. Fungal infections of *Aspergillus, Candida,* and *Cryptococcus;* pneumonitis due to *Pneumocystitis carinii;* virus infections including hepatitis, herpes simplex and cytomegalovirus; and mycobacterial infections have all been recorded in patients with HCL (Bouza *et al.*, 1978).

Hemorrhage is the cause of death in approximately 13% of patients with HCL. Bleeding is the result of the marked thrombocytopenia often present in these patients. Other less frequent causes of death are those associated with illnesses usually present in patients in the same age groups as those in which HCL occurs (Bouroncle, 1979).

IX. SUMMARY

Hairy cell leukemia is a chronic leukemia, predominantly of middle-age males, characterized by pancytopenia, splenomegaly, and the presence of a distinctive cell with long protoplasmic projections. Since the therapy and clinical course of this disease differ from other similar-appearing lymphoproliferative disorders, it is necessary to identify HCL correctly.

REFERENCES

Baker, C. R., Burns, G. F., Cawley, J. C., and Hayhoe, F. G. J. (1976). *Lancet* **1**, 1303.

Bertino, J. R. (1979). *Blood* **54**, 297.

Boldt, D. H., Speckart, S. F., MacDermott, R. P., Nash, G. S., and Valeski, J. E. (1977). *Blood* **49**, 745-757.

Bouroncle, B. A. (1979). *Blood* **53**, 412-436.

Bouroncle, B. A., Wiseman, B. K., and Doan, C. A. (1958). *Blood* **13**, 609-630.

Bouza, E., Burgaleta, C., and Golde, D. W. (1978). *Blood* **51**, 851-858.

Braylan, R. C., Jaffe, E. S., Triche, T. J., Nanba, K., Fowlkes, B. J., Metzger, H., Frank, M. M., Dolan, M. S., Yee, C. L., Green, I., and Berard, C. W. (1978). *Cancer* **41**, 210-227.

Burke, J. S., Byrne, G. E., and Rappaport, H. (1974). *Cancer* **33**, 1399-1410.

Catovsky, D. (1977). *Clin. Haematol.* **6**, 245-268.

Catovsky, D., Pettit, J. E., Galton, D. A. G., Spiers, A. S. D., and Harrison, C. V. (1974). *Br. J. Haematol.* **26**, 9-27.

Cawley, J. C., Burns, G. F., Nash, T. A., Heggy, K. E., Child, J. A., and Roberts, B. E. (1978). *Blood* **51**, 61-68.

Daniel, M. T., and Flandrin, G. (1974). *Lab. Invest.* **30**, 1-8.

Davey, F. R., Dock, N. L., Terzian, J., Bala, R., and Gottlieb, A. J. (1979). *Arch. Pathol. Lab. Med.* **103**, 433-436.

Davey, F. R., Dock, N. L., and Wolos, J. A. (1980). *Br. J. Haematol.* **45**, 29-39.

Debusscher, L., Bernheim, J. L., Collard-Rongé, E., Govaerts, A., Hooghe, R., Lejeune, F. J., Zeicher, M., and Stryckmans, P. A. (1975). *Blood* **46**, 495-507.

Fu, S. M., Winchester, R. J., Rai, K. P., and Kunkel, H. G. (1974). *Scand. J. Immunol.* **3**, 847-851.

Golde, D. W., Stevens, R. H., Quan, S. G., and Saxon, A. (1977). *Br. J. Haematol.* **35**, 359-365.

Golomb, H. M. (1978). *Cancer* **42**, 946-956.

Golomb, H. M., and Mintz, U. (1979). *Blood* **54**, 305-309.

Golomb, H. M., and Vardiman, J. (1978). *Ca* **28**, 265-277.

Golomb, H. M., Catovsky, D., and Golde, D. W. (1978). *Ann. Intern. Med.* **89**, 677-683.

Haak, H. L., DeMan, J. C. H., Hijmans, W., Knapp, W., and Speck, B. (1974). *Br. J. Haematol.* **27**, 31-38.

Haegert, D. G., Cawley, J. C., Collins, R. D., Flemans, R. J., and Smith, J. L. (1974). *J. Clin. Pathol.* **27**, 967-972.

Higgy, K. E., Burns, G. F., and Hayhoe, F. G. J. (1978). *Br. J. Haematol.* **38**, 99-106.

Huber, C., Hsamer, H., Michlmayr, G., and Braunsteiner, H. (1976). *Blut* **32**, 21-28.

Jaffe, E. S., Shevach, E. M., Frank, M. M., and Green, I. (1974). *Am. J. Med.* **57**, 108-114.

Jansen, J., Schuit, H. R. E., VanZwet, T. L., Meijer, C. J. M., and Hijmans, W. (1979). *Br. J. Haematol.* **42**, 21-33.

Katayama, I., and Finkel, H. E. (1974). *Am. J. Med.* **57**, 115-126.

Katayama, I., and Schneider, G. B. (1977). *Am. J. Pathol.* **86**, 163-182.

Katayama, I., and Yang, I. P. (1977). *Am. J. Clin. Pathol.* **68**, 268-272.

King, G., Hurtubise, P. E., Sagone, A. L., LoBuglio, A. F., and Metz, E. N. (1975). *Am. J. Med.* **59**, 411-416.

Leech, J., Roy, R., Flexner, I. M., Glick, A. D., Waldron, J. A., and Collins, R. D. (1975). *Blood* **46**, 1057.

Lewis, S. M., Catovsky, D., Hows, J. M., and Ardalan, B. (1977). *Br. J. Haematol.* **35**, 351-357.

Lusch, C. J., Ramsey, H. E., and Katayama, I. (1978). *Cancer* **41**, 1964-1966.

Moore, J. D., Fay, J., and Logue, G. L. (1977). *Blood* **50**, Suppl. 1, 156.

Naeim, F., Gatti, R. A., Johnson, C. E., Gossett, T., and Walford, R. L. (1978). *Am. J. Med.* **65,** 479–487.

Nanba, K., Soban, E. J., Bowling, M. C., and Berard, C. W. (1977). *Am. J. Clin. Pathol.* **67,** 415–426.

Plenderleith, I. H. (1970). *Can. Med. Assoc. J.* **102,** 1056–1060.

Rieber, E. P., v. Heyden, H. W., Linke, R. P., Saal, J. G., Riethmuller, G., and Waller, H. D. (1976). *Klin. Wochenschr.* **54,** 1011–1019.

Salsano, F., Simonetta, P. S., Ciancarelli, M. P., Pianetelli, M., Lauriola, L., and Musiani, P. (1979). *Acta Haematol.* **61,** 184–193.

Saxon, A., Stevens, R. H., Quan, S. G., and Golde, D. W. (1978). *J. Immunol.* **120,** 777–782.

Schmalzl, F., Huhn, D., Asamer, H., and Braunsteiner, H. (1975). *Acta Haematol.* **53,** 257–276.

Schnitzer, B., and Kass, L. (1974). *Am. J. Clin. Pathol.* **61,** 176–187.

Seshadri, R. S., Brown, E. J., and Zipursky, A. (1976). *N. Engl. J. Med.* **295,** 181–184.

Stewart, D. J., Benjamin, R. S., McCredie, K. B., Murphy, S., and Keating, M. (1979). *Blood* **54,** 298–304.

Trubowitz, S., Masek, B., and Frasca, J. M. (1971). *Blood* **38,** 288–298.

Utsinger, P. D., Yount, W. J., Fuller, R. C., Logue, M. J., and Orringer, E. P. (1977). *Blood* **49,** 19–26.

Yam, L. T., Castoldi, G. L., Garvey, M. B., and Mitus, W. J. (1968). *Blood* **32,** 90–101.

Yam, L. T., Li, C. Y., and Lam, K. W. (1971). *N. Engl. J. Med.* **284,** 357–360.

Yam, L. T., Chaudhry, A. A., and Janckila, A. J. (1977). *Ann. Intern. Med.* **87,** 444–446.

Zucker-Franklin, D., Davidson, M., and Thomas, L. (1966). *J. Exp. Med.* **124,** 533–542.

3
CHRONIC LYMPHOCYTIC LEUKEMIA
Frederick R. Davey

I.	Definition	39
II.	Epidemiology	40
III.	Etiologic Features	40
IV.	Pathologic Observations	41
V.	Pathogenesis	42
VI.	Clinical Features	44
VII.	Laboratory Features	45
VIII.	Differential Diagnosis	47
IX.	Treatment	50
X.	Prognostic Factors	51
XI.	Course of Disease	53
	References	54

I. DEFINITION

Chronic lymphocytic leukemia (CLL) is a malignant proliferation characterized by an accumulation of small lymphocytes (Dameshek, 1967). The malignant lymphocytes involve the peripheral blood and also infiltrate the bone marrow, lymph nodes, spleen, liver, and to a lesser extent, other tissues of the body. Initially the disease is insidious, with only the presence of an absolute lymphocytosis in the blood and an infiltrate in the bone marrow. However, as the disorder progresses, more lymphocytes accumulate in the bone marrow and lymphoreticular tissues, resulting in bone marrow failure, lymphadenopahty, and hepatosplenomegaly.

II. EPIDEMIOLOGY

Chronic lymphocytic leukemia represents 25% of all leukemias in the Western countries (Sweet *et al.*, 1977) but only 2–3% in the Orient (Finch *et al.*, 1969; Wells and Lau, 1960). The median age at diagnosis of patients with CLL is 55 years, with nearly 90% of patients being over age 50 and 67% over 60 (Cutler *et al.*, 1967). Males are more frequently afflicted with this disorder than females. The male-to-female ratio rests between 2:1 and 3:1 (Rundles and Moore, 1978; Zippin *et al.*, 1973).

III. ETIOLOGIC FEATURES

The cause of CLL is not known. Exposure to ionizing radiation is not associated with an increased frequency of this disease (Finch *et al.*, 1969). However, genetic, aging, hormonal, and immunologic factors may influence a person's resistance of susceptibility to CLL.

Genetic factors may render some individuals or populations resistant, whereas others are more susceptible to the development of CLL. For example, the rarity of CLL in Japanese populations in Japan as well as in the United States suggests that a genetic resistance to this disorder may exist.

In contrast, several studies have indicated an increased incidence of CLL among first-degree relatives, including children, siblings, parents, and first cousins (Blattner *et al.*, 1976; Delmas-Marsalet *et al.*, 1974; Gunz and Veale, 1969; Gunz *et al.*, 1975). However, no specific mode of inheritance has been observed.

In one family, a father and four of five siblings developed CLL. In three of the siblings, the peripheral blood leukemic cells shared δ-heavy and κ-light chains as the only detectable surface immunoglobulin, indicating that the CLL observed in these family members may be identical at a molecular level (Blattner *et al.*, 1976).

There is no known association between a specific HLA antigen and susceptibility or resistance with CLL. In familial CLL, however, susceptibility to this disorder may be linked to genes located near the HLA locus (Delmas-Marsalet *et al.*, 1974). In these cases, family members with CLL share a common histocompatibility antigen (HLA) haplotype.

Genetic factors may not be the sole cause of an increased incidence of CLL among family members, since many of the afflicted have a similar environment. In these families, CLL may be a result of a complex interaction between genetically susceptible individuals and some factor(s) in their environment.

Because CLL occurs in the elderly male population and rarely in individuals under age 40, it is possible that the aging process and/or male sexual hormones make individuals more vulnerable to the occurrence of CLL. Lymphocytic response to phytohemagglutinin stimulation (Weksler and Hutteroth, 1974) and serum levels of thymosin (Goldstein *et al.,* 1974) and thymic factor decrease with advancing age. Elderly persons have a higher frequency of anti-smooth muscle, anti-mitochondrial, anti-parietal cell, anti-nuclear, rheumatoid, and lymphocytic antibodies (Diaz-Jouanen *et al.,* 1975; Ooi *et al.,* 1974). These phenomena suggest some alterations in the complex interaction among T cells, B cells, and macrophages of elderly people. In addition, patients with CLL have a higher incidence of autoimmune abnormalities than do control populations (Dameshek, 1967; Lewis and Pegrum, 1978; Pirofsky, 1975). Thus it is possible that the immunologic aberrations observed in elderly populations enhance susceptibility to chronic lymphocytic leukemia.

IV. PATHOLOGIC OBSERVATIONS

CLL is characterized by a persistent absolute lymphocytosis and a lymphocytic infiltrate in the bone marrow. The neoplastic cell is a small mature-appearing lymphocyte with scanty cytoplasm. The nuclear chromatin is clumped and may contain a small nucleolus.

In CLL, there is usually a generalized lymphadenopathy. Secondary pathologic alterations result from the enlargement of lymphoid masses. For example, tonsillar enlargement may result in respiratory obstruction and difficulty in eating. Massive cervical adenopathy leads to problems in the rotation of the neck. Mediastinal adenopathy can result in the compression of respiratory or vascular structures of the chest.

Microscopically, the lymph nodes are diffusely infiltrated by small lymphocytes. Lymphoid follicles with germinal centers usually cannot be identified. Lymphocytes fill the circular and medullary sinusoids and penetrate the capsule and surrounding adipose tissues. In CLL, small lymphocytes characteristically infiltrate the lymph nodes. As a result, the histopathology of CLL is similar to that of well-differentiated lymphocytic lymphoma (Pangalis *et al.,* 1977). However, in many cases of CLL the lymph nodes may contain a moderate to marked number of immature lymphocytes in various foci (Dick and Maca, 1978). These findings were not associated with a more aggressive disease. However, in 3–12% of the lymph nodes from patients with CLL, the characteristically small lymphocyte is replaced by a large anaplastic cell and the histopathology is indisguishable from that seen in histiocytic lymphoma. This finding is associated with advanced and/or terminal disease.

An enlarged spleen is frequently present in CLL. Lymphocytes infiltrate the follicles, periarterial lymphocytic sheath areas, the splenic cords, and the sinuses.

Enlargement of the liver is evident in most cases, but massive hepatomegaly is a rare occurrence. Lymphocytes are prominently distributed in the portal areas. Smaller collections of cells may be observed in the sinusoids. Obstruction of biliary drainage may occur as a result of enlargement of the porta hepatis lymph node (Sweet *et al.*, 1977).

Leukemic skin involvement has been described in 8.3% of patients with CLL (Gunz and Baikie, 1974). Pruritus is the commonest symptom. Scaling exfoliation of the epidermis, as well as single or multiple nodules, may occur (Gates, 1938). Histologically, there is a lymphocytic infiltrate of the upper and middle portions of the dermis. In addition, patients with CLL are prone to the development of herpetic skin lesions.

Chronic lymphocytic leukemia occasionally involves the gastrointestinal tract. The esophagus and colon are rarely infiltrated with leukemia, whereas involvement of the stomach and small bowel are more frequent. Gastric involvement is characterized by thickening of the mucosal folds and occasionally by mucosal ulcerations. Lymphocytes infiltrate the mucosa and submucosa more often than the muscularis and serosal layers. Fungal ulcers of the esophagus and stomach and pseudomembranous enterocolitis are usually terminal events (Prolla and Kirsner, 1964).

Leukemic infiltrates of the lung occur in approximately 30% of advanced cases of CLL (Falconer and Leonard, 1938). The disease appears on radiographs as diffuse, nodular, or miliary lesions. Microscopically, lymphocytes penetrate perivascular and peribronchial tissues and the interstitium of the alveolar spaces. Nodules and tumor masses may form as a result of a large accumulation of lymphocytes. However, pneumonitis is the most common cause of pulmonary dysfunction in patients with CLL.

Hansen (1973) noted that 5% of patients with CLL developed neurologic findings. The neurologic symptoms varied according to the location of the leukemic infiltrate and were usually not clinically severe. Leukemic infiltrates of the central nervous system are not uncommon in postmortem studies (Reske-Nielsen *et al.*, 1974). Lymphocytic infiltrates may be observed in the meninges, along lymphatic spaces of cranial nerves, and occasionally within the substance of the brain in a perivascular pattern (Gétaz and Miller, 1979).

Leukemic infiltrates are also observed in postmortem examinations within the tissues of the genitourinary tract, endocrine system, and skeleton. However, it is unusual for leukemic infiltrates of these organs to result in clinically significant dysfunction.

V. PATHOGENESIS

The basic abnormality in CLL is the massive accumulation and proliferation of lymphocytes. The production rate of individual lymphocytes is low. When a continuous 7-day infusion of tritiated thymidine was administered intravenously to two patients with CLL, only 0.5% labeled and consequently new cells appeared in the blood each day. However, because of the large total number of lymphocytes in these patients, the absolute production rate of blood lymphocytes was markedly increased (Theml *et al.*, 1973).

Evidence suggests that the life span of the neoplastic cells in CLL is prolonged (Stryckmans *et al.*, 1977; Theml *et al.*, 1973). Approximately 90% of blood lymphocytes have a turnover time in excess of 1 year. However, these studies deal with the life span of a single clone of B cell from patients with CLL, and caution must be used in comparing them with the survival of multiple clones of lymphocytes from normal persons. In the latter, the majority of lymphocytes are T-dependent cells.

In CLL, recirculation of lymphocytes from the blood through the lymph nodes, thoracic duct, and back to the blood does not proceed normally. The data suggest that CLL lymphocytes recirculate slowly. It is not clear if this abnormality is the result of the leukemic or of the B-cell nature of the circulating lymphocytes, the excessive number of lymphocytes, or the anatomical alterations of the crowded lymphoid tissue (Stryckmans *et al.*, 1977).

Neoplastic cells from 75 to 90% of the cases of CLL are B lymphocytes. These lymphocytes have monoclonal surface immunoglobulins (Grey *et al.*, 1971; Preud'homme and Seligmann, 1972; Rowlands *et al.*, 1974), Fc (Dickler *et al.*, 1973) and C_3 receptors (Pincus *et al.*, 1972), and Ia antigens (Schlossman *et al.*, 1976). Lymphocytes from CLL patients synthesize surface membrane immunoglobulin (Preud'homme and Seligmann, 1972). In most cases the surface immunoglobulin consists of either IgM or IgD. These CLL cells lack receptors for nonimmune rosettes with sheep erythrocytes (a T-cell property), phagocytic properties, and nonspecific esterases (macrophage characteristics). In those who are afflicted with CLL and are also heterozygous for glucose-6-phosphate dehydrogenase (G-6-PD), a single G-6-PD isoenzyme has been observed in the patient's B lymphocytes, but not in other hemic cells or T lymphocytes. This information suggests that CLL arises from a lymphocyte committed to B-cell differentiation (Fialkow *et al.*, 1978).

Neoplastic lymphocytes from approximately 5% of the cases of CLL are T cells (Brouet *et al.*, 1975; Reinherz *et al.*, 1979). These lymphocytes form nonimmune rosettes with sheep erythrocytes and react with anti-T-cell sera but lack surface immunoglobulin, Fc, and C_3 receptors. Brouet *et al.* (1975) observed that the reactivity of leukemic T lymphocytes with three different heteroantisera to T cells differed among patients, but was homogeneous in individual cases. These findings indicate that the leukemic lymphocytes probably belong to a single subset of T cells.

Neoplastic cells from the remaining cases do not exhibit any cell-surface markers (Foa *et al.*, 1979; Piessens *et al.*, 1973). Therefore, these cases have been listed as ''null'' cell (non-T, non-B) proliferations.

In CLL, immunoglobulin usually cannot be demonstrated within the cytoplasm of the proliferating cell by direct immunofluorescence staining (Preud'homme and Seligmann, 1974). In a rare case, however, intracytoplasmic crystalline inclusions bodies have been demonstrated as a monoclonal immunoglobulin (Gordon and Smith, 1979; McCann et al., 1978).

The high frequency of hypogammaglobulinemia in patients with CLL suggests some difficulty in the production or secretion of immunoglobulin by neoplastic B lymphocytes. It is possible that the neoplastic cells from patients with CLL are blocked at an early stage of differentiation and cannot transform into immunoglobulin-producing cells. In support of this hypothesis, Maino et al. (1977) showed that lymphocytes from three of seven patients with CLL did not secrete increased amounts of immunoglobulin after CLL lymphocytes were incubated with phytohemagglutinin (PHA). Although lymphyocytes from four patients secreted immunoglobulin, the secreted protein consisted predominantly of free light chains with only small amounts of intact immunoglobulins. Thus, an abnormality of immunoglobulin synthesis and/or secretion was suggested in each case. Similar impairment in synthesis of immunoglobulin was also observed when lymphocytes from CLL patients were incubated with pokeweed mitogen (Chen and Heller, 1978). However, other studies indicate that the lack of B-cell differentiation into immunoglobulin-producing plasma cells may be the result of a decrease in T helper lymphocytes rather than an intrinsic abnormality of neoplastic B cells (Chiorazzi et al., 1979; Fu et al., 1978).

Thus CLL, like other lymphocytic malignancies, is a heterogeneous disorder. Most cases of CLL are B-cell proliferations, but a small minority are either T-cell or null-cell neoplasias. In addition, the neoplastic cell present in the B-cell CLL appears to be blocked from terminal differentiation.

VI. CLINICAL FEATURES

In approximately 10–25% of the patients, the onset of CLL is insidious, with no specific symptoms attributable to the disease. These patients are identified by the presence of an absolute lymphocytosis in the peripheral blood and a lymphocytic infiltrate in the bone marrow. Other patients complain of fatigue or the presence of enlarged lymph nodes. It is unusual for patients to present initially with hemorrhagic symptoms, weight loss, or fevers in the absence of infections (Boggs et al., 1966; Galton, 1966).

Enlarged lymph nodes are observed in approximately 85% of patients, whereas splenomegaly is found in 75% and hepatomegaly in 50% of patients with CLL. Lymph nodes are usually nontender and discreet. Enlarged spleens are rarely massive (Sweet et al., 1977).

As the disease progresses, the blood lymphocyte count increases, more lymph nodes are involved, and the spleen and liver enlarge. In more advanced stages, patients may experience easy bruising and pallor. Recurrent infections are frequent. Patients with CLL have an increased susceptibility to bacterial, viral, and fungal infections. Skin, respiratory, and genitourinary tract infections are common. Susceptibility to infections is probably related to a neutropenia and monocytopenia. In addition, a defect in the humoral and cellular immune systems may also contribute to an increased rate of infections.

Collagen vascular disorders such as systemic lupus erythematosus, rheumatoid arthritis, and Sjögren's syndrome have been occasionally associated with CLL (Dameshek, 1967). Marked hypersensitivity reactions to insect bites and to drugs occasionally occur in patients with CLL (Cameron and Richmond, 1971; Weed, 1965). In addition, a second malignancy occurs with increased frequency among patients with CLL (Hansen, 1973; Moertel and Hagedorn, 1957).

VII. LABORATORY FEATURES

The diagnosis of CLL is usually made when there has been a persistent absolute lymphocytosis extending for a period of 2 weeks to 2 months in an individual over age 40. Although some investigators (Han *et al.,* 1967; Ezdinli and Stutzman, 1965; Silver *et al.,* 1978; Rai *et al.,* 1975; Phillips *et al.,* 1977) have accepted an absolute lymphocytosis of $15,000 \times 10^6$/liter as a minimum requirement, others (Bogg *et al.,* 1966; Galton, 1966) have accepted a lower number of peripheral blood lymphocytosis. In addition, Rudders and Howard (1978) noted a monoclonal B-cell proliferation in patients with lymphocyte counts lower than $15,000 \times 10^6$/liter. These findings suggest that despite the paucity of clinical and laboratory findings, early CLL can be readily distinguished from benign lymphocytosis by the use of lymphocyte cell markers.

The peripheral smear usually indicates that 80–90% of the nucleated cells are small lymphocytes. Smudge cells are common, suggesting that they have an increased mechanical fragility. The lymphocytes in the stained smears are usually homogeneous. They are small, and size variation is minimal. The nuclear chromatin is coarsely condensed and a slight amount of cytoplasm is usually evident. Sometimes nucleoli are present in many of the cells.

Lymphocytes from patients with CLL differ in several characteristics from normal peripheral blood lymphocytes. The neoplastic lymphocyte in CLL tends to have more periodic acid Schiff-positive material than normal peripheral lymphocytes (Quaglino and Hayhoe, 1959). CLL lymphocytes contain less surface membrane immunoglobulin per cell than normal peripheral blood B lymphocytes (Ternynck *et al.,* 1974). In addition, CLL B lymphocytes stimulate poorly in a allogeneic or autologous mixed lymphocyte reaction (Smith *et al.,* 1977; Wolos and Davey, 1980). Since no suppressive factors or suppressor cells were detected, it is possible that the poor proliferative response observed in these cultures is the result of an intrinsic defect in the CLL B lymphocyte (Wolos and Davey, 1979).

A variety of enzymes is found in decreased concentration in lymphocytes of patients with CLL. These enzymes include 5'-nucleotidase (Lopes *et al.*, 1973), terminal deoxynucleotidyl transferase (McCaffrey *et al.*, 1975), purine nucleoside phosphorylase (Borgers *et al.*, 1978), adenosine deaminase (Tung *et al.*, 1976), acid phosphatase, and β-glucuronidase (Douglas *et al.*, 1973). Since many of these enzymes are characteristically present in T lymphocytes, the differences observed in CLL may simply reflect the B-cell lineage of these malignant cells.

Twenty to forty percent of patients have an anemia at the time of presentation (Phillips *et al.*, 1977). The anemia in CLL is a result of several factors. In many patients a hypoproliferation of erythrocyte precursors occurs following the infiltration of more than 50% of bone marrow by lymphocytes. Erythrocyte survival may be reduced as a result of sequestration and destruction of red cells by an enlarged spleen. In addition, 10–20% of patients with CLL have a positive direct antiglobulin reaction leading to premature destruction of erythrocytes in the reticuloendothelial system. The antibody is usually an IgG immunoglobulin (Pirofsky, 1975). In one study (Hoffman *et al.*, 1978) of T cell CLL, the malignant lymphocytes suppressed erythroid colony formation. Thus, in this case it appeared that the anemia was the result of malignant T cells inhibiting erythropoietin-responsive stem cells.

Thrombocytopenia is frequently slight, but as the disease progresses it may become severe. In most cases the thrombocytopenia is secondary to a decreased number of bone marrow megakaryocytes and a diminished production of platelets (Phillips *et al.*, 1977). However, thrombocytopenia may also be the result of an immune-mediated process with platelet sequestration and/or destruction in the spleen (Kaden *et al.*, 1978).

During the early stages of the disease, the bone marrow contains only a slight to moderate lymphocytosis, and examination of the marrow aspirate smears may be equivocal. In these cases, examination of the histologic sections of aspirated particles or biopsy often proves helpful. However, at least 40% of the nucleated marrow cells on the aspirate smear must be lymphocytes. In addition, there should be no more than 5% lymphoblasts in either the blood or bone marrow. In more advanced stages of CLL, the marrow is diffusely infiltrated with lymphocytes. This is usually accompanied by a decrease in megakaryocytic, granulocytic, and erythroid elements.

Hypogammaglobulinemia occurs in 50–70% of patients with CLL, and all classes or immunoglobulin may be involved. In one study, IgA was the most severely affected (Foa *et al.*, 1979). However, in a second report IgM immunoglobulin was most frequently depressed (Scamps *et al.*, 1971). In 5% of cases, there is a paraproteinemia usuallv consisting of a monoclonal IgM immunoglobulin. Cryoglobulinemia also occurs in a small number of patients.

Hyperuricemia occurs in 30% of the cases of CLL. Gouty arthritis, however, is unusual. Uric acid nephropathy may occur in these patients, especially if they become well dehydrated prior to treatment with allopurinol (Kritzler, 1958). In contrast, hypercalcemia is infrequent (Sweet *et al.*, 1977).

VIII. DIFFERENTIAL DIAGNOSIS

The persistence of small lymphocytes in excess of $15,000 \times 10^6$/liter in an adult is good evidence for CLL. Microscopic examination of the bone marrow should confirm the diagnosis by showing the presence of lymphocytes representing more than 40% of the marrow cellularity. In children ill with infectious lymphocytosis or pertussis, a transient absolute lymphocytosis of small lymphocytes may exist.

CLL can be differentiated from most cases of lymphosarcoma cell leukemia (LSL). In the latter, the cells are generally larger, contain more abundnt cytoplasm, and display a prominent nucleolus. Nuclear clefts or indentations are

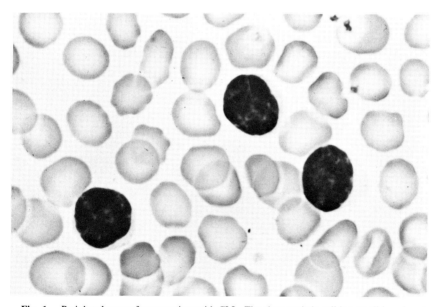

Fig. 1. Peripheral smear from a patient with CLL. The characteristic cell is a small lymphocyte with a high nucleus-to-cytoplasm ratio, clumped nuclear chromatin, and scanty cytoplasm (Wright-Giemsa, ×1000).

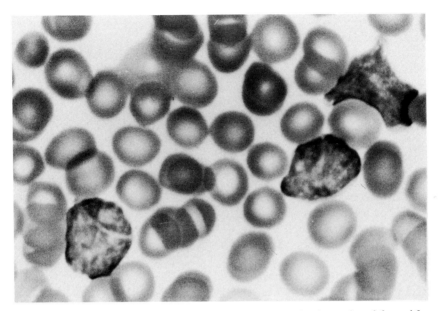

Fig. 2. Cells from patients with lymphosarcoma cell leukemia showing nuclear clefts, and frequently containing nucleoli. The cells of LSL are usually larger than those seen in patients with CLL (Wright-Giemsa, ×1000).

characteristic. (See Figs. 1-4.) The sex ratio and the degree of lymphadenopathy and liver and spleen involvement are similar in CLL and LSL. The mean lymphocyte count is lower in LSL than in CLL (Galton *et al.*, 1974). In addition, the mean survival time of patients appears less in LSL than CLL (Table I).

Prolymphocytic leukemia is usually differentiated from CLL by the presence of excessive lymphocytes (mean of 350,000 × 10^6/liter) massive splenomegaly, moderate hepatomegaly, and minimal lymphadenopahty (Galton *et al.*, 1974). The prolymphocytes represents the majority of cells in the peripheral blood throughout the course of the disease. The cells contain a large vesicular nucleolus and condensed chromatin. The amount of cytoplasm is greater than that of the CLL lymphocyte. In one study (Galton *et al.*, 1974), the mean survival of patients with prolymphocytic leukemia was only 11 months.

The differentiation between hairy cell leukemia (HCL) and CLL is usually not difficult. Most patients with HCL are pancytopenic. The spleen is massively enlarged, the liver is of normal size or only slightly enlarged, and there is no peripheral lymphadenopathy. The neoplastic cells usually contain multiple protoplasmic projections, the nuclear chromatin is clumped, and the cytoplasm is abundant. Cytochemically, the cytoplasm stains positively with acid phosphatase, which is resistant to the inhibitory action of tartrate (Catovsky, 1977).

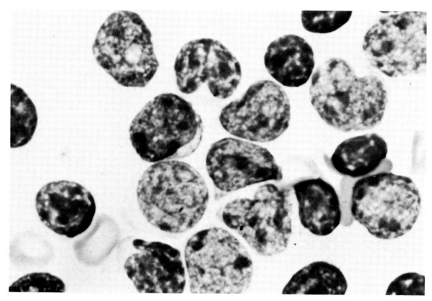

Fig. 3. In prolymphocytic leukemia, the cell contains a large vesicular nucleus, a prominent nucleolus, and a moderate amount of pale blue cytoplasm. (Wright–Giemsa, ×1000).

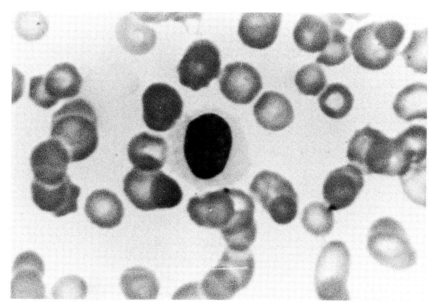

Fig. 4. Characteristic cell from a patient with HCL containing abundant cytoplasm with protoplasmic projections. The nuclear chromatin is usually clumped or slightly vesicular. (Wright–Giemsa, ×1000).

TABLE I

Comparison of Chronic Lymphocytic Leukemia (CLL), Prolymphocytic Leukemia (PL), Lymphosarcoma Cell Leukemia (LSL), and Hairy Cell Leukemia (HCL)[a]

	CLL	PL	LSL	HCL
Age	55	65	60	50
Male:female	2:1	6.5:1	2.5:1	4:1
Initial mean lympho- cyte count per ml	90,000	350,000	40,000	Usually pancytopenia
Lymphadenopathy	Moderate	Mild	Moderate	Usually mild
Splenomegaly	Moderate	Frequently massive	Moderate	Frequently massive
Hepatomegaly	Moderate	Moderate to massive	Moderate	Mild
Response to therapy	Good	Poor	Fair	Good
Survival				
Median	6 years	4 months	3 years	3 years
Mean	6 years	11 months	3 years	5 years

[a] Modified from Galton et al. (1974).

IX. TREATMENT

There is at present no known cure for chronic lymphocytic leukemia. Patients in the early stages of CLL usually do not require chemotherapy. In most centers, indications for chemotherapy in patients with CLL include persistent unexplained depression in performance status, weight loss, fever, progressive enlargement of lymph nodes or spleen, the appearance of new nodes, painful splenomegaly, cytopenia due to bone marrow infiltration, or cytopenias secondary to autoimmune mechanisms (Huguley, 1962; Wiltshaw, 1977).

Several studies have demonstrated the usefulness of alkylating agents in the treatment of CLL (Ezdinli and Stutzman, 1965; Galton et al., 1961). Chlorambucil is the most frequently used drug, and 0.1–0.2 mg/kg is given on a daily basis until the lymphocyte count reaches $10,000 \times 10^6$/liter (Wiltshaw, 1977). Cyclophosphamide has also been employed. In most cases, this type of therapy will produce a reduction in the size of the lymph nodes, spleen and, at times, an increase in the hemoglobin. Some patients require chemotherapy only once or twice a year to remain in control; others require continuous therapy.

Steroids have been used in the treatment of CLL for many years. Prednisone in doses of 30–60 mg daily is particularly helpful in the treatment of autoimmune hemolytic anemia or thrombocytopenia. Treatment is usually continued until the hemoglobin or platelet count rises. Prednisone should then be gradually reduced and alkylating agents initiated. An initial rise in the leukocyte count should be anticipated with steroid therapy. Large doses of prednisone given for a prolonged period of time may predispose a patient to an infection by an opportunistic organism. In addition, prednisone may be helpful in the management of patients with bone marrow failure (Wiltshaw, 1977).

Radiotherapy has been used mainly to treat massively enlarged spleens or bulky lymphadenopathy (Cook and Romano, 1962). Fractionated total-body irradiation has led to some favorable results (Johnson, 1977) in previously untreated cases of CLL. Some success has also been obtained in the management of cytopenic patients using intensive leukophoresis (Cooper et al., 1979).

Few new chemotherapeutic agents of outstanding value have been introduced for the treatment of CLL during the past 10 years (Rundles and Moore, 1978). Vincristine has little usefulness in treatment of the early stages of uncomplicated CLL. Single-drug therapy of CLL has not resulted in prolonged remissions of advanced stages of this disease. However, one report indictes that the combination of cyclophosphamide, vincristine, and prednisone (COP) may be effective for advanced stages of CLL (Liepman and Votaw, 1979). In this study, COP was administered at 3-week intervals, with doses modified according to degree of marrow involvement and thrombocytopenia.

In general, treatment is reserved for patients with persistent systemic complaints, rapidly rising lymphocyte count, and bulky localized disease.

X. PROGNOSTIC FACTORS

Various clinical parameters have been correlated with survival and response to therapy. Rai and co-workers (1975) have devised a staging system for CLL (Table II) based on the degree of lymphocytosis, hemoglobin level, number of platelets in the blood, lymphadenopathy, and presence of hepatosplenomegaly. A significant relationship exists between the stage of disease and survival (Table III). Several studies have now determined that no real differences in survival exist between stages III and IV (Phillips et al., 1977). Perhaps stages III and IV should be combined to include patients with either anemia or thrombocytopenia and a new stage IV considered for patients with anemia and thrombocytopenia.

Phillips et al. (1977) determined that the age of patients was inversely related to prognosis. When age was adjusted for stage and sex, the difference in survival among patients was no longer significant. Although Hansen (1973) and Binet et al. (1977) noted that women patients tended to live longer than men, other investigators (Boggs et al., 1966; Phillips et al., 1977) could not substantiate these conclusions. The level of the lymphocyte count is inversely related to the survival of patients with CLL. Patients with a lymphocyte count less than 50,000 $\times$ 10^6/liter survive longer than those with higher lymphocyte counts (Binet et

TABLE II

Staging System for Chronic Lymphocytic Leukemia[a]

Stage 0	Absolute lymphocytosis with lymphocytes $> 15,000 \times 10^6$/liter with 40% or more lymphocytes in the marrow
Stage I	Absolute lymphocytosis plus lymphadenopathy
Stage II	Absolute lymphocytosis plus an enlarged liver and/or spleen. Lymphadenopathy may or may not be present.
Stage III	Absolute lymphocytosis with anemia (hemoglobin less than 11 gm/dl or hematocrit less than 33%). Lymph nodes, spleen, or liver may or may not be enlarged.
Stage IV	Absolute lymphocytosis with thrombocytopenia (platelet count less than 100,000/dl). Anemia and organomegaly may or may not be present.

[a] From Rai et al. (1975).

al., 1977; Phillips et al., 1977). However, the latter patients tend also to be in a more advanced stage of their disease.

One study has indicated that lymphocyte diameter and the fraction of lymphocytes containing nucleoli were inversely correlated with survival (Dubner et al., 1978). In contrast, Peterson et al. (1975) collected data indicating that survival in patients with large lymphocytes may be longer than in those with small lymphocytes.

Bone marrow lymphocytosis of greater than 80% is a poor prognostic finding. However, hypogammaglobulinemia may not be a significant prognostic factor (Phillips et al., 1977).

Chandra et al. (1979) demonstrated that total body potassium was related to

TABLE III

Median Duration of Survival for Each Stage of Diagnosis as Determined in Various Series (CLL)[a]

Stage of diagnosis	Rai's series		Bogg's series		Hansen's series		Present series	
	No. of patients	Median survival (months)	No. of patients	Median survival (months)	No. of patients	Median survival (months)	No. of patients	Median survival (months)
0	22	>150	3		6	180	11	150
I	29	101	7	130	52	60	25	84
II	39	71	41	108	23	47	60	48
III	21	19	13	9	32	26	29	24
IV	14	19	20	42	39	20	32	24

[a] From Philips, Kempin, Passe, Miké, and Clarkson (1977).

the stage of disease. Following therapy and the reduction of leukemic cell mass, a concomitant reduction in total body potassium was also observed.

Simonsson *et al.* (1978) noted that lymphocytes from CLL patients with progressive disease had glucocorticoid receptors, whereas all patients without glucocorticoid receptors had inactive disease. In contrast, no correlation was found between the level of glucocorticoid receptors and the stage of disease (Homo *et al.*, 1978). However, a significant difference was observed between stage-0 and stage-III/IV patients regarding the *in vitro* inhibitory effect of dexamethosone on tritiated uridine incorporation. In the advanced stages of CLL the inhibition of steroids on the incorporation of tritiated uridine was more pronounced.

XI. COURSE OF DISEASE

The clinical course in CLL is variable (Galton, 1966). Some patients may experience an indolent chronic disorder with few symptoms. However, others have a more aggressive course. The mean survival time varies from 2 to 9 years (Hansen, 1973; Wintrobe and Hasenbush, 1939), and the median survival extends from 1.5 to 7 years (Feinleib and MacMahon, 1960; Hill *et al.*, 1964). Approximately one-third of the patients live longer than 10 years.

As the disease progresses, more lymphocytes accumulate in the lymphoreticular tissues, bone marrow, and peripheral blood. This change is usually associated with neutropenia, thrombocytopenia, and anemia. At this time, the disease may be refractory to chemotherapy. Many patients develop serious infections and die as a result of sepsis. Occasionally patients succumb to hemorrhagic complications within the brain. In rare cases, the terminal stage is characterized by significant weight loss, persistent fever, lymphadenopathy, dysglobulinemia, and a morphologic transition into large pleomorphic cells (Richter, 1928; Long and Aisenberg, 1975). Armitage *et al.* (1978), however, described the development of histiocytic lymphoma in 3.3% of patients with CLL. No consistent laboratory abnormalities were observed in these patients, and it was unclear whether the histiocytic lymphoma in these cases represented a second malignancy or a transitional phase of CLL. Enno *et al.* (1979) described seven cases of CLL whose disease became aggressive and refractory to treatment. This transition was accompanied by the presence in the peripheral blood of a population of immature lymphocytes resembling prolymphocytes. Finally, Kough and Makary (1979) described two patients who developed multiple myeloma late in the course of chronic lymphocytic leukemia. Since lymphocyte surface-marker studies were not performed initially on the CLL lymphocytes, a transition of CLL lymphocytes into multiple myeloma plasma cells was not documented.

REFERENCES

Armitage, J. O., Dick, F. R., and Corder, M. P. (1978). *Cancer* **41**, 422–427.

Binet, J. L., Leporrier, M., Dighiero, G., Charron, D., D'Athis, P., Vaugier, G., Beral, M. H., Natali, J. C., Raphael, M., Nizet, B., and Follezou, J. Y. (1977). *Cancer* **40**, 855–864.

Blattner, W. A., Strober, W., Muchmore, A. V., Blaese, R. M., Broder, S., and Fraumeni, J. F. (1976). *Ann. Intern. Med.* **84**, 554–557.

Boggs, D. R., Sofferman, S. A., Wintrobe, M. M., and Cartwright, G. E. (1966). *Am. J. Med.* **40**, 243–254.

Borgers, M., Verhaegen, H., DeBrabander, M., DeCree, J., DeCock, W., Thone, F., and Geuens, G. (1978). *Blood* **52**, 886–895.

Brouet, J. C., Flandrin, G., Sasportes, M., Preud'homme, J. L., and Seligmann, M. (1975). *Lancet.* **2**, 890–893.

Cameron, S. J., and Richmond, J. (1971). *Scott. Med. J.* **16**, 425–427.

Catovsky, D. (1977). *Clin. Haematol.* **6**, 245–268.

Chandra, P., Sawitsky, A., Chanana, A. D., Chikkappa, G., Cohn, S. H., Rai, K. R., and Cronkite, E. P. (1979). *Blood* **53**, 594–603.

Chen, Y., and Heller, P. (1978). *Blood.* **52**, 601–608.

Chiorazzi, N., Fu, S. M., Montazeri, G., Kunkel, H. G., Rai, K. R., and Gee, T. (1979). *J. Immunol.* **122**, 1087–1090.

Cook, J. C., and Romano, W. (1962). *Am. J. Roentgenol., Radium. Ther. Nucl. Med.* **88**, 892–901.

Cooper, I. A., Ding, J. C., Adams, P. B., Quinn, M. A., and Brettell, M. (1979). *Am. J. Hematol.* **6**, 387–398.

Cutler, S. J., Oxtell, L., Axtell, L., and Heise, H. (1967). *J. Natl. Cancer Inst.* **39**, 993–1026.

Dameshek, W. (1967). *Blood* **29**, 566–584.

Delmas-Marsalet, Y., Hors, J., Colombani, J., and Dausset, J. (1974). *Tissue Antigens* **4**, 441–445.

Diaz-Jouanen, E., Strickland, R. G., and Williams, R. C. (1975). *Am. J. Med.* **58**, 620–628.

Dick, F. R., and Maca, R. D. (1978). *Cancer* **41**, 283–292.

Dickler, H. B., Siegal, F. P., Bentwich, Z. H., and Kunkel, H. G. (1973). *Clin. Exp. Immunol.* **14**, 97–100.

Douglas, S. D., Cohnen, G., König, E., and Brittinger, G. (1973). *Blood* **41**, 511–518.

Dubner, H. N., Crowley, J. J., and Schilling, R. F. (1978). *Am. J. Hematol.* **4**, 337–341.

Enno, A., Catovsky, D., O'Brien, M., Cherchi, M., Kumaran, T. O., and Galton, D. A. G. (1979). *Br. J. Haematol.* **41**, 9–18.

Ezdinli, E. Z., and Stutzman, L. (1965). *J. Am. Med. Assoc.* **191**, 444–450.

Falconer, E. H., and Leonard, M. E. (1938). *Am. J. Med. Sci.* **195**, 294–296.

Feinleib, M., and MacMahon, B. (1960). *Blood* **15**, 332–349.

Fialkow, P. J., Najfeld, V., Reddy, A. L., Singer, J., and Steinmann, L. (1978). *Lancet* **2**, 444–446.

Finch, S. C., Hashino, T., Itoga, T., Ichimaru, M., and Ingram, R. (1969). *Blood* **33**, 79–86.

Foa, R., Catovsky, D., Brozovic, M., Marsh, G., Ooyirilangkumaran, T., Cherchi, M., and Galton, D. A. G. (1979). *Cancer* **44**, 483–487.

Fu, S. M., Chiorazzi, N., Kunkel, H. G., Halper, J. P., and Harris, S. R. (1978). *J. Exp. Med.* **148**, 1570–1578.

Galton, D. A. G. (1966). *Can. Med. Assoc. J.* **94**, 1005–1010.

Galton, D. A. G., Wiltshaw, E., Szurwz, L., and Dacie, J. V. (1961). *Br. J. Haematol.* **7**, 73–97.

Galton, D. A. G., Goldman, J. M., Wiltshaw, E., Catovsky, D., Henry, K., and Goldenberg, G. J. (1974). *Br. J. Haematol.* **27**, 7–23.

Gates, O. (1938). *Arch. Dermatol.* **37**, 1015–1027.

Gétaz, E. P., and Miller, G. J. (1979). *Cancer* **43**, 1858–1861.

Goldstein, A. L., Hooper, J. A., Schulof, R. S., Cohen, G. H., Thurman, G. B., McDaniel, M. C., White, A., and Dardene, M. (1974). *Fed. Proc., Fed. Am. Soc. Exp. Biol.* **33**, 2053-2056.

Gordon, J., and Smith, J. L. (1979). *Br. J. Haematol.* **43**, 155-158.

Grey, H. M., Rabellino, E., and Pirofsky, B. (1971). *J. Clin. Invest.* **50**, 2368-2375.

Gunz, F., and Baikie, A. G. (1974). "Leukemia" 2nd ed. Grune & Stratton, New York.

Gunz, F. W., and Veale, A. M. O. (1969). *J. Natl. Cancer Inst.* **42**, 517-524.

Gunz, F. W., Gunz, J. P., Veale, A. M. O., Chapman, C. J., and Houston, I. B. (1975). *Scand. J. Haematol.* **15**, 117-131.

Han, T., Ezdinli, E. Z., and Sokal, J. E. (1967). *Cancer* **20**, 243-253.

Hansen, M. M. (1973). *Scand. J. Haematol., Suppl.* **18**, 9-144.

Hill, J. M., Loeb, E., and Speer, R. J. (1964). *J. Am. Med. Assoc.* **187**, 106-110.

Hoffman, R., Kopel, S., Hsu, S. D., Dainiak, N., and Zanjani, E. D. (1978). *Blood* **52**, 255-260.

Homo, F., Duval, D., Meyer, P., Belas, F., Debré, P., and Binét, J. L. (1978). *Br. J. Haematol.* **38**, 491-500.

Huguley, C. M. (1962). *Cancer Chemother. Rep.* **16**, 241-244.

Johnson, R. E. (1977). *Clin. Haematol.* **6**, 237-244.

Kaden, B. R., Rosse, W. F., and Hauch, T. W. (1978). *Blood* **52**, 545-551.

Kough, R. H., and Makary, A. Z. (1979). *Blood* **52**, 532-536.

Kritzler, R. A. (1958). *Am. J. Med.* **25**, 532-540.

Lewis, C. M., and Pegrum, G. D. (1978). *Br. J. Haematol.* **38**, 75-84.

Liepman, M., and Votaw, M. L. (1978). *Cancer* **41**, 1664-1669.

Long, J. C., and Aisenberg, A. C. (1975). *Am. J. Clin. Pathol.* **63**, 786-795.

Lopes, J., Zucker-Franklin, D., and Silber, R. (1973). *J. Clin. Invest.* **52**, 1297-1300.

McCaffrey, R., Harrison, T. A., Parkman, R., and Baltimore, D. (1975). *N. Engl. J. Med.* **292**, 775-780.

McCann, S. R., Whelan, A., and Greally, J. (1978). *Br. J. Haematol.* **38**, 369-372.

Maino, V. C., Kurnick, J. T., Kubo, R. T., and Grey, H. M. (1977). *J. Immunol.* **118**, 742-748.

Moertel, C. G., and Hagedorn, A. B. (1957). *Blood* **12**, 788-804.

Ooi, B. S., Orlina, A. R., Masaitus, L., First, M. R., and Pollak, V. E. (1974). *Transplantation* **18**, 190-191.

Pangalis, G. A., Nathwani, B. N., and Rappaport, H. (1977). *Cancer* **39**, 999-1010.

Peterson, L. C., Bloomfield, C. D., Sundberg, R. D., Gajl-Peczalska, K. J., and Brunning, R. D. (1975). *Am. J. Med.* **59**, 316-324.

Phillips, E. A., Kempin, S., Passe, S., Miké, V., and Clarkson, B. (1977). *Clin. Haematol.* **6**, 203-222.

Piessens, W. F., Schur, P. H., Moloney, W. C., and Churchill, W. H. (1973). *N. Engl. J. Med.* **288**, 176-179.

Pincus, S., Bianco, C., and Nussenzweig, V. (1972). *Blood* **40**, 303-310.

Pirofsky, B. (1975). *Clin. Haematol.* **4**, 167-180.

Preud'homme, J. L., and Seligmann, M. (1972). *Blood* **40**, 777-794.

Preud'homme, J. L., and Seligmann, M. (1974). *Prog. Clin. Immunol.* **2**, 121-174.

Prolla, J. C., and Kirsner, J. B. (1964). *Ann. Intern. Med.* **61**, 1084-1104.

Quaglino, D., and Hayhoe, F. G. J. (1959). *J. Pathol. Bacteriol.* **78**, 521-552.

Rai, K. R., Sawistsky, A., Cronkite, E. P., Chanana, A. D., Levy, R. N., and Pasternack, B. S. (1975). *Blood* **46**, 219-234.

Reinherz, E. L., Nadler, L. M., Rosenthal, D. S., Moloney, W. C., and Schlossman, S. F. (1979). *Blood* **53**, 1066-1075.

Reske-Nielsen, E., Petersen, J. H., Sogaard, H., and Jensen, K. B. (1974). *Lancet* **1**, 211-212.

Richter, M. N. (1928). *Am. J. Pathol.* **4**, 285-292.

Rowlands, D. T., Daniele, R. P., Nowell, P. C., and Winzel, H. A. (1974). *Cancer* **34**, 1962-1970.

Rudders, P. A., and Howard, J. P. (1978). *Blood* **52**, 25-35.

Rundles, R. W., and Moore, J. O. (1978). *Cancer* **42**, 941-945.

Scamps, R. A., Streeter, A. M., and O'Neill, R. J. (1971). *Med. J. Aust.* **1**, 535-536.

Schlossman, S. F., Chess, L., Humphreys, R. E., and Strominger, J. L. (1976). *Proc. Natl. Acad. Sci. U.S.A.* **73**, 1288-1292.

Silver, R. T., Sawitsky, A., Rai, K., Holland, J. F., and Glidewell, O. (1978). *Am. J. Hematol.* **4**, 343-358.

Simonsson, B., Nilsson, K., Terenius, L., and Glimelius, B. (1978). *Scand. J. Haematol.* **21**, 379-389.

Smith, J. B., Knowlton, R. P., and Koons, L. S. (1977). *J. Natl. Cancer Inst.* **58**, 579-585.

Stryckmans, P. A., Debusscher, L., and Collard, E. (1977). *Clin. Haematol.* **6**, 159-168.

Sweet, D. L., Jr., Golomb, H. M., and Ultmann, J. E. (1977). *Clin. Haematol.* **6**, 185-202.

Ternynck, T., Dighiero, G., Follezou, J., and Binet, J. L. (1974). *Blood* **43**, 789-795.

Theml, H., Trepel, F., Schick, P., Kaboth, W., and Begemann, H. (1973). *Blood* **42**, 623-636.

Tung, R., Siber, R., Quagliata, F., Conklyn, M., Gottesman, J., and Hirschhorn, R. (1976). *J. Clin. Invest.* **57**, 756-761.

Weed, R. I. (1965). *Blood* **26**, 257-268.

Weksler, M. E., and Hutteroth, T. H. (1974). *J. Clin. Invest.* **53**, 99-104.

Wells, R., and Lau, K. S. (1960). *Br. Med. J.* **1**, 759-763.

Witlshaw, E. (1977). *Clin. Haematol.* **6**, 223-235.

Wintrobe, M. M., and Hasenbush, L. L. (1939). *Arch. Intern. Med.* **64**, 701-718.

Wolos, J. A., and Davey, F. R. (1979). *Clin. Immunol. Immunopathol.* **14**, 77-85.

Wolos, J. A., and Davey, F. R. (1980). *Cancer* **45**, 893-898.

Zippin, C., Cutler, S. J., Reeves, W. J., Jr., and Lum, D. (1973). *Blood* **42**, 367-376.

4
CHRONIC MYELOCYTIC LEUKEMIA
Kanti R. Rai and Arthur Sawitsky

I.	Special Characteristics	57
	A. Influence of Radiation	57
	B. Incidence with Age	58
	C. Marker Chromosomal Abnormality	58
	D. Clonal Origin	59
II.	Clinical Features	59
	A. Definition	59
	B. Diagnostic Criteria	59
III.	Clinical Course	60
	A. Chronic Phase	60
	B. Phase of Metamorphosis (MET)	64
IV.	Summary and Conclusions	67
	References	68

I. SPECIAL CHARACTERISTICS

There are several special features of chronic myelocytic leukemia (CML), also called chronic granulocytic leukemia, that distinguish this disease from all other forms of leukemia. A study of these special features, which are listed below, provides a glimpse of some of the more interesting observations in recent medical research, as well as some of the most frustrating and difficult questions in current medicine.

A. Influence of Radiation

The incidence of chronic myelocytic leukemia was found to be 30–60 times greater among the survivors of the atomic bombs dropped on Nagasaki and Hiroshima than in the population not exposed to radiation. Acute leukemia is the most common form of leukemia among the bomb survivors, whereas the incidence of chronic lymphocytic leukemia was not affected at all. More than one-

CANCER AND CHEMOTHERAPY, VOL. II

third of the leukemias in the exposed Japanese population was CML. This increased incidence of CML was first noted 1 year postradiation and more than 80% of the CML, presumed due to this radiation, occurred in the following 10 years, suggesting a preclinical or induction phase in CML with a range from 1 to 10 years (Stryckmans *et al.*, 1977).

B. Incidence with Age

Typically, but not exclusively, CML is a disease of the adult. Unlike chronic lymphocytic leukemia, which has never been reported to occur in childhood and is almost always diagnosed after the fifth decade of life, CML has been observed among children (albeit rarely) as well as adults. In children there are two forms of CML that are easily distinguishable; a short survival "infantile" form more frequent in infants and toddlers (mean 9 months), and an "adult" form which is clinically similar to that seen in the adult and most frequently in children of 10 to 12 years of age. The incidence of CML is considered to be about 2% of all childhood leukemia, with equal frequency in the infantile and adult forms. However, in the adult over 30 years of age, CML accounts for 20% of all leukemia (Gunz, 1977).

C. Marker Chromosomal Abnormality

A marker chromosome has been sought in all the leukemic disorders, but only in CML has there been a consistent and proved chromosomal abnormality recorded. The abnormal chromosome is called the Philadelphia chromosome and is abbreviated as Ph[1]. The abnormality is found in one chromosome of the autosomal pair of the G group, on chromosome number 22, and consists of deletion of a piece from its long arm (22q−). More sophisticated banding techniques of chromosome analysis using fluorescence of quinacrine or staining with Giemsa have demonstrated that the missing piece of chromosome 22 is translocated to the distal end of the long arm of a number 9 chromosome from the C group. Thus, the Ph[1] abnormality can be precisely defined as 22q−, 9q+ (Rowley, 1973). In some patients the translocation has been found to occur to a C-group chromosome other than number 9. A few patients with acute lymphoblastic leukemia have been found to show the Ph[1] chromosome (Peterson *et al.*, 1976; Beard *et al.*, 1976), but the bulk of evidence supports the notion that this abnormality is most often associated with CML. A minority of patients (approximately 9%) have all the features of CML but are without a demonstrable Ph[1] chromosome. The Ph[1]-negative patients have a significantly shorter survival than the "typical" CML Ph[1]-positive patient (Ezdinli *et al.*, 1970). In children, the Ph[1] chromosome is absent in the infantile form of CML but is found in the adult form (Lawler, 1977).

D. Clonal Origin

The Ph[1] chromosome has been observed in the peripheral blood and bone marrow of CML patients in the precursor cells of granulocytes, erythrocytes, and platelets, as well as in the monocyte–macrophage series. However, this marker chromosome has not been demonstrated in lymphocyte precursors or in fibroblasts (Lawler, 1977). A study of glucose-6-phosphate dehydrogenase (G-6-PD) isoenzymes in CML patients found to be heterozygous for the isoenzymes type A and B in their skin fibroblasts and other non-hematopoietic tissue revealed that the myeloid precursor cells and other cells of myeloid origin in these same individuals stained only for one isoenzyme, either A or B (Fialkow *et al.*, 1967; Fialkow, 1979; Singer *et al.*, 1979). This information supports the concept that the origin of CML is clonal in nature, affecting the myeloid precursor stem cell.

II. CLINICAL FEATURES

A. Definition

The most pronounced feature in CML is cell hyperproduction involving all myeloid cells; an increase in peripheral blood red cells and platelets is common, and a persistent leukocytosis is required for diagnosis. The entire spectrum of the granulocytic series is seen, with a preponderance of the later and more mature forms. As the disease progresses, anemia and thrombocytopenia appear or become more pronounced.

B. Diagnostic Criteria

A patient at the time of initial presentation may or may not be symptomatic. Although no abnormalities may be noted on physical examination, splenomegaly is usually present. A diagnosis of CML is suspected when a persistent leukocytosis is observed. Leukocytosis consists of an increase in the blood stream of absolute numbers of granulocytes, metamyelocytes, and myelocytes. This leukocytosis must not be explainable as a leukemoid reaction to infection or other stress. Other hematological parameters—e.g., erythrocyte count, hemoglobin, platelets, etc.—may or may not be abnormal. Thrombocytosis is present in as many as one-third of the pateints with early CML, and occasionally even an elevated hemoglobin concentration and hematocrit are seen. Anemia and thrombocytopenia are characteristic of the more advanced stages of the disease. Examination of bone marrow aspirate smears as well as of biopsy specimens reveals increased marrow cellularity with a reduction in the amount of marrow fat.

III. CLINICAL COURSE

This disease is noted for two main clinical phases, each of which can be further subgrouped according to the following scheme, which is a modification of that proposed by Spiers (1979).

A. Chronic Phase
    1. Phase at diagnosis or at relapse of a stable phase
    2. Stable disease
    3. Clinical and hematologic remission
B. Phase of Metamorphosis (MET)
    1. Blast phase
    2. Accelerated myeloproliferative phase
    3. Phase of extramedullary leukemia without marrow compromise

At diagnosis, most patients are in the age range of 30–60 years, and about 80–90% will show the Ph^1 chromosome in their leukemic cells. The Ph^1-positive patients differ as a group from those in whom no Ph^1 chromosome is found. The latter patients are somewhat older, show a male predominance (3:1), a mild-to-moderate anemia and thrombocytopenia, and more prominent splenomegaly. Although the initial response to chemotherapy is good in both groups, the duration of response and median survival time is about half (18 months) of that of the Ph^1-positive patient group (median survival 42 months). In both types of CML, the initial and the stable disease phase of variable duration passes on to the phase of metamorphosis which is almost invariably followed by death 6–8 months later.

A. Chronic Phase

The following discussion pertains to the usual clinical picture of the chronic phase at diagnosis or at relapse after stable disease. There are no clinical findings of any abnormality during remission phase except for the persistence of Ph^1 chromosome.

1. Symptoms

The usual symptoms are the following: easy fatigability, loss of appetite or a feeling of being full after eating small amounts of food, weight loss, shortness of breath, and an increased abdominal girth. Some patients may have night sweats, increased appetite, gouty arthritis, and pain over the left side of the abdomen.

2. Physical Findings

Enlargement of the spleen to a variable degree is the most common abdominal finding. Other findings include subcutaneous nodules with a bluish discoloration similar to that of a bruise. Rarely, enlargement of lymph nodes and fever may be noted at the time of initial diagnosis. Tenderness over the sternum or of the other marrow-forming areas is common. Splenic infarction manifested by left upper quadrant pain and a friction rub is usually self-limiting and does not produce severe consequences.

3. Examination of Blood

The hemoglobin level and platelet cound may be normal, elevated, or decreased at initial diagnosis. The total leukocyte count is almost invariably increased at the time of diagnosis but the range of this elevation may be extreme, from 10,000 to 500,000/μl. The differential white cell pattern may reveal 0–5% blasts and promyelocytes, 20–30% myelocytes, 5–10% metamyelocytes, 50–60% segmented neutrophils, 3–6% basophils, 1–2% eosinophils, 5–10% lymphocytes, and 1–3% monocytes. Thus, in addition to the leukocytosis and shift to the left, some degree of absolute basophilia is also observed.

Neutrophil alkaline phosphatase activity is absent or markedly decreased in the Ph^1-positive patient, but may be normal where no Ph^1 chromosome is present. The serum uric acid level is usually high, a fact that must be borne in mind so that these patients should be treated with allopurinol and adequate hydration before antileukemia therapy is instituted. It is necessary to stress that these patients are at an increased risk for developing uric acid nephropathy. Serum levels of vitamin B_{12} and vitamin B_{12}-binding capacity are elevated because leukocyte-associated transcobalamin is increased with the increased numbers of blood leukocytes. The bone marrow picture has already been described in Section II,B.

4. Cell Kinetics

In the chronic phase disease seen initially at diagnosis or at relapse following a stable phase, the total blood granulocyte pool is increased by a factor of 10–100 over the normal (Stryckmans et al., 1977). The average half life ($T_{1/2}$) in the peripheral blood of CML granulocytes is 5–10 times longer than of normal granulocytes, and the effective production of granulocytes is markedly increased. It has been suggested that the increased total body granulocytic cell pool probably disturbs the normal mechanism of granulocyte release from the bone marrow to the peripheral blood, which may explain the presence of numbers of immature cells (myelocytes and metamyelocytes) in the blood during relapse and their relative absence during the stable and remission phases. When the total body granulocyte mass is markedly increased, a traffic of granuloyctes from blood to marrow and to spleen as well as from spleen to blood can be demonstrated (Stryckmans *et al.*, 1977). The proliferative activity of myeloblasts is generally decreased when the peripheral leukocyte concentration is greater than 40,000/μl; this marrow proliferative activity is normal during the remission phase.

5. *Natural History (Chronic Phase)*

At the time of diagnosis a patient is not usually placed on any therapy immediately, but instead is observed at about 2- to 4-week intervals. During this period the presence of symptoms is noted, the size of the spleen is recorded, and the blood count is monitored. About 20% of patients show an initial period of stable disease for 3–6 months, with few or no symptoms, no significant further increase in the size of the spleen beyond that noted at diagnosis, and no significant increase in blood leukocyte numbers. These patients are usually not anemic and have a normal platelet count. Such patients need not be given any antileukemia therapy, and observation is continued.

About 50% of patients, however, have some symptomatology, with a slow but progressive increase in spleen size and peripheral blood leukocyte count. After a period of observation it is possible to establish the pattern of increasing spleen size or leukocyte count for the individual patient. Patients who exhibit a slow rate of increase of these parameters are not treated with antileukemia agents but continue to be observed. Those patients, on the other hand, who show a rapid rate of increase in leukocyte count or of spleen size are treated promptly. These patients are at risk for developing serious complications such as leukostasis, which may result in catastrophic thrombotic–hemorrhagic phenomena in the brain, massive infarcts of the spleen, or infarcts in other organs. There is no critical number of threshold or leukocyte count above which leukostasis will occur, but in our experience, patients with leukocyte counts over 200,000/μl are at significant risk.

Following drug therapy and/or radiotherapy, almost all patients in the chronic phase of CML show a prompt response, with a decline in leukocyte count and a reduction in spleen size. The nature of the response to therapy depends, in part, on the aggressiveness of the treatment plan chosen. Conventional therapy usually results in stable disease with control of the peripheral blood counts and reduction of splenomegaly.

If the therapy chosen is intensive—and such a plan might include splenectomy or splenic irradiation followed by multiple-agent combination chemotherapy—a significant number of patients respond with a full clinical and hematological remission. This remission is characterized by normalization of the blood count, reduction in spleen size to normal, and a normal bone marrow picture. However the Ph[1] abnormality is still demonstrable, although the proportion of myeloid cells positive for the Ph[1] chromosome may be significantly lower than pretreatment values (Cunningham *et al.*, 1979). Usually, neutrophil alkaline phosphatase activity continues to be absent or very low. It should be understood that this type of aggressive combined modality treatment is at present experimental. It remains to be proved whether this approach will delay or prevent the eventual onset of MET or prolong survival to a significant degree.

After a variable period of the chronic or stable phase (which can be as short as 2–3 months or as long as 5–7 years, median 40 months) the disease passes on to the phase of metamorphosis.

6. Treatment

a. Chemotherapy. There are several drugs (Cline and Haskell, 1980) that have been used in the treatment of the chronic phase of CML; one of these, busulfan, has proved to be more effective than others and is usually the first drug chosen. Other drugs that have been tried, but with less effectiveness, are chlorambucil, phenylalanine mustard (melphalan), cyclophosphamide, and 6-mercaptopurine. Dibromomannitol was found to be nearly as effective as busulfan for reducing blood leukocyte counts, but was less well tolerated by patients and the duration of improvement was shorter. Hydroxyurea is as effective as busulfan and may be in more popular usage in the future because of good patient acceptance and freedom from certain toxic effects of the latter.

The side effects of the prolonged use of busulfan are increased skin pigmentation, weakness, anorexia, nausea (mimicking adrenocortical insufficiency), amenorrhea, and premature cataract formation. In addition, an unusual sensitivity of the host tissue to the drug has occasionally precipitated extensive pulmonary fibrosis, which may be fatal. Another less frequent side effect is probably idiosyncratic and consists of prolonged bone marrow aplasia. Busulfan is administered orally, and the usual dosage is 0.06 mg/kg/day. Frequent monitoring of peripheral blood counts is mandatory to prevent overtreatment.

b. Splenic Irradiation. Splenic irradiation is an effective treatment when splenic enlargement is massive and causes symptoms of local pressure. The usual dose is 500–1500 rads delivered over a period of 2–3 weeks. Althouth the spleen size is reduced, the overall disease control is not as satisfactory with splenic irradiation as with busulfan therapy. Occasionally, bone marrow aplasia has been noted following splenic irradiation.

c. Other Treatments. Among other treatments there are four that have been used with no unequivocal benefit but should be mentioned here: (1) splenectomy; (2) leukophoresis; (3) immunotherapy with bacillus Calmette–Guérin and irradiated blast cells (Sokal, 1977); and (4) intensive chemotherapy as given in acute leukemia (Cunningham *et al.*, 1979).

B. Phase of Metamorphosis (MET)

1. Definition

The terminal phase of CML consists of unremitting, aggressive disease ending in death, usually within 6 months. In 1968, Karanas and Silver proposed certain criteria that heralded the onset of terminal phase of CML. These criteria are manifold but essentially take into consideration the percentage of myeloblasts and promyelocytes in peripheral blood, anemia, fever of unexplained origin, thrombocytopenia, and blood leukocyte counts above a certain threshold. The terminal phase of CML has been described in the past also as acute transformation phase, blast crisis, refractory phase, etc. We believe that the term ''phase of metamorphosis'' (MET), introduced by Baikie (1969), covers all these features. Gunz and Baikie (1974) and Spiers (1979) have further clarified the nomenclature of the terminal phase of CML.

2. Overall Clinical Picture

The symptoms, signs and laboratory data may reflect (1) the picture of *de novo* acute leukemia with preponderance of blasts in the peripheral blood and bone marrow and associated with an absence of normal marrow function; (2) the picture of myelofibrosis or refractory anemia or thrombocytopenia (accelerated myloproliferative phase of MET); or (3) extramedullary leukemia with lymphadenopathy, splenomegaly, and subcutaneous nodules with leukemic infiltration in association with peripheral blood and bone marrow findings of the chronic-phase CML. The last form of transformation is usually followed within a few weeks to a few months by an overt blast phase. Eighty percent of patients with CML eventually die because of their leukemia and nearly all of these deaths occur following MET.

3. Symptoms and Signs

The symptoms are varied but usually include severe malaise, loss of appetite, weight loss and fatigue, drenching night sweats, and bone pain. Infection and bleeding diathesis may become prominent. Previously stable splenomegaly frequently worsens.

4. Blood and Bone Marrow Findings

The laboratory findings in the peripheral blood and bone marrow depend upon the type of MET. In the blastic phase, blasts appear in peripheral blood and may constitute 30–90% of the nucleated cells; myelocytes decrease and basophil numbers are elevated initially but may disappear later on. Marked and progressive anemia and thrombocytopenia are usually seen. Bone marrow study discloses a paucity of erythroid elements and of megakaryocytes. Bone marrow biopsy sections (and smears of aspirates) reveal clusters of blast cells, with some increase in fibrosis. In some patients entering the MET phase, the neutrophil alkaline phosphatase activity may suddenly increase and signal the biologic metamorphosis of the disease.

In the accelerated myeloproliferative phase, there is usually anemia and thrombocytopenia, with increasing leukocytosis. A falling leukocyte count in the absence of therapy should arouse the physician's suspicion that MET has occurred. The leukocyte differential pattern may show an increase in blast cells, but the red blood cells invariably have teardrop forms with obvious anisocytosis and poikilocytosis. Giant and bizarre platelet forms may also be seen. Bone marrow study may vary, from a "dry tap" on aspiration and a biopsy section showing marked fibrosis in which clusters of blast cells are seen, to a highly cellular sample with a pattern of mixed granulocyte and erythroid precursor cells consistent with that seen in refractory anemia (i.e., a picture of ineffective erythropoiesis).

In the phase of extramedullary leukemia, the peripheral blood and bone marrow findings are those of the chronic phase of the disease, but a surgical biopsy or needle aspirate of subcutaneous nodules or of enlarged lymph nodes demonstrates sheets of blast cells.

5. Cytogenetics

In 80% of patients, MET is accompanied by additional adnormalities in chromosome preparations besides the presence of the Ph[1] chromosome. Each of the following abnormalities may occur with a frequency of about 20%: (1) a second Ph' chromosome; (2) hyperdiploidy; (3) an isochromosome 17q; or (4) other chromosomal rearrangements and translocations (Lawler, 1977).

6. Cell Kinetics

When blast cells are abundant in the peripheral blood and bone marrow, there are signs of concomitant maturation defects and longer cell generation times are obtained in both *in vivo* and *in vitro* studies (Stryckmans *et al.*, 1977).

7. Lymphoid Characteristics of Blasts

An exciting development was the suggestion that in some patients with MET (approximately one-third), the blast cells may be lymphoid rather than myeloid in origin (Boggs, 1974). The findings in support of the lymphoid nature of these blast cells include:

1. Blast cell reactivity with an antiserum obtained with blast cell antigen from patients with null-cell (Janossy *et al.*, 1976a,b) acute lymphocytic leukemia (ALL)
2. The presence of the enzyme terminal deoxynucleotidyl transferase (TdT) which occurs in thymocytes, bone marrow prothymocytes, and blast cells from T-cell and null-cell ALL (McCaffrey *et al.*, 1975; Marks *et al.*, 1978)

3. The morphology of the blast cells studied by light and electron microscopy have lymphoid characteristics.
4. The drugs used for the treatment of ALL have a greater likelihood of effectiveness in patients with TdT-positive blast cells in MET phase than in TdT-negative MET-phase patients (Canellos, 1977; Marks *et al.*, 1978).

8. Natural History (MET)

Most patients with MET have a known history of CML in the chronic phase for a varying period, but in a small minority the first diagnosis of CML is made when the phase of MET is already overtly manifest. Whether the latter patients have had an unrecognized preclinical CML or represent a variant of *de novo* acute leukemia with Ph[1] chromosome is still an unsettled issue. Once MET has set in the prognosis is poor. Several patients have a fulminant course with no response to any therapy except for toxicity, and death usually occurs within 6 weeks.

Among the MET patients with lymphoblastic features, nearly half may respond to treatment generally effective in ALL, and these patients revert to the chronic phase of CML. However, nearly all these responses are short-lived and MET relapse recurs, followed by a period of refractoriness to all treatment and an early death. The duration of life of such patients from the time of first onset of MET averages about 3 months. Patients in the accelerated myeloproliferative phase of MET have an overall survival of 6–8 months, the median being about 2–3 months. Terminally, all patients present a clinical picture reflecting the repeated courses of therapy and resultant toxicity and complications, which may include profound weakness and severe anemia, requiring frequent red cell transfusions. Muscle wasting and cachexia are commonly seen, along with a protuberant abdomen from the enlarged, at times masive, spleen. The usual causes of death are intracranial or other hemorrhage, systemic infections and, more rarely, complications of leukostasis.

9. Treatment of MET

Most therapeutic decisions are made on individual patient problems. For the blastic phase of MET a number of drugs have been used with sporadic reports of success but with no evidence of consistent beneficial response. These drugs, in various combinations, include hydroxyurea, 6-mercaptopurine, steroids, vincristine, daunorubicin, cytosine arabinoside, bischloronitrosourea, thioguanine, methotrexate, cyclophosphamide, and L-asparaginase (Canellos, 1977; Coleman *et al.*, 1980). Response rates vary between 30–40%, and responses last only a few weeks to a few months. Subsequent treatment is even less effective. Patients in the accelerated myeloproliferative phase of MET are maintained with red cell transfusion therapy; cytotoxic drugs, androgens, and corticosteroids have been used with no significant success. Those patients with extramedullary leukemic infiltrates have been treated by local excision where a nodule is single and accessible; X-ray treatment and cytotoxic drugs may be used but without long-term benefit.

One promising approach in therapy that has not yet been sufficiently tested consists of cryopreservation of autologous patient leukocytes and bone marrow elements while the patient is in the chronic phase or in clinical remission, and subsequent retransfusion of these autologous cells into the patient who has undergone the metamorphosis phase (Canellos, 1977; Goldman *et al.*, 1979).

IV. SUMMARY AND CONCLUSIONS

Chronic myelocytic leukemia is a disease of myeloid proliferation. It is somewhat unique among the malignant diseases in that there is a marker chromosomal abnormality 22q−, 9q+, called the Philadelphia chromosome, which is seen in nearly 90% of patients with CML. The disease appears to be a clonal expansion of the myeloid stem cell. The chronic phase of the disease may initially be deceptively benign in nature and responds with relative ease to primary treatment with oral busulfan or other alkylating drugs. However, such therapy does not prolong the overall survival of patients. The median life expectancy in CML remains about 48 months from the time of initial diagnosis. At about 40 months from diagnosis, the disease takes a turn toward an aggressive phase, which may be associated with either acute blastic transformation, myeloid metaplasia with myelofibrosis, cellular marrow with refractory anemia, or extramedullary leukemia. All these terms are now covered under the common label, the phase of metamorphosis, or MET.

There is presently no method for postponing or preventing the onset of MET. Once MET has set in there is no satisfactory treatment for this phase, and although the course of these patients may vary in severity and duration, almost invariably death supervenes within 8 months. Some patients in the acute blast phase of MET have leukemic cells in the peripheral blood and bone marrow that carry lymphoid cell surface markers, suggesting that the transformation has been to an acute lymphoblastic leukemia (ALL). These patients respond to therapy usually reserved for patients with ALL, but even so, responses are short-lived. Research efforts are being directed toward the postponement of prevention of the onset of the MET phase. One such study proposes the cryopreservation of peripheral blood leukocytes and bone marrow cells while the patient is in the chronic phase and the autologous retransfusion of these cells to patients in whom MET has supervened.

ACKNOWLEDGMENTS

The authors gratefully acknowledge the helpful comments of Willa Gartenhaus, M.D. We also wish to thank Ms. Melanie Nordman for her patience and secretarial skills.

    Grant support was received from the National Cancer Institute (CA-11028), the Helena Rubinstein Foundation, Inc., the United Leukemia Fund, the National Leukemia Association, and the Wayne Goldsmith Leukemia Foundation.

REFERENCES

Baikie, A. G. (1969). *Proc. Congr. Asian Pac. Soc. Hematol. 4th*, p. 197.
Beard, M., Durrant, E. J., Catovsky, D., Wiltshaw, E., Amess, J. L., Brearley, R. L., Kirk, B., Wrigley, P. F. M., Janossy, G., Greaves, M. F., and Galton, D. A. G. (1976). *Br. J. Haematol.* **34,** 169–181.
Boggs, D. R. (1974). *Blood* **44,** 449–453.
Canellos, G. P. (1977). *Clin. Haematol.* **6,** 113–128.
Cline, M. J., and Haskell, C. M. (1980). "Cancer Chemotherapy," 3rd ed., pp. 267–286. Saunders, Philadelphia, Pennsylvania.
Coleman, M., Silver, R. T., Pajak, T. F., Cavalli, F., Rai, K. R., Kostinas, J. E., Glidewell, O., and Holland, J. F. (1980). *Blood* **55,** 29–36.
Cunningham, I., Gee, T., Dowling, M., Chaganti, R., Bailey, R., Hopfan, S., Bowden, L., Turnbull, A., Knapper, W., and Clarkson, B. (1979). *Blood* **53,** 375–395.
Ezdinli, E. Z., Sokal, J. E., Crosswhite, L., and Sandberg, A. A. (1970). *Ann. Intern. Med.* **72,** 175–182.
Fialkow, P. J. (1979). *Annu. Rev. Med.* **30,** 135–143.
Fialkow, P. J., Gartler, S. M., and Yoshida, A. (1967). *Proc. Natl. Acad. Sci. U.S.A.* **58,** 1468–1471.
Goldman, J. M., Catovsky, D., Hows, J., Spiers, A. S. D., and Galton, D. A. G. (1979). *Br. Med. J.* **1,** 1310–1313.
Gunz, F. W. (1977). *Clin. Haematol.* **6,** 3–20.
Gunz, F., and Baikie, A. G. (1974). "Leukemia," 3rd ed., pp. 330–336. Grune & Stratton, New York.
Janossy, G., Greaves, M. F., Revesz, T., Lister, T. A., Roberts, M., Durrant, J., Kirk, B., Catovsky, D., and Beard, M. E. J. (1976a). *Br. J. Haematol.* **34,** 179–192.
Janossy, G., Roberts, M., and Greaves, M. F. (1976b). *Lancet* **2,** 1058–1061.
Karanas, A., and Silver, R. T. (1968). *Blood* **32,** 445–459.
Lawler, S. D. (1977). *Clin. Haematol.* **6,** 55–75.
McCaffrey, R., Harrison, T. A., Parkman, R., and Baltimore, D. (1975). *N. Engl. J. Med.* **292,** 775–780.
Marks, S. M., Baltimore, D., and McCaffrey, R. (1978). *N. Engl. J. Med.* **298,** 812–814.
Peterson, L. C., Bloomfield, C. D., and Brunning, R. B. (1976). *Am. J. Med.* **60,** 209–220.
Rowley, J. D. (1973). *Nature (London)* **243,** 290–293.
Singer, J. W., Fialkow, P. J., Steinman, L., Najfeld, V., Stein, S. J., and Robinson, W. A. (1979). *Blood* **53,** 264–268.
Sokal, J. E. (1977). *Clin. Haematol.* **6,** 129–139.
Spiers, A. S. D. (1979). *Br. J. Haematol.* **41,** 1–7.
Stryckmans, P. A., Debusscher, L., and Collard, E. (1977). *Clin. Haematol.* **6,** 21–40.

5

THE LYMPHOMAS
John M. Bennett

I.	Introduction	69
	A. Drug Reactions	70
	B. Angioimmunoblastic Lymphadenopathy	71
	C. Malignant Localized Lymphadenopathy	71
II.	Hodgkin's Disease	71
	A. Clinical Features	71
	B. Histopathologic Diagnosis	73
	C. Classification	75
	D. Bone Marrow Biopsy	78
	E. Treatment	80
	F. Chemotherapy	81
III.	Non-Hodgkin's Lymphomas	82
	A. Clinical Features	82
	B. Pathology	83
	C. Large Cell Lymphoma (Histiocytic Type)	86
	D. Malignant Lymphoma, Diffuse, Burkitt's Type	87
	E. Nodular Lymphomas	88
	F. Clinical Presentations	89
	G. Therapy	89
IV.	Conclusion	94
	References	94

I. INTRODUCTION

The discovery of lymphadenopathy without an apparent cause confronts the physician with a vexing problem. Enlarged lymph nodes may result from (1) antigen-induced lymphocyte proliferation; (2) suppurative or granulomatous inflammatory reaction in lymph nodes; (3) malignant proliferation of cells that constitute the normal morphology of lymph nodes; and (4) growth of metastatic carcinoma or sarcoma cells in lymph nodes. Any enlargement of a lymph node or

Copyright © 1981 Academic Press, Inc.

group of lymph nodes that persists without an obvious explanation for longer than 4–8 weeks warrants surgical biopsy. In addition to a careful physical examination, a thorough evaluation of the peripheral blood smear is mandatory, since atypical lymphoid cells or frankly neoplastic lymphoid cells may circulate in the peripheral blood and lead to the diagnosis of malignant lymphoma or its leukemic counterpart.

Approximately 50% of lymph node biopsies result in a diagnosis of either malignant lymphoma or carcinoma. These statistics are a function of the accuracy of the pathologist, the timing of biopsy, and the selection of patients. It suggests however that the diagnosis of malignant disease is a common outcome of biopsy of lymph node enlargement in the absence of a clinical diagnosis (Sinclair *et al.*, 1974).

In the differential diagnosis of regional nonmalignant lymphadenopathy, one should consider acute suppurative lymphadenitis secondary to bacterial organisms such as *Staphylococcus aureus* and *Streptococcus hemolyticus*, mycobacterial infection, viral infections such as cat scratch disease (Warrick, 1976), or vaccination reactions such as seen with smallpox, tetanus, typhoid, or diptheria toxoid injections. Veneral disease is an important cause of regional lymphadenopathy secondary to lymphogranuloma venereum or syphilis.

When patients present with generalized lymphadenopathy, the urgency for diagnosis is not as great as when a solitary or regional group of nodes becomes enlarged. The reason for this is that if the cause of the lymphadenopathy turns out to be a lymphoma, by definition it is already advanced and a delay in diagnosis is not as critical as it might be in a patient with earlier disease. Included in the differential diagnosis of generalized lymphadenopathy would be the viral exanthems such as rubella and roseola, infectious mononucleosis—which can mimic malignant lymphoma because of the presence of symptoms including fever, weight loss, malaise, and often prominent splenomegaly—toxoplasma mononucleosis, cytomegalovirus mononucleosis, and certain chronic infections including mycobacterium tuberculosis, brucellosis, and the secondary stage of syphilis. Some of the collagen vascular disorders such as systemic lupus erythematosus can present with lymphadenopathy. Superficial lymph node enlargement is a feature of over half of those patients diagnosed as having sarcoidosis. This adenopathy may persist for many months. The most common finding is bilateral hilar nodes noted on chest X ray.

A. Drug Reactions

Lymphadenopathy may also occur secondary to drug-hypersensitivity reactions. The hydantoin derivatives used in the treatment of epilepsy may produce generalized lymphadenopathy. This syndrome usually recedes quickly with the proscription of the drug. In a few instances, features of malignancy may be present in the lymph node biopsy, but the findings revert to normal after cessation of the drug (Saltstein and Ackerman, 1969). On rare occasions bonafide lymphoma has occurred in association with the long-standing use of hydantoin derivatives (Hyman and Sommers, 1966).

B. Angioimmunoblastic Lymphadenopathy

This is an unusual lymphoproliferative disorder without apparent cause that is associated with fever, night sweats, a skin rash, polyclonal hypergrammaglobulinemia, anemia, and often a positive Coombs' test. The pathology is difficult to interpret since there is often obliteration of the lymph node architecture. However, the population of cells is pleomorphic, consisting of lymphoid cells, plasma cells, and immunoblasts. In addition there is a marked vascular proliferation. The clinical course is variable, with some patients having a prolonged survival but others progressing to a frank immunoblastic sarcoma (Lukes and Tindle, 1975).

C. Malignant Localized Lymphadenopathy

Metastatic Carcinoma

Enlargement of regional lymph nodes may be secondary to involvement either with solid tumors of epithelial origin, or by lymphomas. For example, one can find either squamous cell carcinoma in a cervical node—which usually indicates an origin of the tumor from either the nasopharynx, larynx, or the lung—or one can find adenocarcinoma in the lower cervical or supraclavicular nodes, representing carcinoma from the lung, breast, or even from organs located below the diaphragm such as the stomach, gastrointestinal tract, or prostate gland. Carcinoma cells in inguinal or femoral nodes should raise the suspicion of a primary site of tumor in the vulva, cervix, or ovary in women, and prostate or bladder in men (Berge and Toremalm, 1969).

II. HODGKIN'S DISEASE

A. Clinical Features

Hodgkin's disease usually presents as asymptomatic superficial lymph node enlargement. It commonly affects people between the ages of 15 and 50. Approximately 40% of patients will manifest some degree of systemic symptoms including fever, night sweats, weight loss, and pruritus. Hodgkin's disease usually appears as an enlargement of a local node or group of nodes. This enlargement tends to be nontender and firm to palpation. Close to 60% of patients have

TABLE I

Frequency of Node Involvement

Location	Stage I/II	Stage III/IV
Superficial		
Cervical	65%	70%
Axillary	15	25
Iliac, femoral	10	15
Deep		
Mediastinal	10	60
Hilar	±	10
Para-aortic	±	35
Spleen	±	35

localized enlargement in one or two superficial lymph node areas. In such patients the most commonly involved areas are the cervical or supraclavicular regions, with the mediastinal nodes being involved about as frequently (Table I). Chest X rays are used to evaluate this area (Fig. 1). For examination of deep lymph node areas below the diaphragm, computerized axial tomography (CAT) or lymphangiography is commonly employed (Figs. 2 and 3). Palpable enlarge-

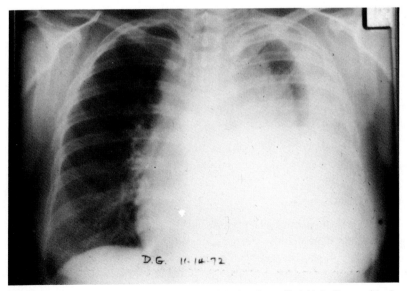

Fig. 1. Chest X ray of patient with mediastinal widening due to Hodgkin's disease and a large pleural effusion.

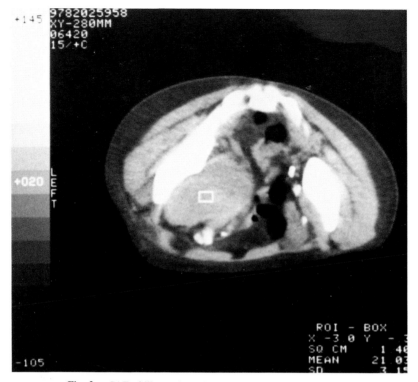

Fig. 2. CAT of iliac nodes enlarged in a patient with lymphoma.

ment of the spleen is uncommon and often is due to a reactive process rather than actual involvement of the spleen by Hodgkin's disease. Similarly, the lung, pleura, liver, or bone marrow are involved in fewer than 10% of patients at presentation (Kaplan, 1972).

In contrast to patients with other forms of lymphoma commonly referred to as non-Hodgkin's lymphoma, frank involvement of the peripheral blood is uncommon. Mild anemia and/or mild neutrophilia and slight monocytosis may occur in approximately 30% of patients, but the finding of neoplastic cells is extremely uncommon.

B. Histopathological Diagnosis

The pathologic diagnosis of Hodgkin's disease has been the identification of an abnormal cell with large inclusion-like nucleoli and polyploidism (Fig. 4). This cell is referred to as a Reed–Sternberg cell, and may well represent an end-stage of other mononuclear malignant-appearing cells that are recognized in

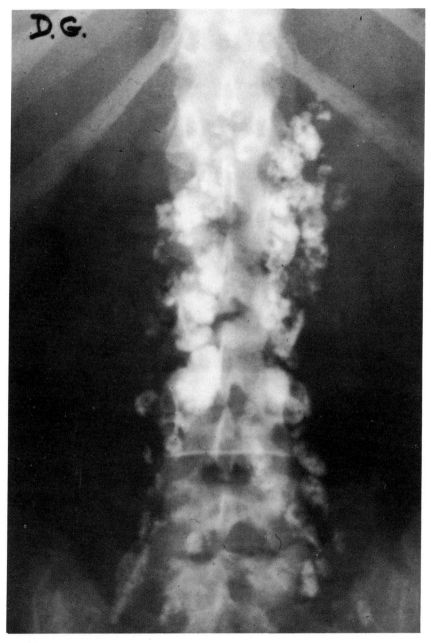

Fig. 3. Bipedal lymphangiogram showing enlargement of retroperitoneal nodes in Hodgkin's disease.

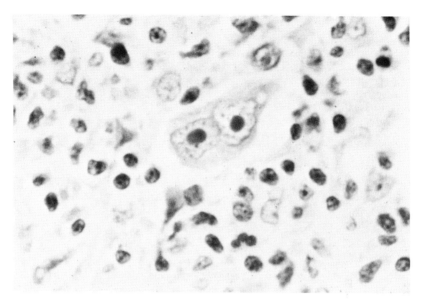

Fig. 4. Classic Reed–Sternberg cell in a patient with mixed-cellularity disease (×480).

this disease. There continues to be considerable debate as to the origin of this cell, some feeling that it may be of lymphoid origin, others feeling that it may be of true monocyte–histiocyte origin. Cells similar to Reed–Sternberg cells have been identified in other conditions such as infectious mononucleosis, histiocytic lymphoma, or undifferentiated metastatic carcinoma. The recognition of this cell in conjunction with other pathologic criteria is considered a prerequisite for the diagnosis of Hodgkin's disease.

C. Classification

Table II illustrates the histological classification of Hodgkin's disease. In the subclassification originally proposed by Parker and Jackson, over 90% of patients fell into the so-called granuloma category. In 1966, Lukes and Butler proposed a new classification that has received widespread acceptance. The major change was the inclusion of two new categories, namely, nodular sclerosis and mixed cellularity (Lukes *et al.*, 1966). In most series, lymphocyte predominance comprises 5% of cases, nodular sclerosis about 50%, mixed cellularity 40%, and lymphocyte depletion 5%. As one progresses from lymphocyte predominance to lymphocyte depletion, the number of giant abnormal histiocytes or Reed–Sternberg cells increases. Table III represents approximate survival figures for Hodgkin's disease, based on pathologic staging and the absence or presence

TABLE II

Histological Classification of Hodgkin's Disease

Parker–Jackson	Lukes–Butler	Reed–Sternberg cells
Paragranuloma (5%)	Lymphocyte predominance (5%)	Rare
Granuloma (90%)	Nodular sclerosis (50%)	Occasional–moderate
	Mixed cellularity (40%)	
Sarcoma (5%)	Lymphocyte depletion (5%)	Moderate–many

of generalized symptoms. It can be seen that the lymphocyte predominance and nodular-sclerosing categories are associated with minimal disease and the absence of symptoms to a much larger degree than mixed cellularity and lymphocyte depletion. This is reflected in the 5-year survival figures.

1. Lymphocyte Predominance

In lymphocytic predominance the predominant cell is a well-differentiated lymphocyte with scattered atypical and normal-appearing histiocytes. Only occasional Reed–Sternberg cells are identified (Fig. 5). In all instances the normal architecture of the lymph node is effaced.

2. Nodular Sclerosis

In the nodular-sclerosing variant the major finding is that of fibrous collagen bands that tend to split the lymph node into well-defined nodular areas. as seen in Fig. 6. These bands frequently arise from a thickened capsular area and extend into the lymph node. In addition, there is a Reed–Sternberg variant cell referred to as a "lacunar" cell. The lacunar cell variant may be the first manifestation of

TABLE III

Survival Figures for Hodgkin's Disease

Pathology[a]	Stage		Symptoms		Five-year survival
	I/II	III/IV	A[b]	B[c]	
L.P. (5%)	90%	10%	100%	0%	85%
N.S. (50%	70%	30%	65%	35%	60%
M.C. (40%)	60%	40%	55%	45%	40%
L.D. (5%)	30%	70%	30%	70%	30%

[a] L.P., lymphocyte predominance; N.S., nodular sclerosis; M.C., mixed cellularity; and L.D., lymphocyte depletion.
[b] A = absence of symptoms.
[c] B = presence of symptoms.

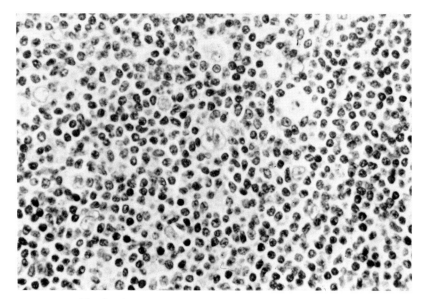

Fig. 5. Lymphocyte predominant: Hodgkin's disease (×240).

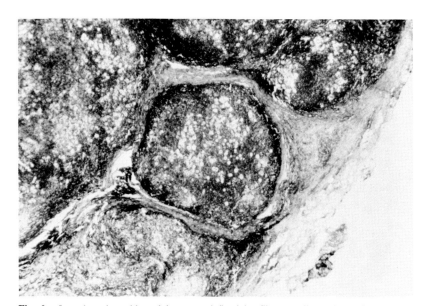

Fig. 6. Lymph nodes with nodular areas defined by fibrous collagen bands in the nodular-sclerosing variant: Hodgkin's disease (×150).

nodular-sclerosing Hodgkin's disease, and may indeed precede the development of the collagen bands.

3. Mixed Cellularity

The mixed-cellularity form of Hodgkin's disease is characterized by diffuse replacement of the normal nodal architecture without an increase in collagen banding. The cytology is much more pleomorphic, with many lymphoid cells, various histiocytes, prominent eosinophils, plasma cells, and moderate numbers of Reed–Sternberg cells (Fig. 7). In integrating the old and new classifications of Hodgkin's disease, it should be noted that the mixed type of the new classification most closely represents the granuloma form of the old classification.

4. Lymphocytic Depletion

The lymphocytic-depletion form of Hodgkin's disease can show either diffuse fibrosis with a general depletion of cells and occasional Reed–Sternberg cells or an extreme proliferation of cells, the majority of which are Reed–Sternberg cells. This latter variant most closely resembles the sarcoma type of the old classification (Fig. 8).

D. Bone Marrow Biopsy

Hodgkin's disease involvement of the bone marrow is being reported more frequently with the use of staging laparotomies and open marrow biopsy as well

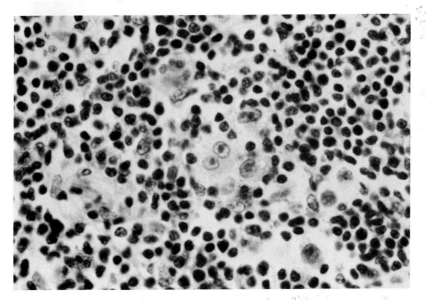

Fig. 7.   Mixed cellularity: Hodgkin's disease (×200).

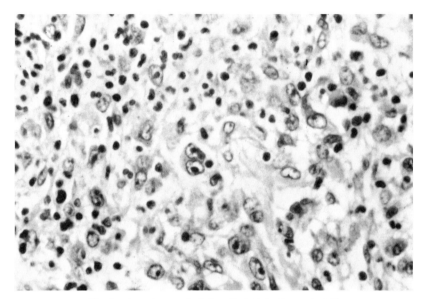

Fig. 8. Lymphocyte depletion: Hodgkin's disease (×240).

as the closed bone marrow biopsy technique. Nevertheless, in contrast to non-Hodgkin's lymphoma, only a small percentage—usually less than 10%—will have focal bone marrow involvement at presentation. Virtually all these patients will have been demonstrated to have had advanced disease—i.e., stage III or IV—prior to the bone marrow biopsy.

Laparotomy

Despite the use of the lymphangiogram and CAT scan, the incidence of false-positive and false-negative results from radiologic technique continues to approach 20–30%. Therefore, accurate diagnosis of the involvement of the liver, spleen, abdominal lymph nodes, or bone marrow may require a staging laparotomy. It is essential to point out that a laparotomy is only done in those instances in which the therapeutic decision may be altered by an assessment of the intro-abdominal structures. Staging laparotomy is not a simple procedure. It produces a morbidity in 5–30% of patients and results in death in approximately 1% of patients. Patients that do not require staging laparotomy include (1) those with stage IV disease proved by percutaneous biopsy; (2) those with a high cervical lymph node enlargement without a palpable spleen, a negative lymphangiogram with either lymphocyte type; (3) those over the age of 65; and (4) most children under the age of 15, where a combined-modality approach including radiation and chemotherapy is often used, regardless of intra-abdominal findings. In most series of patients undergoing staging laparotomy, about 20% of patients have their stage advanced after laparotomy and 15% of patients have the extent of their disease reduced by the procedure.

E. Treatment

Hodgkin's disease is believed to be unicentric in origin and spreads to contiguous nodal sites. Radiation therapy has been demonstrated to be highly effective in permanently eradicating disease in the majority of nodal sites to which it is delivered. The results rest upon the delivery of full doses to involved sites plus extension of fields to include the adjacent uninvolved sites at risk. The field arrangements include the major node-bearing regions on both sides of the diaphragm, and the current techniques have been referred to as "total nodal irradiation" (TNI). For treatment above the diaphragm the technique has been called a "mantle technique," and below the diaphragm an "inverted Y technique" (Fig. 9). The dose to the involved sites is recommended to be 4500 rad, and to uninvolved sites, 3500 to 4000 rad. The overall survival figures have definitely improved (Fig. 10) (Kaplan, 1976). The 40% 5-year survival figures in the

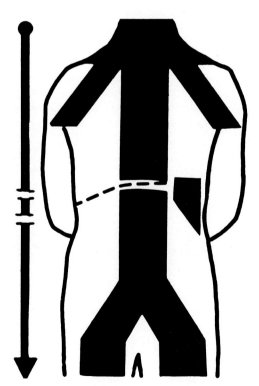

Fig. 9. Diagram of field arrangements in Hodgkin's disease.

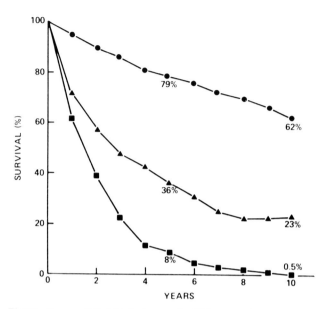

Fig. 10. Therapeutic eras of Hodgkin's disease. ●, 1009 cases, all stages, treated with 6 MEV linear accelerator X ray and/or chemotherapy; ▲, 285 cases, all stages treated by high dose 200 KV X-ray therapy; ■, 754 cases, all stages, with no specific therapy (composite of six reports). From Kaplan (1976), *Cancer Res.* **36**, 3869.

orthovoltage era improved to 75–80% in the megavoltage era. The major gain has been a dramatic improvement in localized stage I and II when the uninvolved lymph node areas were treated fully on the opposite side of the diaphragm.

Recent results reported by Goodman *et al.* (1976) indicate that subtotal nodal irradiation that excludes the pelvis in surgically determined IA and IIA patients results in an 88% relapse-free survival 5 years after initiation of treatment. For patients who fail, it is probable that combination chemotherapy (discussed below) will result in a considerable salvage of at least 50% of these patients, who then will fall into a prolonged survival curve. Another important program using radiation therapy has been that of consolidation radiation in advanced stages after successful induction by combination chemotherapy (Proznitz *et al.*, 1976). This form of treatment may prevent relapses in bulky nodal sites involved prior to chemotherapy.

F. Chemotherapy

Hodgkin's disease is an excellent example of a neoplasm for which the development of effective combination chemotherapy has made a significant difference with regard to the percentage of responses, length of remissions, and prolonged survival. The most successful of the new combinations has been the

TABLE IV

Responses and Survival Using MOPP
Chemotherapy

Number of patients	194
Complete remissions	154 (80%)
5-Year survival	82%
5+-Year survival	66%
10+-Year survival	58% (projected)

four-drug combination termed "MOPP," the acronym for nitrogen mustard, Oncovin , procarbazine, and prednisone (DeVita *et al.*, 1970). The complete remission rate for patients with advanced Hodgkin's disease has been close to 80%, with over 50% of the entire population remaining in complete remission for periods ranging from 5 to 10 years without additional therapy (Table IV) (DeVita *et al.*, 1976). A study by Ziegler *et al.* (1974) demonstrated the effectiveness of the MOPP program in African children with stages I and II disease; radiotherapy was unavailable, yet a 6-year disease-free interval in nine of ten patients was attained. These are truly remarkable events in the history of chemotherapy for malignancies and suggest that a cure for this disease can be accomplished with chemotherapy as well as with radiation treatment.

Since combination chemotherapy appears to be curative in possibly 50% of patients with advanced disease, one can certainly consider that it should be half again as effective for patients with limited disease, producing cure rates of 75-80%. If this is true, then the arena is prepared for the combination of radiation and chemotherapy for localized Hodgkin's disease, with the goal of radiation therapy to sterilize local areas of disease and the goal of chemotherapy to sterilize occult microscopic foci outside of treatment areas.

Finally, we must be prepared to examine carefully the long-term related complications of this aggressive combined modality approach to Hodgkin's disease. The possible development of cardiopulmonary toxicity from Adriamycin (doxorubicin) and bleomycin may affect the quality of life in responding patients. Also, the risk of development of second primary neoplasms may prove to be significant in protocols combining radiotherapy and chemotherapy (Coleman *et al.*, 1977).

III. NON-HODGKIN'S LYMPHOMAS

A. Clinical Features

The non-Hodgkin's lymphomas affect all age groups, but occur most frequently in the elderly. Most patients present with lymph node enlargement in a superficial lymph node group. Lymphomas usually appear as enlargement of cervical, supraclavicular, axillary, or inguinal lymph nodes. Unlike Hodgkin's disease, mediastinal lymph node enlargement is uncommon except in the so-called lymphoblastic lymphoma of adolescence, in which the presenting sign is often that of mediastinal enlargement. Unlike Hodgkin's disease, if the spleen is enlarged it usually contains histopathologic evidence of lymphoma. Extranodal sites involved in descending order of frequency are bone marrow, stomach, small intestine, liver, bone, thyroid, and skin. About 50% of patients have extranodal disease at the time of diagnosis, although this may not be evident with routine diagnostic procedures (Lotz *et al.*, 1976). In contrast to Hodgkin's disease, leukemic manifestations of the non-Hodgkin's lymphomas do occur. Careful examination of the blood in patients with lymphoma may show occasional cleaved lymphocytes even when the leukocyte and lymphocyte counts are normal (Fig. 11). In patients who present with blood and marrow involvement, the distinction between poorly differentiated lymphoma and lymphoblastic leukemia or well-differentiated lymphoma and chronic lymphocytic leukemia becomes a semantic one.

B. Pathology

The Rappaport classification of non-Hodgkin's lymphomas has resulted in a revision of our concepts of these disorders because of the apparent differences of survival among the histologic subtypes, including architectural pattern (nodular versus diffuse) and cell type (lymphocytic or histiocytic) (Rosenberg *et al.*, 1975). These prognostic features are of considerably more value in adults, where close to half of the lymphomas have a nodular pattern, than in children and adolescents, where virtually all the lymphomas have a diffuse pattern (Figs. 12 & 13). Certainly, current available data suggest that nodular lymphomas have a better prognosis overall and a higher survival rate than diffuse lymphomas.

With increasing sophistication in the determinants of the origin of lymphoid cells—i.e., thymus-derived (T cells) or bursal-derived (B cells)—modifications have been proposed in the classification that have proved to be helpful in our understanding of the pathogenesis of these diseases (Lukes and Collins, 1974). The application of "immunological markers" to the study of non-Hodgkin's lymphoma (NHL) has demonstrated that all of the nodular lymphomas and many of the diffuse forms are composed of malignant lymphoid cells of B origin, associated with a leukemic manifestation—i.e., the presence of malignant cells identified in the circulating peripheral blood. The most common forms of NHL under this classification fall basically into three groups: (1) the large cell diffuse lymphomas (formerly called histiocytic lymphomas) which account for approximately 25% of patients; (2) the poorly differentiated lymphocytic lymphomas, nodular, which account for 25% of patients; and (3) the poorly differentiated lymphocytic lymphomas of the diffuse pattern, which account for another 25%.

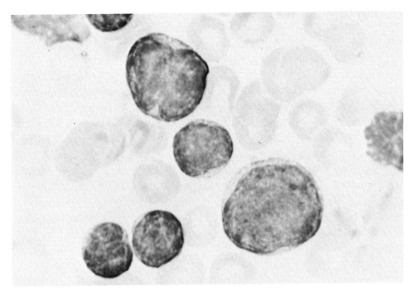

Fig. 11. "Lymphoma cells" in peripheral blood (×500).

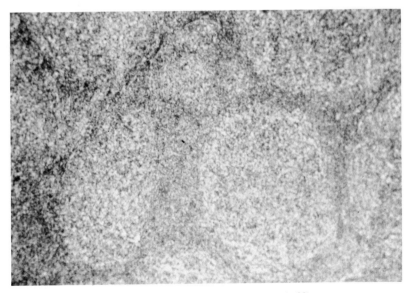

Fig. 12. Nodular lymphoma: low power (×20).

Fig. 13.   Diffuse lymphoma: low power (×20).

mostly of follicular origin. In addition, the vast majority of histiocytic and lymphocytic–histiocytic cell types lack monocyte (macrophage) markers, but have either surface immunoglobulins or have no markers and are therefore referred to as null or non-B–non-T cells.

However, at the present time, the major institutions responsible for conducting combined-modality trials in NHL, including the National Cancer Institute-sponsored multidisciplinary groups, continue to use the Rappaport classification. The non-Hodgkin's lymphomas can be classified as either nodular or diffuse, with a small percentage of patients presenting with both a nodular and diffuse pattern (Table V). Approximately 46% of patients present with a nodular pattern and 54% of patients present with a diffuse pattern. Within each architectural pattern there may occur a variety of different cell types that relate to size and differentiation of the lymphocytic family. In addition, many of the NHLs can be These percentages vary somewhat from series to series, depending upon the interpretation of the size of the malignant population. If, for example, one sees more than three large cells per high power field, then some authorities use the term "mixed-cell lymphoma," either nodular or diffuse pattern. A relatively small percentage of patients present with either undifferentiated lymphomas (Burkitt's type) or non-Burkitt's type, or at the other end of the spectrum, well-differentiated lymphocytic lymphomas, diffuse pattern, accounting for less than 5% of the patient population.

TABLE V

Classification of Non-Hodgkin's Lymphomas

Cell type	Nodular form	Diffuse form	Leukemic form
Histiocytic (large cell)	>5%	30%	Yes
Histiocytic–lymphocytic	5%	5%	Yes
Undifferentiated, Burkitt's	—	<5%	Rare
Undifferentiated, lymphoblastic	—	5%	Yes
Lymphocytic, poorly differentiated	25%	25%	Yes
Lymphocytic, well-differentiated	—	<5%	Yes

C. Large Cell Lymphoma (Histiocytic Type)

In this lymphoma there is usually complete replacement of the lymph node architecture by medium-to-large cells that vary from 18 to 30 μm in size. There are usually several nucleoli present with a variable amount of basophilic or amphophilic cytoplasm (Fig. 14). This tumor more commonly presents in extranodal sites, and bone marrow and liver involvement are less common than in the other forms of NHL. With newer and more aggressive forms of combination

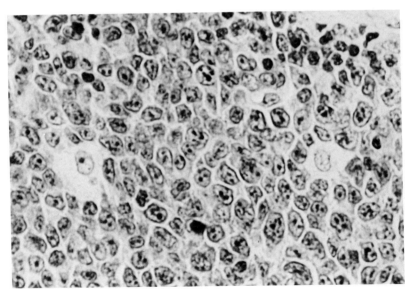

Fig. 14. Histiocytic (large cell) lymphoma: high power (×200).

chemotherapy, the universally poor prognosis for patients with advanced histiocytic lymphoma has been altered, and a significant percentage of these patients may enjoy a protracted remission.

D. Malignant Lymphoma, Diffuse, Burkitt's Type

Although uncommon, this form of lymphoblastic lymphoma is of great interest since it has been found to be associated with a herpes-like virus, and is the most common childhood tumor seen in equatorial Africa. It is seen rarely in the United States but may account for as many as 10% of the lymphoblastic lymphomas recognized in children. With high-dose cyclophosphamide therapy this tumor also can be arrested, with an approximate 25% long-term survival, particularly when it is localized (Ziegler, 1977). It often presents as an extranodal mass involving the jaw in males or the ovary in females. There appears to be a cohesive arrangement of tumor cells, and the cells have round-to-oval nuclei with fine chromatin and prominent nucleoli. Mitotic figures are common, and the cytoplasm is amphophilic. There are often several benign histiocytes contained within the clusters of tumor cells that give it the characteristic "starry-sky" pattern (Figs. 15 , 16). Most of these tumors are found to have bound immunoglobulins of the IgM class on their surface membranes, indicating a probable follicular center origin for this particular lymphoma.

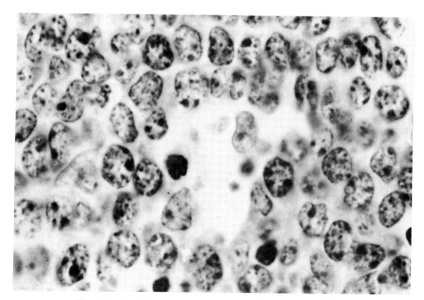

Fig. 15. Burkitt's lymphoma (hematouylin and losin, ×500).

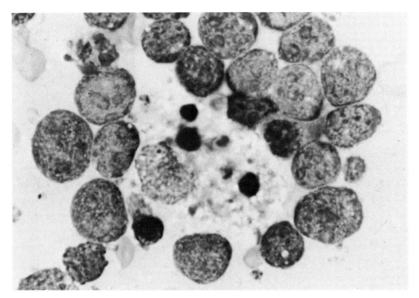

Fig. 16   Burkitt's lymphoma (Wright's stain ×500).

E. Nodular Lymphomas

It is important to differentiate the malignant nodular lymphomas from reactive follicular hyperplasia. The nodular areas are not as sharply demarcated as in the follicular hyperplasias and do not contain the reactive germinal centers with the variety of pleomorphic normal cells. One can recognize certain differences between nodular and diffuse lymphomas, which are summarized in Table VI. Nodular lymphomas are more frequently seen in middle-aged persons, and generally have an indolent course. Extranodal presentations are uncommon and visceral involvement is rare. Diffuse lymphomas are more frequently seen in the

TABLE VI

Nodular and Diffuse Lymphomas

Nodular	Diffuse
Most frequently seen in middle age	Most frequently seen in young and old
Extranodal presentation uncommon	Extranodal presentation frequent
Visceral involvement rare	Visceral involvement frequent
Indolent course	More rapid progression
Very sensitive to chemotherapy	Requires more intensive chemotherapy
Sensitive to irradiation	Less sensitive to irradiation

young and the very old. Extranodal presentation is frequent, and visceral involvement is common. There tends to be a more rapid progression, particularly with the histiocytic and lymphoblastic types, and more intensive chemotherapy is required to produce durable remissions. The large cell or histiocytic lymphomas require therapy with high doses of radiation for control.

F. Clinical Presentations

The vast majority of NHLs have advanced disease on initial presentation. At least 80% of patients, after conventional staging with bone marrow biopsies, liver biopsies, and/or laparoscopy, will be classified as either stage III or IV (Chabner *et al.*, 1976). Of 58 patients referred to the National Cancer Institute as "stage I or stage II" only 5 (6.3%) with nodular lymphoma and 12 of 40 (30%) with diffuse histiocytic lymphoma remained as stage I or II after staging evaluation was complete (Table VII). Therefore, the therapy for non-Hodgkin's lymphoma, with rare exceptions, is designed for systemic rather than regional control.

G. Therapy

1. Single Agents

For at least a decade partial regressions of NHL have been accomplished with a wide range of chemotherapeutic agents, including corticosteroids. These agents fall into several broad categories: alkylating agents (cyclophosphamide, chlorambucil); vinca alkaloids (vincristine, vinblastine); antibiotics (bleomycin, Adriamycin); nitrosoureas (BCNU, CCNU); corticosteroids (prednisone), and miscellaneous agents including procarbazine, streptonigrin, and hexamethylmelamine. For example, a complete remission rate of approximately 15% can be obtained by the use of cyclophosphamide alone. The unique advantage of

TABLE VII

Change in Patient Stage during Workup[a]

	Stage I (%)	Stage II (%)	Stage III (%)	Stage IV (%)
Clinical stage on referral	13	21	42	24
After lymphangiogram	8	15	54	24
After bone marrow	7	13	33	48
After closed liver biopsy	6	11	25	58
After laparotomy	6	8	21	65

[a] From Chabner *et al.* (1976).

TABLE VIII

Dosages of CVP and CV, ECOG Study

	Group I (CVP)	Group II (CV)
Cyclophosphamide	10.0 mg/kg	10.0 mg/kg
Vincristine	0.017 mg/kg	0.017 mg/kg
Prednisone	1.0 mg/kg	—
Course: 8 weeks		

vincristine over vinblastine—significantly less hematologic toxicity—was demonstrated in 1968 (Carbone and Spurr, 1968).

2. Combination Programs

Shortly after the demonstration of the effectiveness of the single agents, several groups used them in a three-drug combination, and the acronym COP or CVP (for cyclophosphamide, Oncovin or vincristine, and prednisone) has become virtually synonymous with the chemotherapy for NHL (Bagley et al., 1972). The importance of prednisone in this three-drug combination was confirmed by the Eastern Cooperative Oncology Group (ECOG), with a larger number of patients achieving complete remission with CVP than with CV (Tables VIII and IX) (Lenhard et al., 1976). From these and other studies complete remissions have ranged from 35–57%, with median durations of 3 to more than 18 months. With the data separated by histological pattern, the complete remission percent was seen to be higher for nodular lymphomas than for diffuse lymphomas. It is important to differentiate relapse-free survival or the disease-free interval from survival. Although overall response rates for lymphomas with nodular and diffuse histologies are similar, median survival is distinctly greater for nodular lymphomas—usually in excess of 6 years, in contrast to 1–2 years for the diffuse type (Rosenberg et al., 1975). Relapse-free survivals for both these major lymphomas are surprisingly similar (Fig. 17).

TABLE IX

Results of Therapy with CVP and CV, ECOG Study

Therapy	Number of patients	Complete remission (%)	Survival (mo)	Partial remission (%)	Survival (mo)
CVP	54	43	57	39	39
CV	59	17	50	53	30

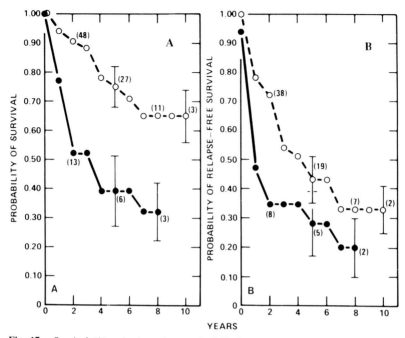

Fig. 17. Survival (A) and relapse-free survival (B) in stage III non-Hodgkin's lymphoma. ○, nodular (51 original patients at risk for entire study); ●, diffuse (17 original patients at risk). Numbers in parentheses indicate the number of patients at risk for the years shown. (Stanford University experience.) From Glatstein *et al.* (1976).

Confirmation of the peculiar biology of nodular lymphomas can be seen in the early results of a prospective study from Stanford University that has demonstrated identical survival rates for three different programs (Portlock *et al.*, 1976). In this study patients were randomized to receive either a single alkylating agent, combination chemotherapy, or combination chemotherapy plus total nodal irradiation. The probability of achieving a remission was identical for all three groups (>80%). Although it did take a longer time to achieve a complete remission with a single agent than with either of the two more intensive programs (40 months versus 16 months), 50% of the patients remained free of disease progression at approximately 3 years, and survival analysis does not suggest prolonged disease-free intervals for a subgroup of patients in remission (Fig. 18).

3. Diffuse Lymphomas

Diffuse histiocytic lymphomas have been viewed as invariably fatal and responsive to chemotherapy only for brief periods. Until several years ago the median survival in most series was approximately 1 year. The importance of obtaining a complete remission can be seen in the results of one study in which

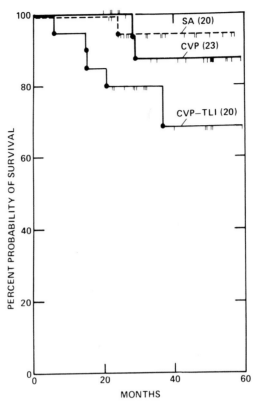

Fig. 18. Survival of patients with nodular lymphoma receiving single-agent therapy (SA), combination therapy (CVP, cytoxan vincristine prednisone), and combination therapy plus radiation (CVP-TLI; TLI, total lymphoid irradiation). From Portlock *et al.* (1976).

the probability of the complete responders living for 2 years was 75%, in contrast to less than 50% for the partial responders and 5% for the nonresponders (Lenhard *et al.*, 1978). The curves of the complete responders have a change in slope suggesting long-term remissions after 60 weeks, with between 20 and 40% of the original group free of disease at 2 years (Fig. 19).

4. Adriamycin and Bleomycin Combinations

The combination of cyclophosphamide, hydroxydaunomycin, Oncovin, and prednisone (CHOP) produces a complete remission rate of close to 70% in diffuse histiocytic lymphoma. It is still too soon to know whether this will translate into a longer disease-free interval for these patients. The addition of bleomycin to the four-drug combination listed above has been referred to as BACOP or CHOP-Bleo. The percentage of complete remissions has not been improved, but for those who achieve complete remission the duration of responses seem to be more durable (Schein *et al.*, 1976).

In the diffuse lymphomas, with the exception of the rare well-differentiated lymphocytic lymphomas, the achievement of complete remission with one of several combination-chemotherapy programs should be the main goal of any treatment program. Without a complete remission the survival for patients with stage III and IV disease is extremely poor. For the nodular lymphomas, present data do not suggest that aggressive induction programs, with or without radiation therapy, alter the survival curves of patients so treated. The goal should be to produce a gradual but continual remission with as little toxicity as possible.

The role of radiation therapy in the advanced lymphomas with particular reference to total body radiation is currently under intense investigation. In a study at the joint Center for Radiation Therapy the 5-year survival figure for nodular lymphomas was 80%, and for diffuse lymphomas 40%, exclusive of histiocytic types that were not included. Relapse-free survivals were 25% and

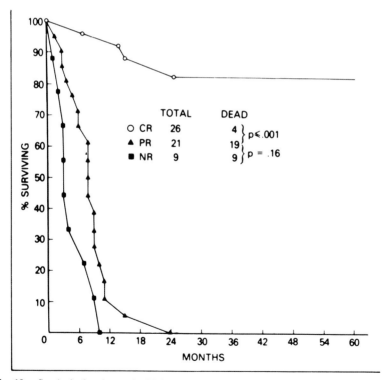

Fig. 19. Survival of patients with histiocytic lymphoma. CR, complete remission; PR, partial remission; NR, no response. From DeVita *et al.* (1975).

10%, respectively, indicating high relapse potential for both groups. These results were not significantly different than a retrospective comparison with a three-drug combination (Hellman *et al.*, 1977).

IV. CONCLUSION

Advances in diagnosis, treatment, and management of the patient with lymphoma have been significant, particularly in Hodgkin's lymphoma. MOPP therapy has produced cures in a large number of patients. However, new and more effective chemotherapy is required to achieve similar results in non-Hodgkin's lymphoma.

ACKNOWLEDGMENT

This work was supported, in part, by USPHS Grants CA-11198 and CA-11083.

REFERENCES

Bagley, C. M., DeVita, V. T., Jr., Berard, C. W., and Cannellos, G. P. (1972). *Ann. Intern. Med.* **76**, 227–234.
Berge, T., and Toremalm, N. G. (1969). *Ann. Otol., Rhinol., & Laryngol.* **78**, 663–670.
Carbone, P. P., and Spurr, C. (1968). *Cancer Res.* **28**, 811–822.
Chabner, D. A., Johnson, R. E., Young, R. C., Cannellos, G. P., Hubbard, S. P., Johnson, S. K., and DeVita, V. T., Jr., (1976). *Ann. Intern. Med.* **85**, 149–154.
Coleman, C. N., Williams, C. J., Flint, A., Glastein, E. J., Rosenberg, S. A., and Kaplan, H. S. (1977). *N. Engl. J. Med.* **297**, 1249–1252.
DeVita, V., Cerpic, A., and Carbone, P. P., (1970). *Ann. Intern. Med.* **73**, 881–895.
DeVita, V. T., Jr., Canellos, G. P., Chabner, B., Hubbard, S. P., Schein, P., and Young, R. C. (1975). *Lancet* **1**, 248–250.
DeVita, V. T., Jr., Canellos, G. P., Hubbard, S. P., Chabner, B., and Young, R. C. (1976). *Proc. Am. Soc. Clin. Oncol.* **17**, 269.
Glatstein, E., Fuks, Z., Goffinet, D. R., and Kaplan, H. S. (1976). *Cancer* **37**, 2806–2812.
Goodman, R. L., Piro, A. J., and Hellman, S. (1976). *Cancer* **37**, 2834–2839.
Hellman, S., Chaffey, J. T., Rosenthal, S., Moloney, W. C., Canellos, G. P., and Skarin, A. T. (1977). *Cancer* **39**, 843–851.
Hyman, G. A., and Sommers, C. (1966). *Blood* **28**, 416–427.
Kaplan, H. S. (1976). *Cancer Res.* **36**, 3863–3877.
Kaplan, H. S. (1972). "Hodgkin's Disease." Harvard University Press, Cambridge, Massachusetts.
Lenhard, R. E., Jr., Prentice, R. L., Owens, A. H., Bakemeir, R., Horton, J. H., Schneider, B. I., Stolback, L., Bernard, C. W., and Carbone, P. P. (1976). *Cancer* **38**, 1052–1059.
Lenhard, R. E., Jr., Ezdinli, E., Costello, W., Bennett, J. M., Horton, J., Amorisi, E. L., Stolback, L., and Coolter, J. (1978). *Cancer* **42**, 41–52.
Lotz, M. J., Chabner, B., DeVita, V. T., Jr., Johnson, R. E., and Bernard, C. W. (1976). *Cancer* **37**, 266–270.

Lukes, R. J., and Collins, R. D. (1974). *Cancer* **34**, 1488–1503.

Lukes, R. J., and Tindle, D. H. (1975). *N. Engl. J. Med.* **292**, 1–8.

Lukes, R. J., Butler, J. J., and Kickes, E. B. (1966). *Cancer* **19**, 317–344.

Portlock, C. S., Rosenberg, S. A., Glatstein, E., and Kaplan, H. S. (1976). *Blood* **47**, 747–756.

Proznitz, L. R., Farber, L. R., Fischer, J. J., Bertino, J. R., and Fischer, D. B. (1976). *Cancer* **37**, 2826–2833.

Rosenberg, S. A., Dorfman, R. F., and Kaplan, H. S. (1975). *Br. J. Cancer* **31**, Suppl. II, 168–173.

Saltstein, S. L., and Ackerman, L. V. (1969). *Cancer* **12**, 164–182.

Schein, P. S., DeVita, V. T. Jr., Hubbard, S., Chabner, B., Canellos, G. P., Bernard, C., and Young, R. C. (1976). *Ann. Intern. Med.* **85**, 417–422.

Sinclair, S., Beckman, E., and Ellman, L. (1974). *J. Am. Med. Assoc.* **228**, 602–603.

Warrick, W. J. (1976). *Prog. Med. Virol.* **9**, 256–301.

Ziegler, J. L., Olweny, C. L. M., Katangoli, E., Bidde, M., Magrath, I., and Kwocka, J. N. (1974). *Lancet* **2**, 1397.

Ziegler, J. L. (1977). *N. Engl. J. Med.* **297**, 75–80.

Part II
Solid Tumors

6

CARCINOMA OF THE BREAST
James F. Holland

I.	Introduction	99
II.	Incidence and Causative Factors	100
III.	Pathology	101
IV.	Clinical Presentation	102
V.	Prognostic Features	102
VI.	Clinical Course of Metastatic Breast Cancer	103
VII.	Surgical Therapy	104
VIII.	Radiation Therapy	105
IX.	Hormonal Therapy	106
X.	Chemotherapy	106
XI.	Discussion	109
	References	110

I. INTRODUCTION

The breast is a secondary sex gland from which mammals take their name. It develops at puberty in the human female under the influence of hypothalamic releasing factors, pituitary hormones, and ovarian estrogen and progesterone. The acini are vestigial in the breast except during pregnancy and lactation. The duct epithelium persists and is susceptible to neoplastic change, however, and carcinoma of the breast, primarily derived from the ductal epithelium, is the most common cancer in the Western female. There now are 106,000 cases per year in the United States, and the incidence rose from 55 per 100,000 in 1940 to 72 per 100,000 in 1965 (Silverberg, 1979).

In areas where breast cancer is common there is a high and accelerating incidence until the age of 50. After 50 the rate of increase slows, but the incidence continues to augment. In areas where breast cancer is uncommon there is a lesser increase in incidence up to the age of 50, but at 50 the incidence

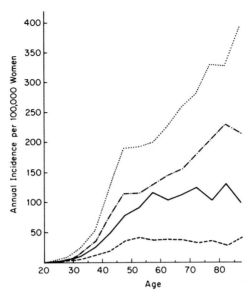

Fig. 1.   Incidence of breast cancer in women versus age in several countries. Dotted line, United States (Connecticut); dotted/slashed line, Norway (rural); solid line, Poland (Warsaw); dashed line, Japan (Osaka). From Saracci and Repetto (1978).

decreases and breast cancer is less frequent in old age (Doll *et al.*, 1966). (See Fig. 1).

II. INCIDENCE AND CAUSATIVE FACTORS

There are cultural and environmental factors that influence breast cancer. Untreated breast cancer, a rarity today in the developed world, leads to death within 5 years in the majority of patients. Spontaneous cure does not occur. Cultural and environmental factors influence the frequency of the disease. The mortality from breast cancer, which correlates well with incidence, is not geographically homogenous in white females in the United States. The disease is disproprotionately frequent in the urban Northeast, less common in the South and Southwest (Mason *et al.*, 1975). Breast cancer in Asia is much less common than in the Western world. It has been demonstrated that when Japanese women migrate to the United States, they gradually assume the U.S. incidence rate (Doll *et al.*, 1966). A principal change is dietary, and this supports the possibility that hormonal changes and imbalances are involved (Miller, 1977).

Several factors protect against breast cancer. Early parity, but not pregnancy that leads to abortion, is protective (MacMahon *et al.*, 1973). The role of lactation has been a source of considerable controversy, but a particular subculture in Asia has been found in which nursing is practiced only with one breast: mothers hold the baby in constant position to be suckled, and if cancer occurs, it is predominantly in the opposite breast (Ing *et al.*, 1977). Oophorectomy prior to menopause is a protective factor, consistent with a role of hormones in the genesis of breast cancer (MacMahon *et al.*, 1971). However, contraceptive pills have not led to an increase in incidence of breast cancer (Vessey *et al.*, 1972). Obesity is positively correlated with breast cancer incidence. This may be related to the role of adipocytes in metabolizing androstenedione and possibly other adrenal steroids to estrogens that could continuously stimulate breast ductal epithelium. The three estrogens estradiol, estrone, and estriol have been studied in the urine of breast-cancer patients. A high concentration of estriol compared to estrone and estradiol appears to protect against breast cancer (MacMahon *et al.*, 1971).

Radiation is an absolute mammary carcinogen. Woman who were repeatedly fluoroscoped in the course of tuberculosis treatment many years ago, or those exposed to radiation from the nuclear explosions in Japan, have an increased incidence of breast cancer (MacKenzie, 1965; Wanebo *et al.*, 1968).

Besides these environmentally and culturally influenced factors, there are familial factors that might be genetic. The risk of breast cancer is increased in sisters and daughters of breast cancer patients (Petrakis, 1977).

Breast cancer in rodents has been shown to be due to infection and transformation events associated with an RNA virus, and this is also suggested in monkeys. Biochemical phenomena associated with such viruses have been detected in human milk, but a causal relationship of virus infection to human breast cancer has not been established (Chopra and Oie, 1972). A proportion of human breast-cancer cells show reactivity with an antiserum against GP52, however. GP52 is a glycoprotein of 52,000 daltons that is also found in the mouse mammary tumor virus (Black, 1977).

III. PATHOLOGY

The duct epithelium of the breast is the predominant site of neoplasia. About 70% of the cancers are of the infiltrating ductal carcinoma type, with lesser frequencies of the papillary and medullary carcinoma histologies. Tubular carcinoma, colloid carcinoma, and lobular carcinoma make up the bulk of the other varieties. Lobular carcinoma is also frequently found as carcinoma *in situ*, not apparently invasive. In this instance the tumor must regress or remain static since the frequency of the *in situ* lesion is disproportionate to the frequency of invasive lobular carcinoma.

IV. CLINICAL PRESENTATION

Breast cancer produces a constellation of symptoms and signs that are relevant for all physicians to know. Although most early breast cancers are painless, the presence of pain does not exclude carcinoma from consideration. Skin retraction is a characteristic feature caused by the fibroblastic proliferation associated with breast cancer. Attachment of fibroblastic extensions to the overlying dermis causes dimpling or indentation when the breast is moved by gravity, by underlying muscle contraction, by arm motion, or by examination in such a way as to move the tumor away from the overlying skin. Asymmetry of the breasts in normal women is common. Change in size or contour is more suggestive of neoplasm. Late in the course of cancer, the affected breast may either increase or decrease in size, depending on epithelial content and fibroblastic response.

Proper examination of the breasts includes inspection, not just in the anatomical position, but with the arms lifted and with the arms akimbo with the hands pressing on the hips to exert pectoral tension. Although retraction is a sign highly suggestive of an underlying cancer, it may also occur with fat necrosis. Edema of the breast is a characteristic finding in advanced breast cancer. *Peau d'orange,* ("skin of an orange"), also called "pigskinning," is due to intracutaneous edema. Inflammation of breast skin correlates with intradermal lymphatic invasion. It conveys a poor prognosis. Paget's disease of the breast constitutes a distortion of the nipple due to neoplastic cells growing out from the major ducts, thence proliferating on the surface of the areola and breast.

V. PROGNOSTIC FEATURES

Breast cancer is a disease that requires treatment. In its untreated state it leads to death. Older criteria of inoperability are changing, and some lesions that once were categorically inoperable are now subject to control by combined modality therapy employing chemotherapy and a regional treatment approach. Size of the breast cancer is a factor of considerable importance in determining prognosis (Fisher *et al.*, 1969). There is an inverse survival gradient. Patients whose tumors are up to 1 cm in size have a 10-year survival of 75%. Those whose tumors are over 10 cm in diameter have only a 25% survival at 10 years. The relationship is not determined by the tumor diameter, per se, but by the propensity for metastasis, which is manifest in axillary and other lymph node metastases.

Lymph node metastases serve as a signal of occult widely disseminated metastatic disease (Fisher *et al.*, 1969). Lymphatic vessel invasion is an unfavorable prognostic sign (Nime *et al.*, 1977). Blood vessel invasion is also an adverse finding, but it is seen primarily in association with multiple lymph node metas-

6

CARCINOMA OF THE BREAST
James F. Holland

I.	Introduction	99
II.	Incidence and Causative Factors	100
III.	Pathology	101
IV.	Clinical Presentation	102
V.	Prognostic Features	102
VI.	Clinical Course of Metastatic Breast Cancer	103
VII.	Surgical Therapy	104
VIII.	Radiation Therapy	105
IX.	Hormonal Therapy	106
X.	Chemotherapy	106
XI.	Discussion	109
	References	110

I. INTRODUCTION

The breast is a secondary sex gland from which mammals take their name. It develops at puberty in the human female under the influence of hypothalamic releasing factors, pituitary hormones, and ovarian estrogen and progesterone. The acini are vestigial in the breast except during pregnancy and lactation. The duct epithelium persists and is susceptible to neoplastic change, however, and carcinoma of the breast, primarily derived from the ductal epithelium, is the most common cancer in the Western female. There now are 106,000 cases per year in the United States, and the incidence rose from 55 per 100,000 in 1940 to 72 per 100,000 in 1965 (Silverberg, 1979).

In areas where breast cancer is common there is a high and accelerating incidence until the age of 50. After 50 the rate of increase slows, but the incidence continues to augment. In areas where breast cancer is uncommon there is a lesser increase in incidence up to the age of 50, but at 50 the incidence

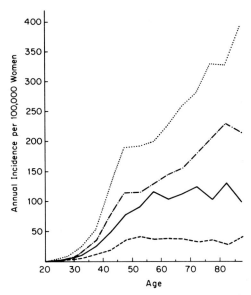

Fig. 1. Incidence of breast cancer in women versus age in several countries. Dotted line, United States (Connecticut); dotted/slashed line, Norway (rural); solid line, Poland (Warsaw); dashed line, Japan (Osaka). From Saracci and Repetto (1978).

decreases and breast cancer is less frequent in old age (Doll *et al.*, 1966). (See Fig. 1).

II. INCIDENCE AND CAUSATIVE FACTORS

There are cultural and environmental factors that influence breast cancer. Untreated breast cancer, a rarity today in the developed world, leads to death within 5 years in the majority of patients. Spontaneous cure does not occur. Cultural and environmental factors influence the frequency of the disease. The mortality from breast cancer, which correlates well with incidence, is not geographically homogenous in white females in the United States. The disease is disproprotionately frequent in the urban Northeast, less common in the South and Southwest (Mason *et al.*, 1975). Breast cancer in Asia is much less common than in the Western world. It has been demonstrated that when Japanese women migrate to the United States, they gradually assume the U.S. incidence rate (Doll *et al.*, 1966). A principal change is dietary, and this supports the possibility that hormonal changes and imbalances are involved (Miller, 1977).

Several factors protect against breast cancer. Early parity, but not pregnancy that leads to abortion, is protective (MacMahon *et al.*, 1973). The role of lactation has been a source of considerable controversy, but a particular subculture in Asia has been found in which nursing is practiced only with one breast: mothers hold the baby in constant position to be suckled, and if cancer occurs, it is predominantly in the opposite breast (Ing *et al.*, 1977). Oophorectomy prior to menopause is a protective factor, consistent with a role of hormones in the genesis of breast cancer (MacMahon *et al.*, 1971). However, contraceptive pills have not led to an increase in incidence of breast cancer (Vessey *et al.*, 1972). Obesity is positively correlated with breast cancer incidence. This may be related to the role of adipocytes in metabolizing androstenedione and possibly other adrenal steroids to estrogens that could continuously stimulate breast ductal epithelium. The three estrogens estradiol, estrone, and estriol have been studied in the urine of breast-cancer patients. A high concentration of estriol compared to estrone and estradiol appears to protect against breast cancer (MacMahon *et al.*, 1971).

Radiation is an absolute mammary carcinogen. Woman who were repeatedly fluoroscoped in the course of tuberculosis treatment many years ago, or those exposed to radiation from the nuclear explosions in Japan, have an increased incidence of breast cancer (MacKenzie, 1965; Wanebo *et al.*, 1968).

Besides these environmentally and culturally influenced factors, there are familial factors that might be genetic. The risk of breast cancer is increased in sisters and daughters of breast cancer patients (Petrakis, 1977).

Breast cancer in rodents has been shown to be due to infection and transformation events associated with an RNA virus, and this is also suggested in monkeys. Biochemical phenomena associated with such viruses have been detected in human milk, but a causal relationship of virus infection to human breast cancer has not been established (Chopra and Oie, 1972). A proportion of human breast-cancer cells show reactivity with an antiserum against GP52, however. GP52 is a glycoprotein of 52,000 daltons that is also found in the mouse mammary tumor virus (Black, 1977).

III. PATHOLOGY

The duct epithelium of the breast is the predominant site of neoplasia. About 70% of the cancers are of the infiltrating ductal carcinoma type, with lesser frequencies of the papillary and medullary carcinoma histologies. Tubular carcinoma, colloid carcinoma, and lobular carcinoma make up the bulk of the other varieties. Lobular carcinoma is also frequently found as carcinoma *in situ*, not apparently invasive. In this instance the tumor must regress or remain static since the frequency of the *in situ* lesion is disproportionate to the frequency of invasive lobular carcinoma.

IV. CLINICAL PRESENTATION

Breast cancer produces a constellation of symptoms and signs that are relevant for all physicians to know. Although most early breast cancers are painless, the presence of pain does not exclude carcinoma from consideration. Skin retraction is a characteristic feature caused by the fibroblastic proliferation associated with breast cancer. Attachment of fibroblastic extensions to the overlying dermis causes dimpling or indentation when the breast is moved by gravity, by underlying muscle contraction, by arm motion, or by examination in such a way as to move the tumor away from the overlying skin. Asymmetry of the breasts in normal women is common. Change in size or contour is more suggestive of neoplasm. Late in the course of cancer, the affected breast may either increase or decrease in size, depending on epithelial content and fibroblastic response.

Proper examination of the breasts includes inspection, not just in the anatomical position, but with the arms lifted and with the arms akimbo with the hands pressing on the hips to exert pectoral tension. Although retraction is a sign highly suggestive of an underlying cancer, it may also occur with fat necrosis. Edema of the breast is a characteristic finding in advanced breast cancer. *Peau d'orange,* ("skin of an orange"), also called "pigskinning," is due to intracutaneous edema. Inflammation of breast skin correlates with intradermal lymphatic invasion. It conveys a poor prognosis. Paget's disease of the breast constitutes a distortion of the nipple due to neoplastic cells growing out from the major ducts, thence proliferating on the surface of the areola and breast.

V. PROGNOSTIC FEATURES

Breast cancer is a disease that requires treatment. In its untreated state it leads to death. Older criteria of inoperability are changing, and some lesions that once were categorically inoperable are now subject to control by combined modality therapy employing chemotherapy and a regional treatment approach. Size of the breast cancer is a factor of considerable importance in determining prognosis (Fisher *et al.,* 1969). There is an inverse survival gradient. Patients whose tumors are up to 1 cm in size have a 10-year survival of 75%. Those whose tumors are over 10 cm in diameter have only a 25% survival at 10 years. The relationship is not determined by the tumor diameter, per se, but by the propensity for metastasis, which is manifest in axillary and other lymph node metastases.

Lymph node metastases serve as a signal of occult widely disseminated metastatic disease (Fisher *et al.,* 1969). Lymphatic vessel invasion is an unfavorable prognostic sign (Nime *et al.,* 1977). Blood vessel invasion is also an adverse finding, but it is seen primarily in association with multiple lymph node metastases. In 15% of patients, breast cancer in the affected breast is histologically multicentric (E. R. Fisher *et al.*, 1975). In patients where there has been contralateral symmetrical biopsy, 15% have had carcinoma *in situ*.

Most of these carcinomas do not go on to become clinically manifest. Indeed, intraductal carcinoma in elderly women may be latent. One study in women over 70 has demonstrated that intraductal cancer *in situ* occurs 19 times more often than clinically evident breast cancer (Kramer and Rush, 1973). This suggests that the rate of progression of intraductal breast cancer in the elderly is frequently too slow to be clinically important, or that many carcinomas *in situ* regress.

Of the local and regional factors that correlate with primary breast cancer curability, by far the most important that can be identified clinically is lymph node metastasis (Fisher *et al.*, 1969). Node metastasis is a measure of host defense in its ability to destroy cells that have arrived at the lymph node. By characterizing survival and recurrence in terms of the amount of lymph node involvement in the dissected axillary specimen, it has been possible to prognosticate, with a high degree of accuracy, the outcome for individual patients. Indeed, B. Fisher and his colleagues (1975) have derived data for patients who relapse at 18 months, at 5 years, or at 10 years. Those who had no lymph node involved in the axillary specimen have a 5% relapse rate at 18 months, an 18% relapse rate at 5 years, and a 24% relapse rate at 10 years. If there are one, two, or three nodes positive in the axilla, the outcome is vastly different. Thirteen percent relapse at 18 months, 50% have relapsed by 5 years, and 65% by 10 years. If there are more than three lymph nodes positive, 52% have already relapsed at 18 months, 79% at 5 years, and 86% at 10 years. Since clinically metastatic breast cancer beyond the nodes still leads to an almost invariably fatal outcome, the prognostic significance of axillary lymph node pathology is apparent. It is easier to understand these findings when node metastasis is regarded not as a mechanical happenstance of floating cells, but rather as the ability or inability of the host to destroy large numbers of cells that get to lymph nodes. Thus it is a manifestation of the level of host defense.

VI. CLINICAL COURSE OF METASTATIC BREAST CANCER

Systemic metastasis occurs by hematogenous dissemination, or by lymphatic spread to axillary, supraclavicular, or internal mammary lymph nodes, with further progression along lymphatic routes to mediastinal nodes. At any point these lymph nodal metastases can give rise to hematogenous spread. Patterns of metastasis assumed to relate to permeation of lymphatic vessels are seen on the skin surrounding the primary tumor site, where microscopic and even gross metastasis in lymphatic vessels can be recognized. When this overlies the breast tumor itself, the breast is spoken of as manifesting inflammatory cancer. Permeation of the lymphatic vessels of the lung retrograde from mediastinal nodes causes a characteristic lymphangitic pattern on X-ray films, with serious compromise of pulmonary function. Lymphatic obstruction may cause edema of the arm. In its most extreme form, lymphatic permeation leads to carcinoma *en cuirassé,* a carapace of tumor eventually encircling the entire thorax.

Vascular invasion may occur in the primary tumor itself, in lymph nodes, or by the return of tumor cells to the venous circulation via the thoracic duct. Hematogenous manifestations of metastasis are commonly seen in the lung (as nodular lesions), in the liver, the skeleton, the ovary, the brain, and the adrenal gland. Permeation of tumor cells from the parietal or visceral pleura may lead to pleural disease with effusion. Peritoneal implantation with or without manifestations of hepatic metastasis may lead to ascites. Vertebral body metastasis is particularly common, in part related to the plexus of vertebral veins allowing for easy spread up and down the vertebral column.

The brain is an increasingly common site of terminal metastatic disease. When chemotherapeutic agents eradicate or suppress metastatic disease in the systemic circulation that might conventionally have led to earlier death, the lower drug concentrations in the cerebral spinal fluid allow central nervous system metastases to become clinically manifest. The morbidity of metastatic breast cancer may be apparent as painful, ulcerative lesions on the homolateral chest, and rarely on the entire thorax and upper abdomen. Lymphedema and occasional invasion of the brachial plexus, producing a useless and painful upper extremity, can also occur. Disordered function of major organs invaded by the neoplasm, including the central nervous system, liver, adrenal gland, and lung, produce the expected syndromes of organ deficiency. Bone pain may often appear before earliest manifestation in X-ray pictures, although radioisotopic skeletal scanning is more sensitive and often can indicate early metastasis. Pathologic fracture is common, particularly in vertebrae and weight-bearing bones.

The mechanisms of death from breast cancer usually involve brain metastasis, pulmonary insufficiency, hepatic insufficiency, hypercalcemia from extensive bone disease, paraplegia from cord compression from vertebral metastasis, cachexia, suicide, or systemic infection during granulocytopenia from treatment or from marrow invasion.

VII. SURGICAL THERAPY

When and what kind of surgery should be performed on a woman with breast cancer? When a patient has a dominant mass in a breast it should be biopsied. A dominant mass is one that is more prominent and usually harder than others, even in the presence of cystic mastopathy. A dominant mass of any kind is a basis for biopsy, and about one in four of such biopsies turns out to be cancer. The cost of missing a diagnosis of breast cancer is clear in terms of the adverse prognosis associated with increased size, because of the correlation with an increased incidence of metastasis.

Optimal methods for controlling the primary tumor are still evolving. Radical mastectomy involves taking the breast, axillary contents, and the pectoralis major and minor. It often entails a skin graft. It was introduced at the turn of the century by Halsted and by others. Modified radical mastectomy is a much better operation in terms of function, and if the tumor is not adherent to the chest wall, an equivalent one in terms of cancer control. Although it takes the entire breast, the lymphatic tissues of the axilla, and often the pectoralis minor muscle, it leaves the pectoralis major intact, allowing for adduction of the arm and better cosmetic status. Total mastectomy without taking any axillary tissue is not advocated, since knowledge of the metastatic status of axillary lymph nodes is valuable. Segmental mastectomy has also been investigated, in which only the tumor and its surrounding breast tissue is removed, leaving much of the breast intact (Veronesi, 1978). Radiotherapy may be administered by electron beam, gamma, or X-irradiation to the remaining breast, with or without implanted radioactive needles. This investigational procedure offers the possibility of salvage of the breast. It is generally held, however, that salvage of life is of such greater significance that it should come before salvage of beauty.

It is incumbent upon all those who advocate procedures less sure than conventional to justify that position by prospective research. The opportunity for plastic reconstruction, or for effective prostheses, allows for preservation of body image and of good appearance in clothing. This is psychologically acceptable to most women as they deal with themselves and with their sexuality. Transplantation of the nipple has been practiced by some to salvage it for later application to a reconstructed breast. Reports of iatrogenic metastasis from occult cancer cells transplanted in the nipple have already appeared.

Before one can advocate the adoption of lesser treatment than modified radical mastectomy, it is important to look at what the cost is in terms of relapse and toxicity, and the implication this has for eventual survival. Formal comparative studies are necessary, particularly today, when the outcome of breast cancer surgery is influenced by adjuvant chemotherapy. Modified radical mastectomy allows an effective external prosthesis for reconstructive surgery and appears to be at least equal to radical mastectomy in its effect against stages I and II disease (National Surgical Adjuvant Project for Breast and Bowel Cancers, 1979).

VIII. RADIATION THERAPY

There is strong advocacy by some physicians for local treatment using radiotherapy because this allows preservation of the breast and a reasonably good cosmetic outcome (Brown *et al.*, 1977; Prosnitz *et al.*, 1977). The data must be viewed primarily in the context of the eventual outcome for life; however, no formal studies have been performed. In the most widely cited radiation report in the United States, with a median follow-up of 33 months, the disease-free outcome is 63% in patients without axillary nodes involved (Prosnitz *et al.*, 1977) versus 85% in a large sequential series of patients followed for nearly twice as long after modified radical mastectomy by a single expert surgeon (Lesnick, 1979). In those who had axillary metastases, radiotherapy resulted in 47% alive without disease after nearly 4 years, whereas after modified radical mastectomy, with all patients observed for at least 5 years, 65% are alive without evidence of disease. Formal comparisons and combination programs with chemotherapy have not been reported.

IX. HORMONAL THERAPY

Upon removing breast tissue it is now good practice to measure some characteristics of its differentiation with respect to sensitivity to hormones. There are separate receptor proteins in breast-cancer tissue that transport estrogens and progestins. The presence of these receptors correlated with response of these tumors to hormonal administration and endocrine organ ablation (McGuire, 1975). They are claimed by some to correlate inversely with sensitivity to chemotherapy (Lippman *et al.*, 1978), but much current opinion does not sustain this view (Kiang *et al.*, 1978 ; (Bonadonna *et al.*, 1979). The administration of hormones does not cure breast cancer. The most dramatic hormonal modification procedure, oophorectomy at the time of mastectomy, did not augment survival (Ravdin *et al.*, 1970). Hormonal factors are probably influential in etiology, but palliative for therapeutic purposes.

X. CHEMOTHERAPY

The possibility of curative breast cancer treatment using cytotoxic chemotherapy at the time of the primary disease is a reality. In advanced metastatic disease, half the patients are dead within a year of initiating chemotherapeutic treatment, and more than 75% are dead at 2 years (Axtell *et al.*, 1976). This is hardly an effective salvage treatment. We have looked at ways of improving this; the advent of Adriamycin has made a slight difference (Tormey, 1975). Multiple drugs, each independently active, have been used in combination chemotherapies. Antimetabolites, alkylating agents, hormones, and interrupters of tubulin assembly are frequent components. Vincristine, prednisone, cyclophosphamide, methotrexate, and fluorouracil (VPCMF) constitute a widely used program known as the Cooper regimen (Cooper, 1969). The last four of these drugs have been shown to be more active than the last three, a popular program because of its simplicity despite its lesser effect (Band *et al.*, 1977). Adriamycin has been substituted for methotrexate in many three- and five-drug programs (Carbone and Tormey, 1977), and has been added to it in one four-drug program (Trunum *et al.*, 1976). Optimal therapy has not yet been achieved, and systemic search for new therapies for metastatic breast cancer continues.

Within 6 weeks, 75% of those who are going to benefit have already shown appreciable tumor regression. In general, a premenopausal woman (under age 50, if menstrual history is unavailable) responds better to chemotherapeutic regimens than a postmenopausal woman, although there is suggestive evidence that this is less an inherent characteristic of the breast cancer than of the lesser ability to tolerate full doses of chemotherapy in the aged. With doses equal to full prescribed protocol, response rates are nearly equal, independent of menopausal status. This is one minor step of slow progress in metastatic breast cancer.

Based on their chemotherapeutic activities in metastatic cancer, the study of drugs given at the time of primary surgery has evolved. Patients with breast cancer with more than three nodes involved have a very adverse prognosis for relapse and survival (Fisher *et al.*, 1969) (Table I). The data of Bonadonna and colleagues (1978, 1979) were gathered in a prospective trial of primary breast cancer treated by surgery alone or surgery plus chemotherapy for women with metastatic breast cancer in axillary lymph nodes (Fig. 2). At 5 years, by life table projection, the probability of being disease-free is significantly less in the control regimen (surgery only) than in the patients who also received chemotherapy with three drugs—cyclophosphamide, methotrexate, and fluorouracil.

The data of R. G. Cooper (1979, unpublished), who first devised the regimen of VPCMF, describe women who had more than three nodes involved with

TABLE I

Treatment Failures 5 and 10 Years after Radical Mastectomy[a]

Nodal status	5 years (%)	10 years (%)
Positive and negative (all patients)	40	50
Negative	18	24
Positive	65	76
One to three nodes	50	65
More than three nodes	79	89

[a] NSABP Protocol B-01 (Fisher and Gebhardt, 1978).

metastatic cancer at the time of surgery. They were treated with the five-drug regimen over a period of 9 months. There is a major difference from the disease-free survival of several groups of women who were treated by surgery alone (B. Fisher *et al.*, 1975). The differences are not appropriate to subject to statistical analysis, however, because they represent studies made at different times by different observers. The same magnitude of difference exists among 21,000 American women studied by the National Cancer Institute (Axtell *et al.*, 1972) (Fig. 3). These women had one or more nodes involved with breast cancer, whereas Cooper's patients had four or more nodes involved, a much worse prognostic characteristic. The reproducible mortality experience for women with one or more nodes involved, treated by surgery alone, is significantly different from the curve plotted for Cooper's patients treated with chemotherapy, who are alive and well without evidence of disease (Cooper *et al.*, 1979).

Women who received adjuvant radiotherapy before chemotherapy sustained little of the improvement that one could ascribe to the chemotherapy. There appears to be an adverse interaction after surgery when radiotherapy is given before chemotherapy (Holland *et al.*, 1980). This interaction might relate to the delay before giving the chemotherapy. It might relate to the damage to the bone marrow that occurs from radiotherapy, thereby compromising the doses of

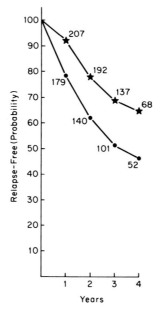

Fig. 2. Surgical adjuvant trials. Probability of disease-free survival for breast cancer patients treated by surgery alone (●—●, radical mastectomy) and by surgery plus CMF chemotherapy (★—★). From Bonadonna *et al.* (1978).

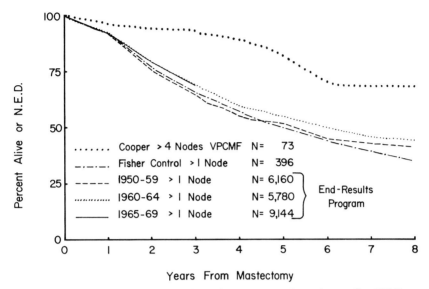

Fig. 3. Survival of breast cancer patients after mastectomy for various studies. N.E.D.

chemotherapy that can be given. It might also relate to the impact of radiotherapy on lymphoid populations. It has been shown that circulating lymphocytes may be depressed for 2 years after radiotherapy (Stjernsward, 1974). In some way this might impair the host's immunologic responses, a third component in the interaction between tumor and chemotherapeutic treatments. Thus, in a host immunodepressed by radiotherapy, chemotherapy may not have the same activity.

We have designed a study testing the five-drug regimen that Cooper described versus the three-drug regimen that Bonadonna described versus the three-drug regimen plus immunotherapy with MER, the methanol extraction residue of bacillus Calmette-Guérin (Tormey *et al.,* 1979). To date some 500 patients have been entered on this study. It is celar that MER adds nothing to this chemotherapeutic program. For women with more than three nodes involved with metastatic breast cancer, CMFVP is significantly superior to CMF ($p = .01$) in terms of disease-free interval. We are continuing to study three drugs versus five drugs in women in which one, two, or three nodes are involved.

XI. DISCUSSION

Emphasis in breast cancer belongs on research, and after etiology and prevention, most of the research should be aimed at treating disseminated disease. Breast cancer is often not a local disease in the breast at the time of diagnosis.

Great emphasis belongs on chemotherapy adjuvant to surgery to control the micrometastatic dissemination present in approximately one-half of patients treated with curative intent. Local control of the breast can usually be effectively carried out with modified radical mastectomy. This is a safe and effective procedure that leads to an acceptable cosmetic result and removes the carcinoma. A breast-sparing procedure, surgical and/or radiotherapeutic, is an entirely appropriate subject of research, under systemic chemotherapy coverage, but should be done as an investigative undertaking with proper safeguards. There is as yet no proof that lesser surgery such as segmental resection or radiotherapy is equal in terms of survival or recurrence.

Nothing would improve the outlook for breast cancer better than early diagnosis. Mammography is a technique that can display tumors before they are palpable. It is particularly valuable in postmenopausal women where the fat content of the breast is relatively high. False-negatives are painfully frequent premenopausally, however, because of the similarity of tumor and normal breast glandular tissue on the X-ray film. Logistically, mammography is not nearly as practical as self-examination. Fewer than 250,000 women in the United States were scheduled for a national mammography screening program. More than 110,000,000 females live in the United States. Mammography becomes an insuperable logistic and economic problem for screening.

However, every women can examine her own breasts without charge. Ninety percent of breast cancer is found by the patient herself, most accidentally during bathing or dressing, when a mass large enough to be found is encountered. A woman who does not systematically examine herself misses the chance to find a breast mass at a smaller size. A woman can get to know the texture of her own breast best. In so doing, she can discover masses that are smaller than 1 cm in size, and these should be brought immediately to the attention of a physician. Under such circumstances one would anticipate that the cure rate using surgery or local destruction by radiotherapy would markedly increase, and our concern with disseminated breast cancer could be much diminished. In the meantime, however, it is incumbent on every physician to teach—and to preach—breast self-examination. Each physician should alert himself to the major impact that chemotherapy has made on breast cancer immediately following effective surgery. With this knowledge put into practice, we can change the high mortality of the western world's most common women's cancer.

REFERENCES

Axtell, L. M., Cutler, S. J., and Meyers, M. H. (1972). "End Results in Cancer," Rep. No. 4, CDMEW Publ. No. NIM 73-272, p. 101. US Govt. Printing Office, Washington, D.C.
Axtell, L. M., Asire, A. J., and Meyers, M. H., eds. (1976). "Cancer Patients Survival," No. 5, DHEW Publ. No. NIH 77-992. US Govt. Printing Office, Washington, D.C.

Band, P. R., Tormey, D. C., and Bauer, M. (1977). *Proc. Am. Assoc. Cancer Res.* **18,** 228.

Black, M. M. (1977). *Contemp. Top. Immunobiol.* **6,** 239–262.

Bonadonna, G., and Valagussa, P. (1980). *In* "Adjuvant Therapy of Primary Breast Cancer in Principles of Cancer Treatment" (S. K. Carter, E. Glatstein, and R. E. Livingston, eds.) (in press).

Bonadonna, G., Valagussa, P., Rossi, A., Zucali, R., Tancini, G., Bajetta, E., Brambilla, C., DiFranzo, G., Banfi, A., Rilke, F., and Veronesi, U. (1978). *Semin. Oncol.* **5,** 450–464.

Bonadonna, G., DeFranzo, G., and Tancini, G. (1979). *Proc. Am. Soc. Clin. Oncol.* **20,** 359.

Brown, G. S., Kramer, S., and Brandy, L. (1977) *Int. J. Radiat. Oncol., Biol. Phys.* **2,** 1145–1148.

Carbone, P. P., and Tormey, D. G. (1977). *In* "Combination Chemotherapy for Advanced Disease" (W. McGuire, ed.), pp. 165–215.

Chopra, H. C., and Oie, H. K. (1972). *J. Natl. Cancer Inst.* **48,** 1059–1065.

Cooper, R. G. (1969). *Proc. Am. Assoc. Cancer Res.* **10,** 15.

Cooper, R. G., Holland, J. F., and Glidewell, O. (1979). *Cancer* **44,** 793–798.

Doll, R., Payne, P., and Waterhouse, J., eds. (1966). "Cancer Incidence in Five Continents. A Technical Report." Springer-Verlag, Berlin and New York.

Fisher, B., Black, N. H., and Bross, I. D. J. (1969). *Cancer* **24,** 1071–1080.

Fisher, B., Slack, N., Katrych, D. L., and Wolmark, N. (1975). *Surg., Gynecol. Obstet.* **140,** 528–534.

Fisher, E. R., and Gebhardt, (1978). *Semin. Oncol.* **5,** 385.

Fisher, E. R., Gregorio, R. M., Fisher, B., Redmond, C., Vellios, F., and Sommers, S. C. (1975). *Cancer* **36,** 1–85.

Holland, J. F., Glidewell, O., and Cooper, R. G. (1980). *Surg., Gynecol. Obstet.* **150,** 817–821.

Ing, R., Ho, J. H. C., and Petrakis, N. L. (1977). *Lancet* **2,** 124–127.

Kiang, D. T., Frenning, D. H., and Goldman, A. L. (1978). *N. Engl. J. Med.* **299,** 1330–1334.

Kramer, W. M., and Rush, B. F. (1973). *Cancer* **31,** 130–137.

Lesnick, G. (1979). *N.Y. State J. Med.* **79,** 41.

Lippman, M. E., Allegra, J. C., and Thompson, E. B. (1978). *N. Engl. J. Med.* **298,** 1223–1228.

McGuire, W. I. (1975). *Cancer* **36,** 638–644.

MacKenzie, I. (1965). *Br. J. Cancer* **19,** 1–8.

MacMahon, B., Cole, P., Brown, J. B., Aoki, K., Lin, T. M., Morgan, R. W., and Woo, N. C. (1971). *Lancet* **2,** 900–902.

MacMahon, B., Cole, P., and Brown, J. (1973). *J. Natl. Cancer Inst.* **50,** 20–42.

Mason, T. J., McKay, F. W., Hoover, R., Blot, W. J., and Fraumeni, J. F., Jr. (1975). "Atlas for Cancer Mortality for U.S. Countries 1950–1969," DHEW Publ. No. NIH 75-780. USDHEW, Washington, D.C.

Miller, A. B. (1977). *Cancer* **39,** 2704–2708.

National Surgical Adjuvant Project for Breast and Bowel Cancers, Pittsburg (1979). "Progress Report." NSABP.

Nime, F. A., Rosen, P. P., Thaler, H., Ashikari, R., and Urban, J. A. (1977). *Am. J. Surg. Pathol.* **1,** 25–30.

Petrakis, N. L. (1977). *Cancer* **39,** 2709–2715.

Prosnitz, L. R., Goldenberg, I. S., and Packard, R. A. (1977). *Cancer* **39,** 917–923.

Ravdin, R. G., Lewison, E. F., Slack, N. H., Dao, T. L., Gardner, B., State, D., and Fisher, B. (1970). *Surg., Gynecol. Obstet.* **131,** 1055–1064.

Saracci, and Repetto, (1978). *Semin. Oncol.* **5,** 342.

Silverberg, E. (1979). *Cancer* **29,** 6–21.

Stjernsward, J. (1974). *Lancet* **2,** 1285–1286.

Tormey, D., Falkson, G., Weiss, R., Perloff, M., Glidewell, O., and Holland, J. F. (1979). *In* "Adjuvant Therapy of Cancer" (S. E. Jones and S. E. Salmon, eds.), pp. 253–260. Grune & Stratton, New York.

Tormey, D. C. (1975). *Cancer Chemother. Rep. Part 3* **6**, 319–327.

Trunum, B., Hoogstraten, B., and Kennedy, A. (1976). *Proc. Am. Soc. Clin. Oncol.* **17**, 242.

Veronesi, U. (1978). *Semin. Oncol.* **54**, 395–402.

Vessey, M., Doll, R., and Sutton, P. M. (1972). *Br. Med. J.* **3**, 719–724.

Wanebo, C. K., Johnson, K. G., Sato, K., and Thorslund, T. W. (1968). *N. Engl. J. Med.* **279**, 667–671.

7
CLINICAL PRESENTATIONS OF GASTROINTESTINAL CANCER
Philip Schein

I. Large-Bowel Carcinoma 113
   A. Etiology 114
   B. Clinical Presentation 115
   C. Diagnosis 116
II. Carcinoma of the Pancreas 117
   A. Etiology 118
   B. Pathology 118
   C. Clinical Presentation 118
   D. Diagnosis 120
III. Carcinoma of the Stomach 121
   A. Etiology 121
   B. Pathology 122
   C. Clinical Presentation 122
   D. Diagnosis 123
   References 123

I. LARGE-BOWEL CARCINOMA

Colorectal carcinoma is a major health problem in the United States. It ranks second to skin cancer in overall incidence, with approximately 102,000 new cases diagnosed each year, representing 13% of all cancer (American Cancer Society, 1978). Approximately 52,000 deaths per year are directly attributable to this disease, or 13% of all cancer mortality—second to lung cancer. Although large-bowel cancer has been one of the most extensively investigated malignancies with regard to therapy, relatively little progress has been made, as is reflected in the static survival statistics over the past three decades. Overall, the incidence in only slightly higher in men than in women, and the mean age is approximately 65 years.

CANCER AND CHEMOTHERAPY, VOL. II

113

A. Etiology

The etiology of this tumor remains undetermined. Several lines of evidence would suggest that dietary factors play a role in causation. Burkitt has developed a hypothesis from epidermiologic data in which he proposed that the Western diet of refined carbohydrate and low fiber content sets the stage for colorectal cancer (Walker and Burkitt, 1976). He has implicated the physical characteristics of the resultant stool, including the low volume, hard consistency, and prolonged transit time. This has been correlated with an increase in the anaerobic flora of the large bowel, and in particular the bacteroides group (Aries and Crowther, 1969). Others have suggested that the high fat content of our diet may be equally important, with an increase in fecal excretion of cholesterol metabolites and bile acids. The latter finding may be of importance since specific secondary bile acids, such as deoxycholic and lithocholic acid, can act as promoters of carcinogens in rat colon (Reddy, 1976). It is possible to interrelate the two theories; the anaerobic bacteria flora, found in populations with a low fiber intake, produce an enzyme, 7α-dehydroxylase, which can degrade the primary bile acids, cholic acid and chenodeoxycholic acid, to the carcinogen-promoting forms. Although a firm recommendation regarding dietary measures for the prevention of colorectal cancer is not possible at present, a diet low in fat and with an ample fiber content appears prudent for many reasons.

We also recognize that specific conditions can predispose to the development of large bowel cancer. One such antecedent is chronic ulcerative colitis. Patients with diffuse involvement of the colorectal mucosa (pan-colitis), which has remained active for 10 or more years, have a high incidence of colon cancer. The risk has been estimated to be 20% per decade after the first 10 years, with a cumulative occurrence of 25–50% by 35 years after the onset of colitis (Moertel, 1973a). The carcinoma that arises in the setting of ulcerative colitis has some special clinical features: it is more likely to involve the right and transverse colon, it has an increased tendency to be multicentric in origin, and it tends to be undifferentiated and scirrhous in histology. In general, the prognosis of such cases tends to be less favorable when compared to the spontaneously occurring tumor in the general population. A similar association has now been described for Crohn's disease of the colon involving patients with an early onset of symptoms and a long history of total colonic involvement (Weedon et al., 1973).

Familial polyposis coli is a rare syndrome, transmitted as an autosomal dominant, and characterized by the development of large numbers of adenomatous polyps on the mucous membrane of the colon and rectum. The condition is usually expressed in adolescence or early adult life, and it almost invariably leads to the development of adenocarcinoma of the bowel. The average age at diagnosis of carcinoma with this condition is about 40, compared with an average of

60 in non-polyposis patients. An additional characteristic is the high incidence of multifocality—48% in the St. Mark's Hospital series, or 15-fold greater than expected (Bussey, 1975). Once the carcinoma is diagnosed, the prognosis is usually grave. Two related disorders are Gardner's syndrome, where the polyposis is associated with sebaceous cysts, subcutaneous tumors, and facial and cranial osteomas, and Turcot's syndrome—polyposis and malignant tumors of the central nervous system.

Villous adenomas of the colon are soft, sessile, velvetlike growths. Their most frequent location is in the rectum. They may produce copious amounts of mucous, which is passed with the morning bowel movement after an overnight accumulation. In extreme cases this condition can result in severe electrolyte imbalances (David *et al.*, 1962). Most villous adenomas are benign, and do not recur if completely excised. However, an estimated 30–40% are malignant, and in particular the larger lesions.

There is considerable controversy as to whether adenomatous polyps of the large bowel are premalignant. The size of the polyp can be used as a crude guide: Lesions of 1.5 cm have a 2–5% probability of malignancy, which increases to approximately 25% for polyps 3.5 cm and larger (Behringer, 1970).

B. Clinical Presentation

The large bowel is not a homogeneous organ in respect to its normal function, or in the pathologic features of the malignancy that may arise is each anatomic region. This has an important bearing on the constellation of symptoms that, as a generalization, tend to characterize tumors of the right colon versus the left colon and rectum (Moertel, 1973a; Woolley, 1976).

1. Right Colon

The right colon, including the cecum and ascending portions, is the primary site of large-bowel cancer in approximately 15% of cases. The principal function of the right colon is the absorption of water and electrolytes secreted from the small intestine. The fecal stream in the right colon is liquid, and is converted to a semisolid state which is then stored in the more distal portions of the large bowel. An additional factor is the caliber and distensibility of the right colon, which is sixfold greater than that of the sigmoid region. Lastly, the tumors that arise in the right colon, though large, tend to be soft fungating masses that do not commonly encompass the entire circumference of the bowel.

Because of these functional and pathologic features, tumors of the right colon are not likely to present with symptoms or signs of obstruction. The possible exceptions are neoplasms that arise in the region immediately adjacent to the ileocecal valve; the resulting symptoms have been mistaken for appendicitis in elderly patients. Tumors of the right colon are insidious in onset. The patient may experience only vague dull abdominal discomfort or colic. Moreover, by the time the tumor is correctly diagnosed, it is palpable as an abdominal mass in as many as 75% of cases. Chronic blood loss is a feature of the disease. The patient may describe stools that are mahogany-red in color, but all too often the bleeding is diagnosed only by occult blood testing. In approximately one-third of patients this problem may be sufficiently long-standing so as to result in symptoms of anemia.

2. Left Colon

Tumors arising in the left colon, including the descending and sigmoid segments, account for approximately 30% of the total. The normal function of this region of the bowel is the storage of the solid stool. When compared to neoplasms of the right colon, tumors of the left tend to be firm, scirrhous, and circumferential. These factors, coupled with the reduced caliber of the left colon, make acute or chronic symptoms of obstruction an important clinical presentation. It has been estimated that as many as 50% of acutely obstructed colons result from carcinoma, and as a possible initial symptom of the disease. More commonly, the clinical manifestations of obstruction are chronic and progressive. The resulting symptoms are protean and include abdominal pain, and a change in bowel habits with constipation at times alternating with diarrhea. There may be a history of recent need for laxatives or enemas, or decreased caliber of stools. In contrast to the right-sided colonic tumors, bleeding when present is more overt, with dark or bright red coating the surface of the stool. The incidence of palpable tumor is less than in the cecum; the literature suggests a range of 26–46% of all cases.

The principal symptoms of rectal cancer include bleeding and changes in stool habit. The latter may present as an increased frequency of stools, tenesmus, as well as the urge to defecate in the morning, so-called morning diarrhea. The tumor may produce substantive amounts of mucous, which if severe may be indicative of an underlying large villous adenoma. Because of progressive obstruction of the bowel lumen, the patient may note a decrease in stool caliber. Pain with rectal cancer is regarded as a late and ominous sign, since it is usually representative of tumor extension into the pararectal tissues, with infiltration of nerve trunks. Malignancies of the rectum constitute 40% of large-bowel tumors, the leading site. Approximately 75% are within the reach of an examining finger.

C. Diagnosis

The diagnosis of colorectal cancer in a symptomatic patient is relatively straightforward, and can be made with a high degree of accuracy with available techniques. The problem rests with the early detection of asymptomatic patients, the Dukes' A and B cases having a high probability for cure with prompt surgery. The use of guaiac-impregnated slides as a screening technique for detecting occult blood from the colorectal carcinoma, the Hemacult test, is now undergoing prospective evaluation. Patients are asked to prepare two slides on three consecutive days. The accuracy of this test, a decrease in false positives and false negatives, can be improved by ensuring that the individual eats a meat-free, high-residue diet for at least 24 hours before the first stool collection. Initial pilot studies have produced promising results, with as many as 85% of those diagnosed pathologically localized, compared to 40% in national figures (Winawer and Sherlock, 1976).

Sigmoidoscopy and the barium enema have been the mainstays in diagnosis. Approximately 55% of colorectal cancer occurs within the range of the 25-cm sigmoidoscope. Although early detection can be achieved with annual screening using this technique, the cost-effectiveness leaves a great deal to be desired. It is estimated that the discovery of each potential curative lesion with screening sigmoidoscopy would exceed $70,000. Nevertheless, the overall diagnostic value of sigmoidoscopy is unquestioned (Winawer and Sherlock, 1976).

The development of the flexible fiberoptic colonoscope has revolutionized our diagnostic capabilities, allowing the entire colonic lumen to be examined. In addition to detecting asymptomatic small lesions missed on barium enema studies, it also provides a means to assess objectively equivocal findings on X ray. It may also be used to search for synchronous colonic tumors, which occur in about 3% of patients (Moertel, 1966).

Between 60 and 85% of patients with advanced stages of colorectal cancer will present with a plasma Carcinoembryonic antigen, CEA, concentration greater than 2.5 ng/ml; marked elevations are frequently recorded with the onset of hepatic metastases. The percentage of abnormal levels in patients with small primary tumors is appreciably lower. The overall lack of sensitivity, as well as the well-known problems in specificity, do not allow this tumor marker to be used in diagnosis.

II. CARCINOMA OF THE PANCREAS

Carcinoma of the pancreas is now estimated to afflict 220,000 individuals per year in the United States (American Cancer Society, 1978). Essentially, all patients with this tumor can be expected to die of the disease, the majority within 1 year of diagnosis. Pancreatic cancer has shown a dramatic increase in incidence during the past 50 years, and now ranks as the fourth most common cause of cancer death in this country. This increase in diagnosis has been most apparent in black males.

A. Etiology

Epidemiologic studies conducted by Wynder (1975), have served to identify several populations that appear to be at significant increased risk for this disease. Most notable are cigarette smokers, not surprising in view of the number of carcinogens that have been demonstrated in cigarette smoke. It has been hypothesized that tobacco carcinogens in bile may reflux into the pancreatic duct or, alternatively, are distributed to the pancreas from the bloodstream. A diet high in fat and/or cholesterol has also been correlated with an increased risk of pancreatic cancer. Surveys of members of the American Chemical Society have emphasized that chemical workers, particularly those who have been exposed to beta-naphthylamine and benzidine, have a higher than expected incidence of this tumor (Wynder, 1975). The role of chemical carcinogenesis is further supported by laboratory studies, which have demonstrated the induction of pancreatic tumors in rodents with a variety of agents such as nitrosamines, nitrosamides, and azaserine (Longnecker and Curphey, 1975; Pour *et al.,* 1975; Reddy and Rao, 1975).

B. Pathology

The pathologic features of human pancreatic epithelial neoplasms have been described in detail by Cubilla and Fitzgerald (1975). The majority of these tumors (95%) are adenocarcinomas, with duct cell adenocarcinomas predominating. It is widely held that the site of origin is the pancreatic ductal system. There is some evidence, however, from studies in rodents to suggest that neoplastic transformation of the pancreatic acinar cell, after exposure to carcinogens, may cause it to take the appearance of ductal epithelium (Reddy and Rao, 1975).

The primary tumor arises in the head region of the pancreas twice as frequently as in the body and tail. Cubilla and Fitzgerald (1975) have emphasized, however, that multifocal neoplasia may also be present in the organ in as many as 19% of the cases, which should have some implications as to the extent of optimal surgical resection.

C. Clinical Presentation

Pancreatic cancer is more common in males than in females, with a sex ratio of 2:1. This is a disease of the elderly, with a peak incidence at age 60. The predominant symptoms of pancreatic cancer result from the direct extension of the tumor into the nerves of the retroperitoneal space, obstruction of the common bile duct, direct invasion of the duodenum as well as other visceral organs, and overt metastatic spread to liver and lung (Gray *et al.,* 1973; Smith *et al.,* 1967; Macdonald *et al.,* 1976).

Pain is the most common presenting problem. Initially it may appear as a vague, poorly localized complaint, but it eventually becomes established as a progressive and persistent problem. There are several general presentations: Epigastric pain predominates; it may be colicky or dull and steady, with some radiation into the lower back. Less commonly, the pain will be confined to the back region, which would suggest a possible orthopedic or neurological condition. There may be a history of paroxysms associated with meals, exacerbation at night, or a partial relief by changes in posture, particularly by sitting or bending forward. The prolonged use of heating pads may leave a telltale discoloration of the skin of the abdomen or back. Pain with pancreatic cancer can be largely explained by the encasement of nerve trunks by the tumor and the prominent desmoplastic reaction. Pain represents one of the most debilitating features of the disease.

A history of recent weight loss can also be elicited from the majority of patients, and may be the only sign of the underlying tumor. This can be explained in most cases by a state of anorexia and the poorly understood cachexia syndrome, which are almost universal accompaniments of the disease. Frequently patients describe specific abnormalities in taste sensation and aversions to certain foods, particularly meat. Pancreatic insufficiency with steatorrhea, as well as diabetes, may result from occlusion of the pancreatic duct or direct destruction of the exocrine and endocrine function of the organ.

Jaundice is an important clinical feature of pancreatic cancer. It is estimated that 75–90% of patients with primary tumors in the head region will become icteric. In the majority of cases, jaundice follows an antecedent period of abdominal pain. However, jaundice may present as the first symptom of the disease, resulting from an early occlusion of the common bile duct as it transverses through the head of the pancreas to the ampulla of Vater. It is important to note that this is the subgroup of patients, albeit limited in number, for whom prompt surgery may have curative potential. In contrast, jaundice associated with primary tumors of the body or tail is a late finding, which signifies advanced metastatic disease to the liver or the porta hepatis.

A change in bowel habit is commonly described, either diarrhea or constipation resulting from anorexia. With invasion of the duodenum, or stomach, there may be symptoms of obstruction, with dysphagia, nausea, and vomiting. Frank gastrointestinal bleeding is rare, whereas occult bleeding is detectable in approximately 50% of the cases. Thrombophlebitis, classically superficial, migratory, and anticoagulant-resistant, has been shown in some series to occur with increased frequency. It may present as the first sign of the disease, and has been correlated with tumors of the body and tail region of the pancreas. Psychiatric disorders have also been described, including depression and anxiety states that may herald the presence of the tumor.

On physical examination there may be signs of generalized cachexia and jaundice. Tenderness to deep palpation of the epigastrium is detectable in approximately 25% of patients, as is the presence of an enlarged and hard liver. A palpable upper abdominal mass, representing a primary tumor in the tail or body of the pancreas, may be present in 10–25% of cases. Obstruction of the splenic vein by tumor encasement can result in splenomegaly, an otherwise uncommon finding with gastrointestinal cancer, with possible hypersplenism. A similar occlusion of the portal vein may produce esophageal varices, and may contribute to the development of ascites. The rare acinar cell carcinoma has been associated with a clinical syndrome of subcutaneous fat necrosis, polyarthralgia, and eosinophilia, as well as elevated serum lipase activity.

D. Diagnosis

It is quite apparent that attempts to obtain an "early diagnosis" of pancreatic carcinoma based upon clinical symptomalogy or signs are destined to be futile. By the time the disorder is suspected it is often quite far advanced and unresectable. On the other hand, to investigate every patient with abdominal discomfort or weight reduction for the possibility of an underlying neoplasm would entail enormous expense, with little return. Nevertheless, if the present dismal survival statistics are to be improved, it will require the detection of this disease at an asymptomatic stage; the number of cases that are candidates for surgical resection for cure would be increased, and other modalities of therapy would have a greater prospect of success.

It is for this reason that there has been a rapid proliferation and evaluation of new diagnostic procedures for pancreatic cancer (Fitzgerald *et al.*, 1978). A relatively high percentage, 70–90%, of true-positive diagnoses have been claimed for each of the procedures, including arteriography, endoscopic retrograde cholangiopancreatography, ultrasonography, and scanning. However, this high success rate has been achieved in symptomatic patients who either were suspected of having the disease or had overt physical signs. It is generally accepted that the present methods of diagnosis are too crude for purposes of screening an asymptomatic population. An example is the current use of the CAT scan, which has been found to have significant limitations (Moertel, 1973b).

The density of the normal pancreas is identical to that of the neoplastic pancreas, and at present there is no means of differential enhancement. As a result, the CAT scan depends upon the detection of areas of enlargement, and the presence several centimeters of tumor mass, containing billions of cancer cells, is required before positive diagnosis can be made. The most promising approach for the future is the development of a sensitive and specific tumor marker. The pancreatic oncofetal antigen (POA), a glycoprotein present in fetal and malignant pancreatic tissue, represents one such attempt (Gelder *et al.*, 1978). Unfortunately this material, like the CEA, has not fulfilled the criteria of a useful screening test. Nevertheless, the overall validity of this approach has been established and it is generally accepted that identification of a tumor-specific produce represents the most promising avenue of research for the early diagnosis of pancreatic cancer.

III. CARCINOMA OF THE STOMACH

It is estimated that there will be 23,000 new cases of gastric carcinoma diagnosed this year, with 15,000 deaths (American Cancer Society, 1978). Ths incidence of this tumor in the United States has demonstrated a striking and continuing decrease during the past four decades, but it still ranks as the sixth most common cause of cancer death. In contrast, the incidence and mortality rates from gastric cancer in Japan and Chile are five times that of this country. Environmental factors are strongly suggested from studies of the incidence of this tumor among Japanese immigrants to the United States; there is a five- and threefold decrease in males and in female Japanese born in California, respectively, compared to natives (MacGregor, 1974). Similarly, the overall decrease in incidence in the United States can not be explained by changes in the genetic pool.

A. Etiology

There is considerable debate as to the importance of possible risk factors for gastric cancer. There is general agreement that pernicious anemia, with its associated severe atrophic gastritis, predisposes to this tumor with estimated occurrence rates of 5–10% (Hoffman, 1970). Chronic atrophic gastritis, independent of pernicious anemia, and adenomatous gastric polyps have been suspected as having premalignant potential, but the evidence is not conclusive. The same can be said for the possible association with blood group A. Several families have been identified that do appear to have an inheritable form of this disease, and gastric cancer after a partial gastrectomy is reported to be significantly increased following an interval of 10–15 years postsurgery for benign disease.

There is evidence that tumors of the stomach can be induced with chemical carcinogens, supporting the conclusions of epidemiologic studies. Asbestos, in addition to its proven role for mesothelioma and lung cancer, has also been associated with gastric cancer. Other suspected etiologic factors include smoked meat (containing carcinogenic hydrocarbons), salted fish, and nitrites which can react with secondary amines to form carcinogenic nitrosamines and nitrosamides. As a correlate, methyl nitro nitrosoguanidine has been well established as a carcinogen for the stomach of rats and dogs (MacGregor, 1974).

B. Pathology

Carcinoma of the stomach is twice as common in men as in women. The average patient is 55–60 years of age at the time of diagnosis, but the disease is known to occur in childhood. The pathology of this tumor is well described. In regard to location within the stomach, the adenocarcinoma arises in the pyloris and antrum in 50% of cases. Primary tumors of the lesser curvature and body each account for 20%, whereas the cardia is the site of origin in 7%, a location that carries a particularly poor prognosis. Carcinomas of the greater curvature are uncommon, accounting for only 3% of the total. The pathologic presentation may take one of four major forms. Ulcerative tumors are the most common (75%), and differentation from a benign ulcer may present a difficult diagnostic problem. Polypoid tumors and the diffusely infiltrating linitis plastica presentation each account for 10%. The superficial spreading carcinoma is less common (Moertel, 1973c).

Once established, the tumor may disseminate by four possible routes. There is direct and contiguous invasion into the greater or lesser omentum, colon, pancreas, esophagus, or liver. The regional lymph nodes are involved early in the disease, and distant metastases to the left supraclavicular (Virchow's node) and the left anterior axillary group are well known. The liver is the most common site for hematogenous metastases, but the lung and bones may also become involved. Lastly, diffuse implantation of the tumor within the peritoneal cavity is observed in a relatively high percentage of cases, and may result in the formation of Blumer's shelf along the rectum, or seeding of the ovaries to form a Kurkenberg's tumor.

C. Clinical Presentation

Cancer of the stomach may produce no discernible symptoms for long periods. The initial complaint is usually mild epigastric discomfort, which may present as only a vague sensation of fullness, gas pains, or with a typical peptic ulcer pattern, partially relieved by antacids. Eventually the pain becomes more prominent, bringing the patient to the attention of a physician after the tumor has had an opportunity to grow to the extent that it may no longer be resectable.

Anorexia, early satiety, and distortion of taste and smell all contribute to common phenomenon of weight loss. Approximately 50% of patients will experience nausea and vomiting, typically with primary tumors of the pylorus, which may progress to partial gastric obstruction. Dysphagia may be the first presenting symptom of a lesion of the cardioesophageal region. Gross hematemesis or melena is very uncommon, whereas anemia from chronic occult blood loss is a frequent finding.

On physical examination, the left supraclavicular and left anterior axillary lymph node regions must be careful examined for adenopathy, which may be present in 5% of patients at the time of diagnosis. Epigastric tenderness is elicited in only 20% of patients. Palpation of the umbilical region may reveal the presence of a subcutaneous nodule. Metastatic disease may be manifested by a hard nodular liver, or the presence of a Blumer's shelf on rectal examination.

Gastric cancer has been associated with a number of paraneoplastic syndromes. It is the most common cancer found in association with acanthosis nigricans and dermatomyositis, as well as microangiopathic hemolytic anemia (Schutt, 1976).

D. Diagnosis

The earliest stages of gastric cancer, mucosal and submucosal, are typically asymptomatic. They can only be diagnosed by routine screening, as is carried out in Japan because of the high incidence, or by accidental discovery. The Japanese have relied on the use of double contrast barium fluoroscopy, which has proved a sensitive diagnostic procedure. This is followed by fiberoptic gastroscopy and biopsy. Gastric analysis demonstrates histamine or pentagastrin-fast achlorhydria in approximately 75% of patients, and CEA may be elevated with advanced disease. However, a sensitive and specific tumor marker, which would allow for cost-effective mass screening of asymptomatic cases, has not as yet been identified.

REFERENCES

American Cancer Society (1978). "Cancer Facts and Figures." Am. Cancer Soc., New York.
Aries, V., and Crowther, J. (1969). Gut 10, 334–335.
Behringer, G. E. (1970). Dis. Colon Rectum 13, 116.
Bussey, H. J. R. (1975). "Familial Polyposis Cell." Johns Hopkins Univ. Press, Baltimore, Maryland.
Cubilla, A. L., and Fitzgerald, P. J. (1975). Cancer Res. 35, 2234–2248.
David, J. R., Seavey, P. W., and Sessions, J. T., Jr. (1962). Ann. Surg. 115, 806–816.
Fitzgerald, P. J., Fortner, J. G., and Watson, R. C. (1978). Cancer 41, 868–879.
Gelder, F. B., Reese, C. J., Moossa, A. R., Hall, T., and Hunter, R. (1978). Cancer Res. 38, 313–324.
Gray, L. W., Crook, J. N., and Cohn, I., Jr. (1973). Proc. Natl. Cancer Conf., 7th, 1972 pp. 503–510.
Hoffman, N. R. (1970). Geriatrics 25, 90.
Longnecker, D. S., and Curphey, T. J. (1975). Cancer Res. 35, 2249–2258.
Macdonald, J. S., Widerlite, L., and Schein, P. S. (1976). J. Natl. Cancer Inst. 56, 1093–1099.
MacGregor, I. L. (1974). J. Am. Med. Assoc. 227, 911–915.
Moertel, C. G. (1966). "Multiple Primary Malignant Neoplasms." Springer-Verlag, Berlin and New York.

Moertel, C. G. (1973a). *In* "Cancer Medicine" (J. F. Holland and E. Frei III, eds.), pp. 1597–1627. Lea Febiger, Philadelphia, Pennsylvania.

Moertel, C. G. (1973b). *In* "Cancer Medicine" (J. F. Holland and E. Frei III, eds.). pp. 1559–1570. Lea Febiger, Philadelphia, Pennsylvania.

Moertel, C. G. (1973c). *In* "Cancer Medicine" (J. F. Holland and E. Frei III, eds.), pp. 1527–1541. Lea & Febiger, Philadelphia, Pennsylvania.

Pour, P., Kruger, F. W., Althoff, J., Cardesa, A., and Mohr, U. (1975). *Cancer Res.* **35,** 2259–2268.

Reddy, B. S. (1976). *Semin. Oncol.* **3,** 351–359.

Reddy, J. K., and Rao, M. S. (1975). *Cancer Res.* **35,** 2269–2277.

Schutt, A. J. (1976). *Clin. Gastroenterol.* **5,** 681–699.

Smith, P. E., Krementz, E. T., Reed, R. J., and Bufkin, W. J. (1967). *Surg., Gynecol. Obstet.* **124,** 1288–1290.

Walker, A. R. P., and Burkitt, D. P. (1976). *Semin. Oncol.* **3,** 341–350.

Weedon, D. D., Shorter, R. G., Ilstrup, D. M., Huizenga, K. A., and Taylor, W. G. (1973). *N. Engl. J. Med.* **289,** 1099–1103.

Winawer, S. J., and Sherlock, P. (1976). *Semin. Oncol.* **3,** 387–397.

Woolley, P. V. (1976). *Semin. Oncol.* **3,** 373–376.

Wynder, E. L. (1975). *Cancer Res.* **35,** 2228–2233.

8

CANCERS OF THE HEAD AND NECK
Montague Lane

I.	Introduction	125
II.	Incidence	127
III.	Etiology	127
IV.	Histopathology and Spread	129
V.	Clinical Manifestations	130
	A. Oral Cavity	130
	B. Nasal Cavity	134
	C. Paranasal Sinuses	135
	D. Nasopharynx	137
	E. Oropharynx	137
	F. Hypopharynx	140
	G. Larynx	141
	H. Salivary Glands	142
VI.	Diagnosis	142
VII.	Clinical Staging	142
VIII.	Management	143
IX.	Conclusions	145
	References	146

I. INTRODUCTION

Head and neck cancers are an important group of malignant neoplasms that arise in anatomically adjacent sites of the upper airways and digestive tract: the oral cavity, the nasal cavity and paranasal sinuses, nasopharynx, oropharynx, hypopharynx, larynx, and salivary glands (Fig. 1A and B). These tumors, excluding those of salivary gland origin, have many similarities of etiology, pathology, mode of spread, and treatment. Nevertheless, there may be major differences between them with respect to presenting symptoms and findings, ease

The material presented in this chapter appears in part in
Cancer—Diagnosis and Management,
by Le Jacq Publishing, Inc., New York.

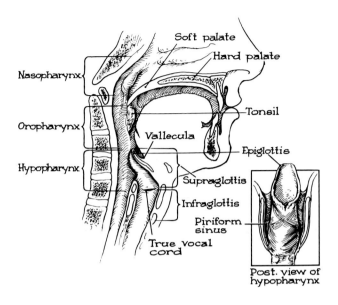

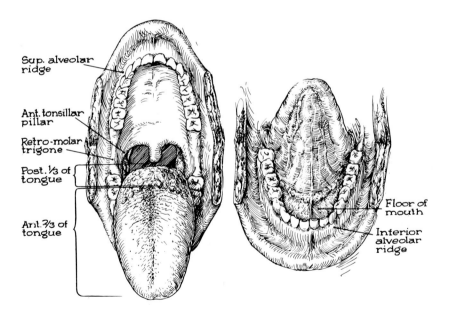

Fig. 1A and B.   Anatomical sites of head and neck cancers. Reprinted with permission from Physicians Programs, Inc.

of detection and diagnosis, clinical evolution, and prognosis. These differences are determined not only by site of the primary but also by the intrinsic biological properties of each tumor. The discussion that follows will place emphasis upon the natural history of head and neck cancers. This information is fundamental for comprehension of the approaches to their diagnosis and treatment. The complexity of head and neck cancers mandates a comprehensive multidisciplinary effort in patient management from the outset.

II. INCIDENCE

Approximately 7% of the malignant cancers other than skin cancers diagnosed annually in the United States arise in the head and neck. Their importance is highlighted by the fact that they have a higher incidence than lymphoma, leukemia, cancers of bone, soft tissue, and the central nervous system, melanoma, and myeloma. Most head and neck cancers are more prevalent in men (American Joint Committee for Cancer Staging and End Results Reporting, 1976); salivary gland tumors occur slightly more often in women. Cancers of the oral cavity constitute the largest anatomical group of head and neck cancers, but the most frequent specific site is the larynx, followed by cancers of the lip and tongue (Axtell, et al., 1972). Treatment results may be excellent or poor depending upon the primary site, extent of disease at diagnosis, and biological behavior of the tumor. Although more than half the patients are cured of their disease with proper treatment, those with incurable head and neck cancer often suffer severe disability and disfigurement and are very difficult therapeutic problems (Fig. 2).

III. ETIOLOGY

Epidemiological factors associated with head and neck cancers are shown in Table I. The two major factors are chronic consumption of tobacco and alcohol (Wynder et al., 1957). Tobacco smoking is consistently incriminated in oral-cavity cancers other than lip and in cancers of the oropharynx and the hypopharynx. Cigarette smoking is related to cancer of the larynx in particular. Concomitant chronic use of alcohol is generally noted, and many patients use both tobacco and alcohol excessively (Rothman and Keller, 1972). Tobacco chewing and snuff dipping are often associated with cancers of the floor of the mouth and buccal mucosa. The practice of chewing betel nuts in combination with tobacco contributes to the high incidence of oral cavity cancer in India and other southeastern Asian countries (Khanolkar, 1959). Cancer of the anterior two-thirds of the tongue has also been related to poor dentition.

The repetitive chronic exposure of the epithelium of the upper airways and

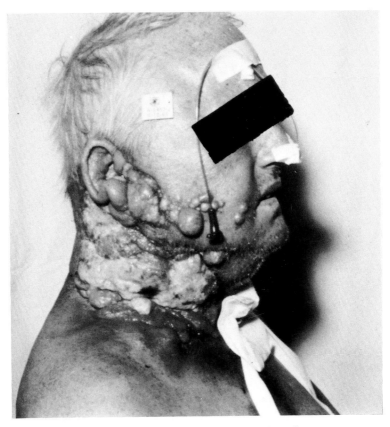

Fig. 2. Patient with advanced cancer of the hypopharynx.

digestive tract to tobacco and alcohol may result in multiple primary cancers of these sites. The oral mucous membranes of many of these patients may reveal leukoplakia with or without malignant change in some sites, carcinoma *in situ* in others, and frank carcinoma as well. Second head and neck primary cancers are common and should always be anticipated by careful examinations of patients who have been successfully treated for one cancer of this region, especially if there is continued exposure to carcinogenic influences. Unlike tobacco, alcohol contains no known carcinogens, yet its influence on head and neck cancer is synergistic with tobacco, not simply additive. Its effects may be mediated through nutritional deficiencies (McCoy, 1978).

Chronic exposure to sunlight appears to be the major factor in lip cancer, which is commonly seen in ranchers and farmers (del Regato and Spjut, 1977). Swedish women have a high incidence of cancer of the hypopharynx, which has been associated with the Plummer–Vinson syndrome. An increased incidence of

TABLE I

Epidemiological Factors

Site	Associated factor
Intraoral cavity, oropharynx, hypopharynx	Tobacco smoking with or without alcohol ingestion
Floor of mouth, buccal mucosa	Tobacco chewing
Oral cavity	Betel nut with or without tobacco chewing
Anterior tongue	Poor dentition
Lip	Sunlight
Hypopharynx	Plummer–Vinson syndrome
Nasal cavity and sinuses	Nickel refining, woodworking, leather working, radium-dial painting, chemical and petroleum work
Nasopharynx	Epstein–Barr virus (?); genetic

nasal cavity and sinus carcinomas has been reported in various industrial groups, including nickel refiners, radium-dial painters, woodworkers, and leather manufacturers. Increases in incidence have also been noted in chemical and petroleum industry workers (Fraumeni, 1975). There is a high frequency of antibodies to Epstein–Barr virus antigen in nasopharyngeal cancer and in Burkitt's lymphoma in Africa, but the etiological role of the virus has not been proved (de-Thé and Geser, 1974). Nasopharyngeal cancer is particularly common in Cantonese men, and this has been related to genetic and environmental factors. Alaskan natives are also at high risk for this tumor.

Most cancers of the head and neck occur predominantly after age 50, but nasopharyngeal cancers have a peak incidence in the fifth decade. For most sites, the age-specific incidence increases progressively from the fifth to the eighth decade, undoubtedly reflecting additive carcinogenic insults. Head and neck cancers also occur in children in a variety of cell types other than squamous cell carcinoma, which is the major type in adults.

IV. HISTOPATHOLOGY AND SPREAD

Most head and neck cancers are squamous cell carinomas that arise from the epithelium lining the upper aerodigestive tract. Some tumors of the tongue, tonsil, nasopharynx, and hypopharynx tend to be poorly differentiated. Histopathological characteristics indicative of lack of cellular differentiation, i.e., increased mitotic activity, increased invasiveness, and lack of plasma lymphocytic response have been related to poor prognosis (Lund et al., 1977).

Malignant tumors of the hard palate usually are adenocarcinomas derived from minor salivary glands, but squamous cell carcinomas also occur. Many other histological types of benign and malignant neoplasms, including metastatic carcinomas, occur in the upper aerodigestive tract, but all are less frequent than squamous cell cancers. Most salivary gland tumors are benign and arise in the parotid gland. The mixed tumor, which may contain several epithelial elements and assumes various patterns, is the commonest benign parotid gland tumor. Malignant salivary gland tumors include mucoepidermoid carcinomas, adenoid cystic carcinomas, adenocarcinomas, and other cellular types.

Epidermoid carcinomas of the head and neck tend to remain localized; with progression there is invasion of adjacent structures, metastases through draining lymphatics to proximal and then to remote lymph nodes, and extension intracranially along peripheral branches of cranial nerves. Some tumors spread superficially and are exophytic or verrucous, whereas others invade deeply with little obvious disturbance of the mucous membranes. Ulceration, secondary infection, bleeding, and foul breath are common, and death often results from infection, inanition, aspiration pneumonia, and hemorrhage. Hematogenous metastases primarily involve the lungs, bones, and liver, and usually occur late in the course of the disease. They are observed most frequently with poorly differentiated to anaplastic carcinomas, which commonly arise in the nasopharynx, tongue, tonsil, hypopharynx, and supraglottic larynx. Death from distant metastases has become more common as treatment advances have improved control of primary tumor sites. The more malignant adenocarcinomas of minor and major salivary gland origin, various sarcomas, and lymphomas have a high incidence of hematogenous metastases.

V. CLINICAL MANIFESTATIONS

Although head and neck cancers share many common characteristics, their clinical manifestations differ significantly (del Regato and Spjut, 1977; Mac-Comb and Fletcher, 1967), depending upon the anatomic location of the primary, the growth rate and biological aggressiveness of the tumor, and the extent of the tumor at the time of diagnosis. These factors have considerable interdependence.

A. Oral Cavity

The oral cavity includes the lips, buccal mucosa, lower and upper alveolar ridges, retromolar gingiva, floor of the mouth, hard palate and anterior two-thirds of the tongue. Intraoral cancers often are asymptomatic until they become quite large or have invaded extensively.

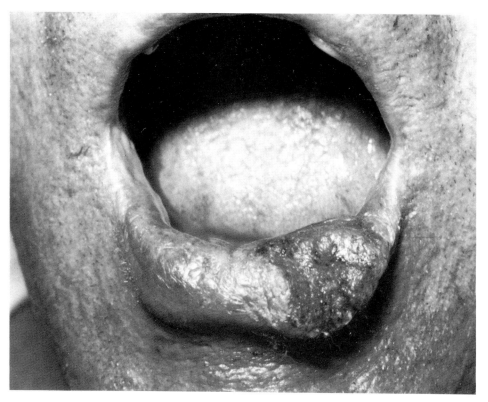

Fig. 3. Cancer of the lower lip.

1. Lip

These cancers may present as a sore that fails to heal, repeatedly ulcerates and crusts over, and gradually increase in size (Fig. 3). The lesion may also assume an exophytic and verrucous form, with enlargement of the involved lip, cracking, and bleeding. Keratinizing tumors often have an associated inflammatory reaction. Spread to submental and submaxillary nodes from either lip and to preauricular and high anterior cervical nodes from the upper lip occur late in the course of lip cancer.

2. Buccal Mucosa

Cancers of this region may become fairly extensive before producing symptoms. In some cases an enlarged submaxillary node may be the first signal of a large intraoral tumor. Leukoplakia is commonly associated with buccal mucosa and other intraoral cancers, and multiple primary lesions are not unusual. Ulcera-

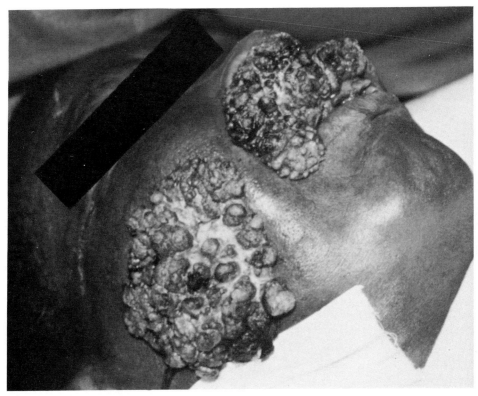

Fig. 4. Cancer of the buccal mucosa with penetration of the cheek.

tive lesions may invade the buccinator muscle and can extend far posteriorly and anteriorly. Pain and bleeding often accompany invasion of the maxilla and the inferior alveolar ridge. Trismus generally is a late symptom and represents muscle invasion. The cheek may become swollen and the tumor can extend through the skin (Fig. 4) and create fistulas. Intraoral exophytic lesions interfere with mastication. Secondary infection is common with ulcerative and exophytic lesions and contributes to the development of inanition. Verrucous carcinomas may be asymptomatic and appear benign until major local advance and tissue destruction have taken place. Infected ulcerative lesions produce a foul breath.

3. Upper and Lower Alveolar Ridge

These cancers, which generally arise in the molar or premolar areas, often are asymptomatic, but may bleed following brushing of the teeth or mastication, or may cause difficulty with dentures bringing them to the attention of a dentist. Upper alveolar ridge cancers may extend into the hard palate, gingivobuccal gutter, and maxillary antrum. Lower ridge lesions may spread to the floor of the mouth and gingivobuccal gutter. Advanced lesions of alveolar bone may cause pain, and there may be unilateral otalgia. The submaxillary nodes are commonly involved in alveolar carcinomas.

4. Retromolar Gingiva

The lesions may cause persistent sore throat and be detected by the patient or on examination by a dentist or physician. These tumors often progress silently until they are large and have spread to the anterior faucial pillar and to the submandibular nodes. They frequently are ulcerative and deeply invasive. With invasion of the mandible they may produce pain, difficulty in chewing, and otalgia.

5. Floor of the Mouth

These cancers may be detected by the patients with their tongues or on self-examination (Fig. 5). Lesions that are large or involve and partially fix the

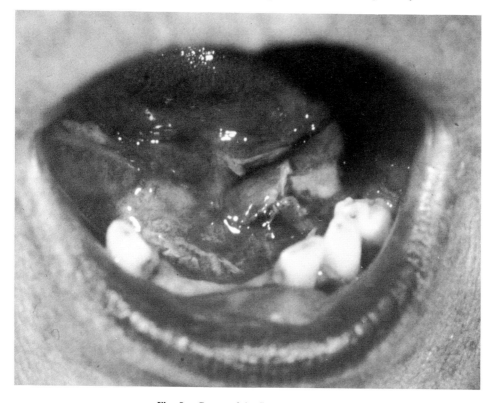

Fig. 5.   Cancer of the floor of the mouth.

tongue may interfere with speech. Bleeding, difficulty with lower dentures, and excessive salivation may also occur. Ulcerated lesions and those involving the mandible may be painful; with infection and necrosis the breath becomes foul. Palpable submandibular adenopathy is frequently present at initial diagnosis. Distant metastases are unusual.

6. Hard Palate

Most tumors of the hard palate are benign and are asymptomatic until large enough to interfere with the passage of food, with speech, or with the fitting of dentures. The malignant minor salivary gland tumors may also evolve slowly and produce late symptoms as above or produce pain and bleeding. Hematogenous metastases to lung, bone, and liver may be present at the time of diagnosis. Local necrosis, ulceration, and infection all contribute to the development of inanition. Squamous cell carcinomas spread to the gums and soft palate and often ulcerate, become infected, and invade bone. Metastases to the upper jugular nodes are present in some cases.

7. Anterior Two-Thirds of Tongue

This is the commonest site of intraoral cancer. Initially, these may be asymptomatic ulcerative or papillary cancers found particularly on the lateral borders adjacent to jagged, carious teeth. Bulky papillary lesions may interfere with speech and mastication, or may bleed easily (Fig. 6). Pain is a common accompaniment of ulceration and infection, and these necrotic infected lesions produce malodorous breath. When the lingual nerve is involved, the patient develops pain referred to the ipsilateral ear via the auriculotemporal branch of the trigeminal nerve. Lateral lesions may spread posteriorly toward the anterior pillar and cause dysphagia. Deep extension toward the floor of the mouth, which often occurs with ventrally located lesions, may limit lingual mobility. Some lesions may cross the midline. Early lymph node invasion occurs in approximately half the patients, with involvement first of the subdigastric nodes in the upper jugular chain. Bilaterally involved nodes are not infrequent. Hematogenous metastases are common late in the course of the disease. However, death most often is related to consequences of the primary lesion.

B. Nasal Cavity

Tumors of this site are uncommon. Squamous cell carcinoma is the most frequent of the malignant tumors. Adenocarcinoma, salivary gland tumors, sarcomas, melanomas, lymphomas, plasmacytomas, and various benign lesions may originate in this site. Nasal obstruction, discharge, and bleeding are common complaints. Tumors that arise in the middle and lower turbinates may produce unilateral swelling of the nose. Unremitting headache and symptoms of sinusitis may result from obstruction of the ostia of the maxillary, frontal, and

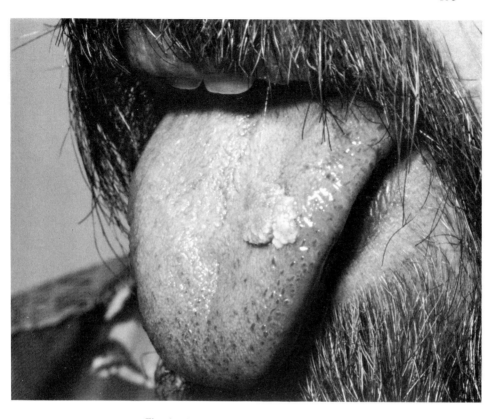

Fig. 6. Papillary cancer of the anterior tongue.

ethmoid sinuses, which may be secondarily infected. Pain may also result from bone destruction and invasion of the sinuses and cranial cavity. Patients may also complain of pain in the upper teeth. Swelling near the inner canthus, displacement of the eye, and frontal headache are late symptoms of tumors arising near the anterior ethmoids. Persistent lacrimation will result from obstruction of the lacrimal duct. Occasionally, the nasal septum may be destroyed. Death generally results from local progression of disease.

C. Paranasal Sinuses

The early symptoms of *frontal sinus cancer* simulate persistent frontal sinusitis because of obstruction and secondary infection. With disease progression there may be unilateral swelling over the sinus, with destruction of the anterior wall and displacement of the eye downward and laterally. The skin may ulcerate. The tumor may extend posteriorly into the anterior fossa.

Ethmoid sinus carcinomas are characterized by epistaxis and unilateral nasal

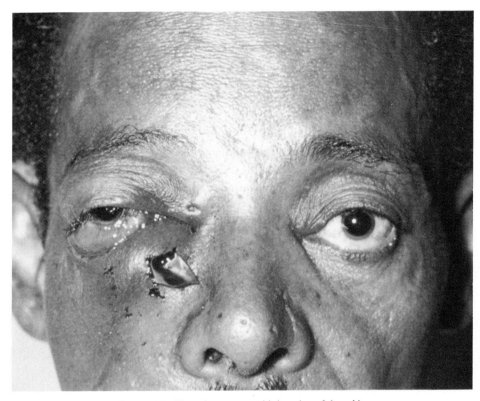

Fig. 7. Maxillary sinus cancer with invasion of the orbit.

discharge, pain, swelling, and ulceration near the inner canthus, destruction of the septum, and flattening of the bridge of the nose. The eye is displaced laterally. Excessive lacrimation occurs if the lacrimal duct is blocked. The tumor may invade the dura in the anterior fossa through the cribriform plate and along the olfactory nerves.

Sphenoidal sinus cancers produce deep retro-orbital or occipital pain and may invade the nasal cavity, nasopharynx, sella, and middle fossa. Fortunately, frontal and sphenoidal sinus carcinomas are rare.

Maxillary sinus carcinoma is the commonest of the paranasal sinus cancers. Symptoms are related to the location of the tumor within the sinus. Inferiorly located lesions produce pain in the upper molars and loosening of the teeth due to alveolar destruction. Involvement of the gums and hard palate may interfere with the fit of dentures. There may be deep pain and trismus, unilateral numbness of the tongue, and otalgia. The middle cranial fossa may be invaded via the fifth cranial nerve. Anterior and lateral wall lesions present with facial pain and swelling. Lesions that extend medially produce nasal obstruction. Superiorly located lesions usually cause epistaxis and malar swelling. The tumor may extend through the orbit and cause diplopia—due to displacement of the eye upward and laterally (Fig. 7)—infraorbital pain, and sensory loss in the cheek and upper lip. Obstruction of the lacrimal duct will produce excessive lacrimation. The tumor may enter the middle cranial fossa through the foramen rotundum, and foramen lacerum, and via perineural extension along branches of the fifth and seventh nerves. Hemianesthesia of the palate may occur. Palpable cervical node metastases, usually to high jugular nodes, are uncommon and occur late with sinus carcinomas. Hematogenous metastases are unusual.

D. Nasopharynx

The commonest presentation of these cancers is cervical lymphadenopathy. A deep node under the upper posterior aspect of the sternocleidomastoid muscle is most characteristically palpable, and there is frequent involvement of the spinal accessory, posterior triangle, mid- and lower jugular, and supraclavicular nodes. Bilateral cervical adenopathy is common. Unilateral symptoms of diminished hearing, a sense of fullness in the ear, or chronic earache may result from obstruction of the eustachian orifice. A serious otitis may be noted. Nasal quality of speech and nasal obstruction occur frequently. Invasion of the base of the skull results in cranial nerve involvement and lateral rectus paralysis, ophthalmoplegia, and blindness, or pain in the distribution of the sensory divisions of the fifth nerve may develop. With extension to the retroparotid space, the tumor may involve the cervical sympathetic nerve and the last four cranial nerves, producing difficulty in swallowing, partial loss of taste, Horner's syndrome, hoarseness, and unilateral paralysis of the trapezius and sternomastoid muscles or the tongue. Death results from progressive local and intracerebral disease or hematogenous metastases to lungs, liver, and bones, which are common.

E. Oropharynx

The major subdivisions of the oropharynx are the palatal arch, including the soft palate and posterior tonsillar pillar, the tonsillar fossa and tonsil, the base of the tongue including the glossoepiglottic and pharyngoepiglottic folds, and the pharyngeal wall, including lateral and posterior walls and posterior tonsillar pillar. The symptoms of oropharyngeal cancer are rather similar, differing primarily at each site in the time of onset relative to the extent of disease and in severity.

1. Palatal Arch and Soft Palate

Local pain and odynophagia occur early, dysphagia is a common complaint, and trismus may develop with extension of cancer into the pterygoid fossa. The high jugular nodes are often involved at presentation and may be bilateral.

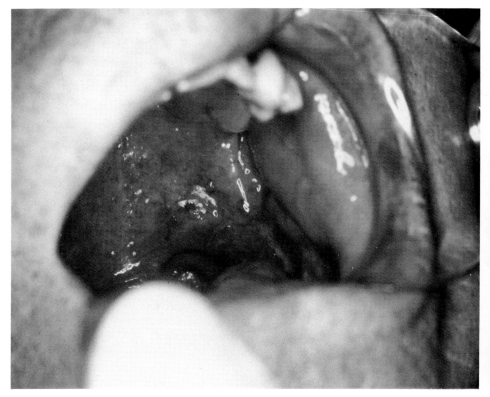

Fig. 8.   Cancer of the left tonsil with extension to the palate.

2. Tonsil

These squamous cell cancers often are asymptomatic, or produce a slight sore throat until they become rather large (Fig. 8). Tonsillar cancers may extend to the soft palate. Extensive tumors may produce unilateral otalgia and dysphagia. High jugular node involvement is common at presentation, and distant metastases are rare except in undifferentiated carcinomas. The undifferentiated tumors produce little local symptomatology, but early cervical node metastases and metastases to the lungs, liver, and bones are common.

3. Base of Tongue

These cancers infiltrate deeply into the tongue and produce pain that becomes severe early in their course. Odynophagia, unilateral otalgia, and dysphagia are common; speech may become nasal in quality, and the patient may have difficulty in protruding the tongue. Pain, hemorrhage, malnutrition, and aspiration are frequent problems. The upper jugular nodes are frequently involved on presentation. The poorly differentiated squamous carcinomas have a high tendency to metastasize hematogenously. Periepiglottic tumors have minimal early symptomatology and frequently are recognized after metastases to mid-jugular and other cervical nodes. With disease progression, patients may complain of odynophagia, unilateral otalgia, dysphagia, cough, and hoarseness; aspiration is a frequent problem.

4. Pharyngeal Walls

Cancers of the lateral and posterior pharyngeal wall (Fig. 9) usually are quite extensive before becoming symptomatic and may present with mid-jugular adenopathy. Spread to the hypopharynx is common, and invasion of the thyroid cartilage may be noted. Dysphagia, otalgia, and painful swallowing are late symptoms. Progressive extension of disease locally may result in exsanguination from penetration of the internal carotid artery.

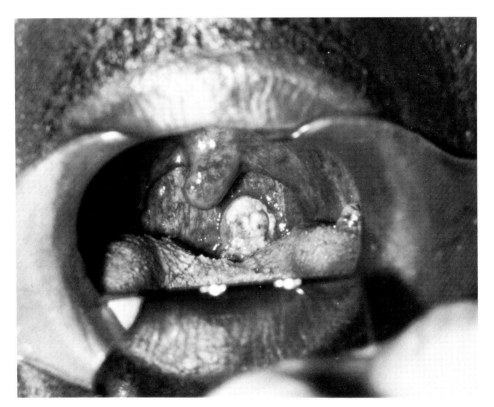

Fig. 9. Cancer of the posterior pharyngeal wall.

F. Hypopharynx

The pyriform sinus, postcricoid area, and posterior pharyngeal wall comprise the hypopharynx. Most of the malignant tumors in this site arise in the pyriform sinus. The evolution of carcinomas of the hypopharynx often is insidious. These squamous carcinomas tend to be less well differentiated. Odynophagia is the most frequent early symptom. Dysphagia becomes severe as the tumors enlarge or infiltrate the hypopharyngeal and esophageal tissues. Unilateral otalgia is common due to the involvement of the glossopharyngeal nerve. Hoarseness results from extension into or edema of the larynx. Pyriform sinus carcinomas invade the thyroid cartilage and produce neck pain and swelling. Mid-jugular adenopathy is common, and may be the presenting sign. Hematogenous metastases are not unusual in patients with controlled primary lesions. Death may result from aspiration, pneumonia, cachexia, or internal carotid artery hemorrhage.

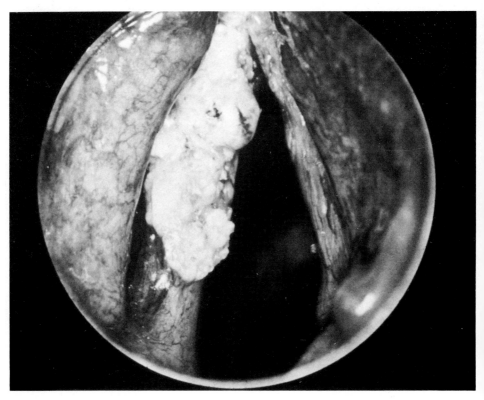

Fig. 10. Mirror view of cancer of the right true vocal cord.

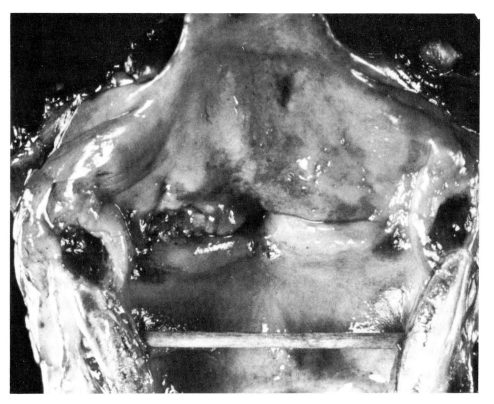

Fig. 11. Posterior view of cancer of the left supraglottis.

G. Larynx

There are three major subdivisions of the larynx: supraglottic, glottic, and subglottic. Glottic cancers (true vocal cord) are the most frequent (Fig. 10). The most common presenting symptom is hoarseness. Initially this may be intermittent, particularly in supraglottic lesions involving the false cords, but it becomes persistent. Hyperplasias and other benign lesions of the glottis may also produce persistent hoarseness; these must be distinguished histopathologically. Cancers of the supraglottis (Fig. 11) may present with continued soreness in the throat, whereas unilateral otalgia can be the first symptom of cancers of the subglottis. These tumors spread primarily by local extension (i.e., spread to both vocal cords, fixation of the arytenoids), and may produce destruction of surrounding cartilage and airway obstruction.

H. Salivary Glands

Malignant salivary gland tumors are characterized by rapidly progressive painful swelling in either the parotid or submaxillary glands, enlargement of adjacent lymph nodes, and early hematogenous metastases to lungs, liver, and bones. Parotid lesions frequently produce peripheral seventh-nerve paralysis and pain in the preauricular region or the angle of the mandible. With invasion of the retroparotid space, palsies of the ninth to twelfth cranial nerves become evident. Adenocarcinomas of the submaxillary glands may evoke severe mandibular pain.

VI. DIAGNOSIS

Head and neck cancers may be discovered in routine dental or medical examinations of asymptomatic individuals. The patient may notice the lesion or lymph nodes on self-examination and seek medical attention, or have dental or denture difficulty and visit the dentist. Most frequently, persistent symptomatology will cause the patient to visit a physician or dentist. In all of these circumstances the diagnosis is likely to be rendered if (1) the physician or dentist is familiar with the natural history and the characteristic gross appearances of these tumors; (2) there is a high suspicion of head and neck cancers in abusers of tobacco and alcohol; and (3) an effort is made to explain persistent symptoms described in the previous sections. The diagnosis must be established by biopsy of the primary site and histopathological confirmation. However, it is essential that a physician skilled in the diagnosis and management of head and neck cancer by consulted when the diagnosis is suspected in order to obtain a thorough examination of the upper airways and digestive system, take appropriate biopsies, and establish the extent of the disease. A team approach will be required from the outset to conduct and interpret a complete diagnostic evaluation and to plan and effect primary therapy, rehabilitation, follow-up, and further therapeutic measures. As a minimum, the team should consist of the primary physician, a surgeon specialist in head and neck cancer, a pathologist, a diagnostic radiologist, a radiotherapist, and a medical oncologist. Other specialists may be required in planning treatment and rehabilitation. In addition, most patients require considerable psychosocial support.

VII. CLINICAL STAGING

When the primary site of a head and neck cancer has been histopathologically confirmed, the extent of disease must be determined (clinical staging). Accurate clinical staging is critical for the development of a treatment plan. There is reasonably good correlation for several sites between stage of disease and prognosis. A widely used system is that developed by the American Joint Committee for Cancer Staging and End Results Reporting (1976), which provides definitions of the extent of primary tumor at each site (T), degree of nodal involvement (N), and presence or absence of distant metastasis (M). The TNM characteristics are then used to define stages I–IV at each site. All patients with distant metastases are classified as stage IV. While staging is extremely useful, other factors such as tumor differentiation, coexistent illnesses, and nutritional status influence prognosis and therapy.

VIII. MANAGEMENT

After a pathological diagnosis has been made, the management of head and neck tumors is predominantly determined by the location of the primary lesion, the histological classification, and the clinical stage. This information is required to establish whether the objective of therapy will be curative or palliative. Other factors to be considered include the presence or absence of significant medical problems such as cardiac or pulmonary diseases, age, nutritional status, and the socioeconomic situation. The patient and his family must have a reasonable understanding of the usual beneficial and adverse consequences of therapeutic alternatives, including symptomatic support only, and of available reconstructive and rehabilitative modalities. The informed patient must be a participant in the treatment program that is selected.

The primary treatment modalities for head and neck cancer are radiation therapy and surgery. Surgical treatment directed at cure is designed to remove completely the primary tumor and involved nodes, with preservation of physiological functions and avoidance of extreme physical and cosmetic defects, unless the latter can be corrected by subsequent reconstructive surgery. A radical neck dissection may be performed in patients with clinically involved cervical nodes at diagnosis, in those whose primary tumor can be controlled by surgery or radiation therapy, or in those patients whose primary tumor has been controlled but who subsequently develop cervical node metastases. This procedure involves unilateral *en bloc* removal of all the lymph nodes and lymphatics of the anterior and lateral neck, the sternohyoid and omohyoid muscles, the internal jugular vein, and the submaxillary gland. In the event that a curative surgical attempt is not feasible or that there has been postoperative recurrence, consideration may be given to palliative surgery for problems of airway or digestive tract obstruction, pain, bleeding, or infected and necrotic lesions.

Radiation therapy is usually delivered by high energy sources (^{60}Co, linear accelerators, betatrons), but interstitial treatment may also be employed. Treatment with radiation alone may be curative in some circumstances and may avoid creation of functional or cosmetic deficits. It is more effective than surgery for nasopharyngeal cancers. Also, it can be utilized if the patient cannot tolerate or refuses surgery. Radiotherapy is often given postoperatively as an adjuvant to surgical therapy. Preoperative radiotherapy may convert some lesions considered "inoperable" to "operable." However, preoperative radiotherapy is generally not administered routinely to patients with operable disease, and the value of this approach is uncertain and is the subject of investigation. Palliative radiotherapy is quite useful for many incurable primary lesions and for recurrent cancers, to reduce tumor bulk and relieve symptoms.

Chemotherapeutic agents have had extensive trial in patients with head and neck cancer. Table II lists several drugs that have been found to have activity in patients with advanced and recurrent lesions. The observed responses usually are partial, though occasionally complete, and often are accompanied by subjective improvement and weight gain. Response rates tend to be higher in patients who have not previously received surgery and radiation therapy. As indicated in the Table, the duration of response tends to be short. Methotrexate has had the most extensive clinical trials, and various routes, schedules, and techniques of therapy have been explored in an effort to improve its efficacy. High-dose methotrexate with leucovorin rescue has been said to be more effective and less toxic than intermittent intravenous therapy with conventional doses. A controlled comparison of these programs was unable to establish this contention (De Conti, 1976). A study in our patients has shown that an induction course of methotrexate followed by weekly maintenance therapy results in continued suppression of immunocompetence, but that treatment at 3-week intervals permits intermittent recovery of immunity. A program of three successive daily intramuscular injections of methotrexate at 3-week intervals has been studied in the Southwest Oncology Group and has resulted in median survivals of approximately 1 year in responding patients, a significant improvement in duration of response.

Mucositis as well as oral and gastrointestinal ulcerations can be caused by methotrexate, bleomycin, fluorouracil, and Adriamycin. Doses of these drugs must be reduced or carefully scheduled when they are used in combination, to prevent augmented mucous membrane toxicities. This is also true if they are

TABLE II

Single-Agent Therapy in Advanced Head and Neck Cancer

Drug	Response rate (%)	Duration (months)
Methotrexate	35–55	3–4
Hydroxyurea	10–25	3
Fluorouracil	10–15	3
Bleomycin	15–20	2–3
cis-Platinum	35–40	3

given concomitantly with radiation therapy. Methotrexate and *cis*-platinum require adequate renal function for their excretion and can impair renal function. Such impairment can increase the systemic toxic effects of the drugs, so that careful scheduling and attention to renal function and drug dosage is mandated when they are given in combination.

A pressing need exists to improve the treatment of head and neck cancer. There is a significant failure rate for stage III and IV lesions of all sites. Although the results are generally good for stage I and II disease, they certainly could be improved. Ideally, it would be desirable to cure these patients without any disfiguring procedures. Although relatively standard practices for radiation therapy have been evolved for head and neck cancer of various stages and sites, research is in progress on techniques of dose fractionation, high linear energy transfer radiations (neutrons, pi-mesons), radiation sensitizers such as metronidazole, simultaneous chemotherapy and radiotherapy, and hyperbaric oxygenation during radiotherapy. These approaches are directed at increasing the response of hypoxic tumor cells to radiation.

Local and systemic hyperthermia are also being examined. Various sequences of chemotherapy, radiation therapy, and surgery are under investigation (Goldberg *et al.*, 1977; Taylor *et al.*, 1977). Chemotherapy is being evaluated as a primary modality to improve operability of advanced lesions, and postoperatively as an adjuvant to prevent local or systemic recurrence. As local therapy has improved and resulted in a higher percentage of patients with controlled primary disease, the percentage of deaths from distant metastases has increased. Thus, the need for effective adjuvant therapy is highlighted. Immunotherapy is also being evaluated as an adjunctive form of treatment. Hyperalimentation and other supportive measures are being used to improve the ability of patients to tolerate surgery, radiation, and chemotherapy, and to improve their immunocompetence. Research on new reconstructive techniques and the development of better prosthetic materials and devices are required to improve post-treatment function and cosmesis.

IX. CONCLUSIONS

There has been progress made in the management of head and neck cancer. Considerable effort should be expended to educate the public to avoid excessive exposure to factors associated with high incidences of these cancers, such as tobacco, alcohol, industrial carcinogens, and sunlight, since most of these tumors could be prevented. Careful attention to early symptoms, detailed physical examination, and the use of modern diagnostic techniques will improve recognition of early stages of these neoplasms, which are amenable to curative therapy. Ongoing research in prevention, diagnosis, staging, surgery, radiotherapy, chemotherapy, immunotherapy, nutrition, and rehabilitation may be expected to have a beneficial impact on this important group of cancers in the future.

ACKNOWLEDGEMENT

The author expresses his appreciation to Dr. Roy B. Sessions and Dr. Melvin Spira for providing several of the clinical photographs shown in this chapter.

REFERENCES

American Joint Committee for Cancer Staging and End Results Reporting (1976). "Staging of Cancer at Head and Neck Sites," Manual, Chapter 8. AJCC, Chicago, Illinois.

Axtell, L. M., Cutler, S. J., and Myers, M. H. (1972). End Results in Cancer. Report No. 4. National Cancer Institute. p. 5. Bethesda, Md.

de-Thé, G., and Geser, A. (1974). *Cancer Res.* **34**, 1196.

De Conti, R. C. (1976). *Proc. Amr. Assoc. Cancer Res. Am. Soc. Clin. Oncol.* **17**, 248.

del Regato, J. A., and Spjut, H. J. (1977). "Cancer." Mosby, St. Louis, Missouri.

Fraumeni, J. F., Jr. (1975). *J. Natl. Cancer Inst.* **55**, 1039–1046.

Goldberg, N. H., Chrétien, P. B., Elias, E. G., Hande, K. R., Chabner, B. A., and Myers, C. E. (1977). *Proc. Am. Assoc. Cancer Res. Am. Soc. Clin. Oncol.* **18**, 292.

Khanolkar, V. R. (1959). *Acta Unio. Int. Contra Cancrum* **15**, 66–77.

Lund, C., Sogaard, H., Jorgensen, K., Elbrond, O., Hjelm-Hansen, M., and Andersen, P. (1977). *Dan. Med. Bull.* **24**, 162–168.

MacComb, W. S., and Fletcher, G. H. (1967). "Cancer of the Head and Neck." Williams & Wilkins, Baltimore, Maryland.

McCoy, D. G. (1978). *Laryngoscope* **1**, Pt. 2, Suppl. 8, 59.

Rothman, K. J., and Keller, A. Z. (1972). *J. Chronic Dis.* **25**, 711–716.

Taylor, S. G., IV, Bytell, D. E., and Sisson, G. A. (1977). *Proc. Am. Assoc. Cancer Res. Am. Soc. Clin. Oncol.* **18**, 346.

Wynder, E. L., Bross, I. J., and Feldman, R. (1957). *Cancer* **10**, 1300–1323.

9
CARCINOMA OF THE LUNG
Robert L. Comis

I.	Introduction	147
II.	Classification	147
III.	Evaluation of Lung Cancer	150
IV.	Management of Non-Small-Cell Anaplastic Cancer	153
	A. Localized Disease	153
	B. Combined Modality Approaches for Potentially Curable Disease	155
V.	Management of Metastatic Non-Small-Cell Anaplastic Lung Cancer	156
VI.	Evaluation and Management of Small-Cell Anaplastic Carcinoma	158
	A. Evaluation	159
	B. Management	159
VII.	Conclusion	163
	References	163

I. INTRODUCTION

Lung cancer is the most common cause of cancer death in the United States and in many other industrialized nations in the world. Overall 5-year survival rates have ranged between 5–7% for the past 30 years, and unless early detection methods become available, or cigarette smoking ceases, death from lung cancer will continue to be a paramount problem.

II. CLASSIFICATION

The four major histological types of lung cancer, their approximate proportions, and yearly incidences are listed in Table I (Silverberg, 1979). The Working Party for Lung Cancer (WPL) and World Health Organization (WHO) histological classifications are presented in Table II. Both epidermoid and small cell anaplastic carcinoma are strikingly related to cigarette smoking, with the relative

TABLE I

Incidence of Lung Cancer by Cell Type

Cell type	Approximate (%)	Approximate yearly cases (1979)
Epidermoid	40	45,000
Large cell anaplastic	22	24,600
Small cell anaplastic	18	20,000
Adenocarcinoma	10	12,000
Bronchioloalveolar	4	4,500

risk of developing these cell types being 25 and 20 times greater than in the nonsmoking population, respectively. The relationship between cigarette smoking and large cell anaplastic carcinoma is intermediate, and adenocarcinoma has a definite but relatively small association with cigarette smoking—i.e., males, 3.0 and females, 1.3 times the nonsmoking population (Harris, 1973).

For cell types other than small cell anaplastic carcinoma, there is a relationship between clinical stage at the time of diagnosis and survival. The classification

TABLE II

Comparison of the WHO and WPL Classifications

WHO classification	WPL classification
I. Epidermoid carcinoma	10. Epidermoid carcinoma
	11. Well differentiated
	12. Moderately differentiated
	13. Poorly differentiated
II. Small cell anaplastic carcinoma	20. Small cell anaplastic carcinoma
1. Fusiform	21. Lymphocyte-like (oat cell)
2. Polygonal	22. Intermediate cell (fusiform,
3. Lymphocyte-like	polygonal, others)
4. Others	
III. Adenocarcinoma	30. Adenocarcinoma
1. Bronchogenic	31. Well differentiated
a. Acinar	32. Moderately differentiated
b. Papillary	33. Poorly differentiated
2. Bronchioloalveolar	34. Bronchioloalveolar/papillary
IV. Large cell carcinoma	40. Large cell carcinoma
1. Solid tumors with mucin	(40/30) with mucin production
2. Solid tumors without mucin	(40/10) with stratification
3. Giant cell	41. Giant cell
4. Clear cell	42. Clear cell

TABLE III

TNM Classification for Lung Cancer American Joint Committee for Staging

T = Primary tumors

T0	No evidence of primary tumor
TX	Tumor proved by the presence of malignant cells in bronchopulmonary secretions but not visualized roentgenographically or bronchoscopically
T1	Tumor 3 cm or less in greatest diameter, surrounded by lung or visceral pleura and without evidence of invasion proximal to a lobar bronchus at bronchoscopy
T2	Tumor more than 3 cm in greatest diameter, or a tumor of any size which, with its associated atelectasis or obstructive pneumonitis, extends to the hilar region. At bronchoscopy the proximal extent of demonstrable tumor must be at least 2 cm distal to the carina. Any associated atelectasis or obstructive pneumonitis must involve less than an entire lung, and there must be no pleural effusion
T3	Tumor any size with direct extension into an adjacent structure such as the chest wall, the diaphragm, or the mediastinum and its contents; or demonstrable bronchoscopically to be less than 2 cm distal to the carina; any tumor associated with atelectasis or obstructive pneumonitis of an entire lung or pleural effusion

N = Regional lymph nodes

N0	Demonstrable metastasis to regional lymph nodes
N1	Metastasis to lymph nodes in the ipsilateral hilar region (including direct extension)
N2	Metastasis to lymph nodes in the mediastinum

M = Distant metastasis

M0	No distant metastasis
M1	Distant metastasis such as in scalene, cervical, or contralateral hilar lymph nodes, brain, bones, lung, liver, etc.

and staging established by the American Joint Committee for Staging and reviewed by Mountain (1976) are presented in Tables III and IV. The approximate median and 5-year survival rates for localized or regionally spread lung cancer, excluding small cell anaplastic, are presented in Table V. For T1 and T2 disease independent of nodal status, epidermoid carcinoma is associated with a longer median and higher 5-year survival rate than adenocarcinoma or large cell anaplastic cancer. The same median and 5-year survival advantage for epidermoid carcinoma also exists for N0 and N1 disease independent of T status. No apparent relationship was noted between the proposed staging system and survival in patients with small cell anaplastic carcinoma.

Performance status is another factor that appears particularly significant in determining survival in lung cancer patients with metastatic or advanced localized or regional disease. Survival may increase 100–200% within cell types and stage, when patients who are initially nonambulatory are compared to those who are ambulatory (Zelen, 1973).

TABLE IV

Lung Cancer, American Joint Committee Staging Classification

Stage	TNM
0 (Occult carcinoma)	TX N0 M0
I	T1 N0 M0
	T1 N1 M0
	T2 N0 M0
II	T2 N1 M0
III	T3 with any N or M
	N2 with any T or M
	M1 with any T or N

III. EVALUATION OF LUNG CANCER

The presenting signs and symptoms of lung cancer differ according to cell type (Table VI). Small cell anaplastic carcinoma and adenocarcinoma both have a propensity for early dissemination, whereas epidermoid carcinoma, in particular, and large cell anaplastic cancer, to a lesser degree, present with local symptoms and signs (Cohen, 1974).

Most patients with lung cancer are diagnosed because of the presence of signs, symptoms, and an abnormal chest X ray that suggest malignancy. In addition to different presenting signs and symptoms, different cell types tend to present with different radiological patterns. In general, epidermoid carcinoma and small cell anaplastic cancer tend to present as central lesions on X ray, whereas adenocarcinoma and large cell anaplastic cancers present as peripheral lesions in 50–70% of cases.

TABLE V

Approximate Median and 5-Year Survival for Localized and/or Regional Lung Cancer[a]

Stage	TNM	Survival	
		Median (months)	Five-year (%)
I	All	22	38
	T1 N0 M0	32	40
	T2 N0 M0	20	34
	T1 N1 M0	18	34
II	T2 N1 M0	10	10
III	Any T, N	—	10
	T3 N0 M0	12	16
	T3 N1 M0	8	8

[a] Excluding small cell anaplastic carcinoma.

TABLE VI

Origin of Symptoms and Signs in Patients with Bronchogenic Cancer[a]

Cell type	Primary tumor	Intrathoracic spread	Distant metastases
Epidermoid	* * *	* *	*
Large cell anaplastic	* * *	* *	* *
Small cell anaplastic	* *	* *	* * *
Adenocarcinoma	*	*	* * *

[a] * = occasionally; ** = frequently; *** = very frequently.

A microscopic diagnosis of carcinoma of the lung can be made from samples obtained from a cytology examination of sputum or from tissue specimens obtained by bronchoscopic biopsy. The latter is more reliable in evaluating cell type. The yield of positive sputum cytologies increases asymptotically from 40% to approximately 90% of histologically confirmed cases as the number of early-morning deep-cough specimens increases from one to five consecutive daily collections (Erozan and Frost, 1970). In the hands of an experienced cytopathologist, a cytopathological diagnosis of malignancy is rarely incorrect (≤ 1% false-positive rate). On the other hand, the accuracy with which a specific cytological cell-type diagnosis correlates with the ultimate histological diagnosis varies with the degree of differentiation of the tumor. The cytological diagnosis of well-differentiated squamous cell carcinoma is correct about 95% of the time. Small cell anaplastic carcinoma is correctly diagnosed by sputum cytology in 75-90% of cases. When poorly differentiated tumors are diagnosed cytologically, including adenocarcinoma and squamous cell carcinoma, the correlation with histological findings is correct in only 20-25% of cases (Lukeman, 1973).

Mediastinoscopy is an important procedure in determining the potential for curative resection (Goldberg et al., 1974). It is generally accepted that contralateral mediastinal nodal involvement or high ipsilateral mediastinal nodal involvement (N2 disease) contraindicates radical surgery. The incidence of positive mediastinal node disease at mediastinoscopy and the character of spread differ according to histological type (Table VII).

The majority of lung cancer patients present with advanced localized, regional, and/or metastatic disease. Autopsy data from Matthews (1974) confirm a relatively high incidence of "early" metastatic spread, even in patients who appear to have had resectable disease (Table VIII). Twenty-four percent of patients dying from postoperative complications within 1 month after a "curative resection" were shown to have distant metastases. The presence of persistent or disseminated disease varied with cell type. Forty percent of patients with adenocarcinoma had distant disease, whereas 14 and 17% of patients with large

TABLE VII

Lung Carcinoma: Mediastinal Spread

Pathology	Number of patients	Mediastinoscopy			
		Positive	Ipsilateral	Contralateral	Bilateral
All cell types	179	86 (48%)	35 (41%)	8 (9%)	43 (50%)
Squamous cell	64	10 (16%)	7 (70%)	2 (20%)	1 (10%)
Large cell	74	47 (68%)	17 (36%)	6 (13%)	24 (51%)
Small cell	23	17 (70%)	5 (30%)	—	12 (51%)
Adenocarcinoma	18	12 (66%)	6 (50%)	—	6 (50%)

TABLE VIII

Autopsy Findings in Patients Dying within One Month of "Curative" Resection

Cell type	Number of patients	Number with persistent disease	Number with distant metastases
Epidermoid	131	44 (33%)	22 (17%)
Small cell	19	13 (70%)	12 (63%)
Adenocarcinoma	30	13 (43%)	12 (40%)
Large cell	22	3 (17%)	3 (14%)
Total	202	73 (35%)	49 (24%)

TABLE IX

Preferred Metastatic Sites of Lung Cancer by Cell Type Autopsy Data

Site	Cell type (% involvement)			
	Epidermoid	Adenocarcinoma	Large cell	Small cell
Liver	25	41	48	74
Bone	20	36	30	37
CNS	—	37	25	29
Adrenals	23	50	59	55

cell anaplastic and epidermoid cancer, respectively, had demonstrable metastases outside the chest. Over 30% of patients with distant disease had liver metastases.

Matthews (1976) has also cited autopsy data indicating the propensity of poorly differentiated tumors (epidermoid and adenocarcinoma) to spread more widely than more differentiated tumors. This prediliction for metastases is particularly striking for epidermoid carcinoma, where 52% of patients with well- or moderately differentiated tumors had disease limited to the thorax, whereas no patient with poorly differentiated cancer had disease confined to the chest. The preferred sites of metastases of the various cell types at autopsy are presented in Table IX. Although these are autopsy data, it can be seen that three of the four preferred sites—i.e., liver, bone, and brain—could conceivably be accurately assessed preoperatively by currently available noninvasive radiological and radionuclide techniques.

IV. MANAGEMENT OF NON-SMALL CELL ANAPLASTIC CANCER

A. Localized Disease

A flow diagram of a theoretical group of 100 lung cancer patients is presented in Fig. 1. The data are presented in this fashion to illustrate that the minority of all patients diagnosed as having lung cancer fall into a potentially curative category. Only about 7% of all patients will survive 5 years, free of disease.

Approximately 20–30% of all patients with lung cancer are candidates for a potentially curative resection. Presently, surgery is the only modality with well-

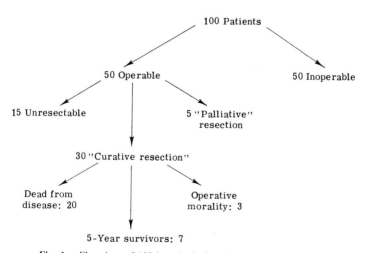

Fig. 1. Flowchart of 100 hypothetical patients with lung cancer.

documented curvative potential for stage I and II lung cancer. There is general agreement that patients with stage I and II disease should receive an appropriate pulmonary resection, either lobectomy or pneumonectomy. To evaluate the stage of disease appropriately, patients must have had bronchoscopy and mediastino-scopy prior to surgery. Adjunctive studies to evaluate the patient for metiastatic disease should be performed before radical surgery, particularly in patients with poorly differentiated tumors. Finally, the patient must have adequate pulmonary reserve to tolerate a pulmonary resection. Table X shows a proposed pretreat-ment evaluation with the accompanying theoretical data derived from these studies which relate to the ''absolute'' or ''relative'' contraindications to surgery. It must be recognized that such criteria are subject to variations within institutions and among individual surgeons. The operative mortality in properly selected cases ranges from 5 to 10% at most major institutions.

The 5-year survival after a curative resection for all stages of non-small cell anaplastic lung cancer is approximately 20–30%. Expectedly, there is a dif-ference within cell types and within stage. Surgical results adapted from data presented by Mountain (1977; Mountain et al., 1974) are shown in Table XI. Even in these highly selected cases, 50–90% of patients resected for cure die with recurrent or disseminated disease.

Radical radiotherapy is not an adequate alternative to radical surgery as a ''curative'' approach to stage I and II lung cancer. A randomized study by Morrison et al. (1963) compared radical surgery to supervoltage radiotherapy (4500 rads in 4 weeks) as the primary treatment for potentially resectable lung

TABLE X

Steps in Evaluating Patient for "Curative Surgery"

Evaluation method	Unresectability	
	Relative	Absolute
Bronchoscopy	Lesion ≤ 2 cm from tracheal bifurcation	Disease in carina small cell carcinoma
Mediastinoscopy	High ipsilateral mediastinal nodes	Contralateral tracheal nodes
Metastatic evaluation (all poorly differentiated tumors)	—	Positive
Medical evaluation		
FEV_1[a] or FVC[b]	—	<1 liter
Maximum breathing capacity	—	<40%
Pa_{CO_2}	—	>40 mm Hg

[a] Forced expiratory volume in 1 sec.
[b] Forced vital capacity.

TABLE XI

"Curative" Resection: Approximate 5-Year Survival (Percentage)
by Cell Type and Stage

	Stage		
Cell type	I	II	III
Epidermoid	47	32	13
Adenocarcinoma	50	15	2
Large cell	36	19	11

cancer. The 4-year survival rate was 30% and 6% for surgery and radiotherapy, respectively. Radiotherapy should be considered in cases in which nonpulmonary medical complications contraindicate surgery. Radical radiation therapy (5000–6000 rads in 5–6 weeks) causes a severe radiation pneumonitis, resulting in a functional pneumonectomy. Therefore, the pulmonary medical contraindications to radical surgery hold for radical radiation therapy with curative intent.

It is generally accepted that radiotherapy is the modality of choice for advanced lung cancer localized to the chest or ipsilateral supraclavicular nodes. The 5-year survival rate for patients with advanced unresectable, clinically localized lung cancer ranges from 3 to 6% in most series (Lee, 1974). Roswit et al. (1968), in a randomized, controlled study, showed no significant survival gain for a group of patients receiving radiotherapy when compared to a control group treated with supportive care only. This study is generally challenged because of the relatively low dose of radiation employed. The fact remains, though, that in the only well-controlled study available there was no difference in survival for treated or untreated groups.

B. Combined Modality Approaches for Potentially Curable Disease

To date, there is no conclusive evidence indicating a mean, median, or overall survival advantage for potentially curable patients treated with a combination of pre- or postoperative radiotherapy, chemotherapy plus surgery, or chemotherapy plus radiotherapy. Most (15 of 20) of the reported adjuvant chemotherapy studies have employed low-dose single-agent treatment of relatively short duration (Legha et al., 1977). Most of the studies have not been well designed and have not stratified cases according to cell type or stage. There are several studies in progress employing intensive multiagent chemotherapy as an adjuvant to surgical resection. These studies should establish whether currently available chemotherapeutic programs are capable of significantly altering survival in resectable patients.

A study is in progress employing an intrapleural instillation of BCG (Bacille Calmette-Guérin) postoperatively in patients with resectable lung cancer, stages I–III (McKneally et al., 1976). The rationale for this approach is based upon a reported increase in disease-free survival observed in patients who develop an empyema after surgical resection (Ruckdeschel et al., 1972). The study includes a randomly allocated control group that receives isoniazid alone. Currently, there appears to be a disease-free survival advantage for BCG-treated patients with stage I disease. There appears to be no advantage for patients with stage II or III disease. This appears to be a promising avenue of research, but cannot be considered "standard" therapy at the present time. Another study is being conducted comparing a placebo to intrapleural BCG, with or without levamisole, in resectable lung cancer in an attempt to verify these results.

V. MANAGEMENT OF METASTATIC NON SMALL-CELL ANAPLASTIC LUNG CANCER

Except for moderately to well-differentiated squamous cell carcinoma of the lung, most lung cancers kill as a result of widespread extrathoracic dissemination. The median survival for patients with metastatic epidermoid, large cell, or the adenocarcinomas type of cancer has been reported to be 9.4, 11.1, and 6.9 weeks, respectively, in patients treated with a placebo by the Veterans Administration (V.A.) Lung Group (Zelen, 1973).

Metastatic epidermoid, large cell anaplastic, and adenocarcinomas are among the most chemotherapy-resistant diseases. Recent review articles have cited objective response rates of 20–30% for a variety of drugs, including the alkylating agents, nitrosoureas, and antimetabolites. There is no single agent to date that has been shown to give a consistent objective response rate of greater than 25%. Complete responses are virtually nonexistent. Even high intermittent-dose cyclophosphamide, which is often discussed as being an active single agent, has yielded only a 0–15% objective response rate in recent studies that employ currently accepted criteria of objective response (Livingston, 1977).

The majority of the recent literature on the chemotherapy of non-small cell lung cancer includes the use of aggressive combination chemotherapy. Most of the data arise from single-institution studies. Some studies employing combination chemotherapy have reported 30–45% objective response rates, and a significant survival advantage for responders to combination chemotherapy over those treated with minimally active single agents (Eagan et al., 1977; Brittell et al., 1978; Bitran et al., 1976; Chahinian et al., 1977). A comprehensive analysis of many of these studies has been presented by Livingston (1977). In general, broadening the scope of single-institution studies to include patients from a variety of institutions has failed to document the reported activity. Interpretation

TABLE XII

Prognostic Factors: Non-Small-Cell Anaplastic Lung Cancer

Performance status
Pretreatment weight loss ($\geqslant 6\%$ or $\geqslant 10$ lb)
Disease stage
Cell type
Intact delayed hypersensitivity
Prior therapy
? Sex (female > male)

of most studies is hampered by the use of historical controls and/or the lack of a precise definition of the prognostic variables known to effect response and, most importantly, survival. These factors are presented in Table XII.

A general analysis of several randomized studies comparing single agents, or less intensive combination chemotherapy regimens, to more intensive regimens is presented in Table XIII. Only one study (Hansen *et al.*, 1976) has reported a survival advantage for all patients with metastatic adenocarcinoma treated with intensive combination chemotherapy compared to less intensive therapy. Unfortunately, these data have not been reproduced by others.

TABLE XIII

Randomized Chemotherapy Trials in Non-Small-Cell Anaplastic Lung Cancer[a]

Investigator	Regimen[b]	Adenocarcinoma	Large cell	Squamous
Hansen *et al.*, 1976	HN$_2$ or CTX + CCNU vs. HN$_2$ or CTX + CCNU + Mtx	+++	−	−
Bodey *et al.*, 1977	CTX vs. COMB	o	o	−
Alberto *et al.*, 1976	Mtx, CTX, VCR, PCZ simultaneous vs. sequential	o	o	−
Edmonson *et al.*, 1976a	HN$_2$ or CTX + CCNU vs. HN$_2$ or CCNU	−	−	−
Livingston, 1977	BACON vs. NAC	o	o	−
Eagan *et al.*, 1977	DAG vs. CAP	++	++	++
Brittell *et al.*, 1978	P vs. P-CA vs. CAP	++	o	o

[a] +++, Significant increase in objective response and overall survival; ++, Significant increase in objective response; responders survive longer than nonresponders; no increase in overall survival; o, Data not available or inadequate patient numbers; −, No increase in survival, objective response or response duration for more intensive versus less intensive therapy.

[b] CTX, cyclophosphamide; A, Adriamycin; B, bleomycin; DAG, dianhydrogalactitol; N or HN$_2$, nitrogen mustard; Mtx, methotrexate; P, *cis*-platinum; PCZ, procarbazine; M, methyl CCNU; O or VCR, vincristine; C, CCNU in BACON and NAC or cyclophosphamide in CAP.

The impact of current combination chemotherapeutic regimens on the overall survival of treated groups is questionable, at best, and the true implications of existing data will depend upon the results of properly designed and executed Phase III studies in large patient populations.

VI. EVALUATION AND MANAGEMENT OF SMALL-CELL ANAPLASTIC CARCINOMA

Small cell anaplastic carcinoma is the most aggressive type of lung cancer. Placebo-treated patients from the V.A. Lung Group studies with disease outside of one hemithorax and/or the ipsilateral supraclavicular node (extensive disease) had a 1.4-month median survival. Placebo-treated patients with limited disease (disease confined to one hemithorax and/or the ipsilateral supraclavicular node) had a 3.0-month median survival (Zelen, 1973).

Although the precise cell of origin of small cell anaplastic carcinoma is unknown, it is postulated that the disease arises from the granule containing basal lining cells of the bronchial epithelium (K cells). Data supporting this hypothesis include the prevalent finding of electron-dense granules by electron microscopy in small cell anaplastic carcinoma, and the well-known association of small cell anaplastic carcinoma with ectopic polypeptide hormone production, including ACTH, antidiuretic hormone, and melanocyte-stimulating hormone. These points have been reviewed by Tischler (1978). Small cell anaplastic carcinoma has one of the highest mean labeling indices, calculated growth fractions, and calculated volume-doubling times of any major solid tumor (Muggia et al., 1974).

There has been increasing interest in the histological variations within the general class of small cell anaplastic lung cancers. The three major variants are (1) the lymphocyte-like or classic "oat cell" carcinoma; (2) the polygonal variant; and (3) the fusiform variant. The latter two types are termed "intermediate" in the WPL classification (Table II). One of the purposes of the subclassification is to determine whether the variants of the classic oat cell carcinoma differ in their clinical presentation or response to therapy. Most data indicate that there is no difference in clinical presentation or response to therapy when the classic oat cell carcinoma is compared to the intermediate types (Matthews et al., 1978). Another recent clinicopathologic observation has been the detection of significant alterations in the morphology of small cell anaplastic carcinoma after aggressive antitumor therapy when autopsy material is compared to the original biopsy specimen. At autopsy, there can be a marked tendency for the small cell anaplastic tumors to form glands, tubules, squamous nests, anaplastic large cells, and/or giant cells after treatment with chemotherapy and/or radiation therapy (Matthews, 1979).

A. Evaluation

As mentioned previously, there is no significant difference in survival at 2 years when the TNM staging system (Tables III,IV) is applied to small cell anaplastic carcinoma (Mountain, 1978). These data indicate the propensity of this disease to disseminate early, independent of the apparent anatomic distribution of definable intrathoracic disease. The preferred sites of metastases include the liver, brain, bone, and bone marrow. Bone marrow involvement occurs in about 23% of cases. In 1977, Hirsch *et al.* reported a 50% increase in yield of positive bone marrow examinations by employing bilateral iliac crest bone marrow biopsies and aspirates, as opposed to unilateral procedures. The propensity of this disease for bone, bone marrow, liver, and brain metastases mandates that appropriate radiologic and radionuclide studies be performed in all patients prior to making a therapeutic decision. Bilateral bone marrow aspirates and biopsies increase the yield of positive evaluations with no significant increase in morbidity. Peritoneoscopy with directed liver biopsy appears to be the most sensitive means to evaluate hepatic involvement (Margolis *et al.*, 1975), and should be strongly considered as an adjunct to noninvasive staging when significant differences in therapy attend the diagnosis of disseminated versus clinically limited disease.

B. Management

1. Surgery, Radiotherapy

Prior to the advent of effective combination chemotherapy, the 5-year survival rate in patients having disease clinically limited to the thorax had ranged from 0 to 5%. A randomized study comparing surgery to "radical" radiation therapy performed by the British Medical Research Council showed no 5-year survivors in the surgically treated group, and a 5% survival in patients treated with radical radiation therapy (Fox and Scadding, 1973). Thus, in the era of single-modality treatment, surgery appeared inferior to radiotherapy for patients with limited disease. More important, this study demonstrated the inability of local modalities to control the entire disease process, since 96% of all treated patients initially thought to have localized disease were dead within in 5 years.

Regarding the conventional role of surgery in the therapy of small cell carcinoma, it should be mentioned that one study has reported a 36% 5-year survival rate in a highly selected group of patients having a solitary pulmonary nodule ($\leq$ 6 cm), which could not be diagnosed prior to thoracotomy, and which was histologically shown to be small cell anaplastic carcinoma (Higgins *et al.*, 1975).

Small cell anaplastic carcinoma is the most radiotherapy-responsive type of lung cancer. The objective response rate is over 90%, and response appears to be dose-dependent (Choi and Carey, 1976). Radiotherapy is therefore an effective modality in palliating localized symptoms secondary to the primary or metastatic disease, as well as being a possibly useful adjunct to aggressive systemic therapy.

2. Single-Agent Chemotherapy

Small cell carcinoma is the most chemotherapy-responsive lung cancer cell type. Several years ago the V.A. Lung Group Study reported an increase in median survival of 1.4 to 4.0 months in patients treated with a placebo versus those treated with cyclophosphamide, respectively (Zelen, 1973). Livingston (1978) has reviewed the single-agent activity of a variety of drugs in small cell anaplastic carcinoma. An adaptation of these data is presented in Table XIV. The listing includes most of the drugs that are used in current combination-chemotherapy programs. The most recent additions to the list of active drugs have been two plant alkaloids, vincristine and VP-16 (4-dimethyl-epipodophyllotoxin ethylidene glucoside, VP16-213), and Adriamycin_. Although single drugs can induce a reasonably high overall objective response rate, the response duration is short, and the number of complete responses is negligible. In addition, the response rates cited are cumulative data from several studies. Generally such cumulative data overestimate objective response, particularly for older drugs such as cyclophosphamide and methotrexate.

3. Combination Chemotherapy and Combined Modality Studies

Prior to the advent of intensive combination chemotherapy or combined modality treatment, we, and particularly the patient, were confronted with a situation in which the disease was highly responsive, yet the duration of palliative effects was short and the possibility for cure was virtually nonexistent. The application of the principles of combination chemotherapy and combined-

Table XIV

Single Agents in Small Cell Carcinoma[a]

Drug	No. of patients	Response (%)	CR (%)
Cyclophosphamide	189	52 (28%)	4
Adriamycin	36	11 (31%)	—
Methotrexate	73	22 (30%)	—
Vincristine	43	18 (42%)	7
VP-16	167	75 (45%)	9
CCNU	76	11 (14%)	4
Hexamethylmelamine	69	21 (30%)	7
HN$_2$	55	24 (44%)	—

[a] Adapted from Livingston (1978).

modality treatment has drastically altered this outlook and has raised the possibility for better palliation and cure.

Randomized studies by Edmonson *et al.* (1976b), Lowenbraun *et al.* (1975), and Alberto *et al.* (1976) comparing combination chemotherapy to single-agent, or a series of single-agent, treatments have established the superiority of combination chemotherapy over single-agent therapy in this disease. There has been a veritable explosion of combination-chemotherapy and combined-modality studies in small cell anaplastic carcinoma. A review of the hundreds of studies is beyond the scope of this chapter, but several excellent general reviews are available (Bunn *et al.*, 1977; Broder and Selawry, 1977; Greco and Einhorn, 1978).

Even in the era of intensive combination chemotherapy, one of the most powerful prognostic factors in predicting a significant response is clinical stage. There is a highly significant difference in complete response rate, median response duration, and long-term survival when patients with limited and extensive disease are compared. For limited-disease patients, the complete response rate is generally about 60%, whereas the complete-response rate found in patients with extensive disease is generally less than 25%. The median survival for all limited- and extensive-disease patients is now approximately 51 weeks and 33 weeks, respectively (Bunn *et al.*, 1977).

An analysis of long-term survival from our institution (Ginsberg *et al.*, 1979) employing a regimen including CCNU, cyclophosphamide and vincristine (CCV), and modifications of CCV designed to incorporate Adriamycin and intensify the dose of all drugs, has yielded only 1/36 (9%) long-term survivors with extensive disease (3.5 years) and 7/34 (21%) 2–4-year survivors with limited disease. Of the nine patients who appeared to be disease-free at 16–18 months after extensive restaging procedures, only one (11%) has relapsed after discontinuing chemotherapy. The median time off therapy is presently 17 months, and the median overall disease-free survival is 36 months. These data, implying the possibility for cure in small cell anaplastic lung cancer, are consistent with other studies of intensive combination chemotherapy and combined-modality studies available in the literature (Greco and Einhorn, 1978). Implicit in this possibility for cure is the requirement for a complete response.

Since clinical stage is such an important factor in predicting response, it is important that refinements in the definition of extensive and limited disease be made. Studies have clarified the effect of the presence of a malignant pleural effusion and contralateral supraclavicular nodal involvement on response to therapy and survival. Livingston *et al.* (1978) have shown that the median survival of patients with a malignant pleural effusion as the only site of extension is identical to those with classically defined extensive disease. Furthermore, they have shown that contralateral supraclavicular nodal involvement, previously defined as extensive disease, does not adversely affect prognosis.

In addition to clinical stage, performance status is a very important factor in determining response to therapy and survival. When patients are divided into ambulatory versus nonambulatory status, there are striking differences in complete response, with half as many complete responses seen in the more impaired patients within both the limited and extensive disease categories (Livingston *et al.*, 1978). Patients in bed more than 50% of the waking hours have a median survival of only 6 months versus 12 months for patients who are ambulatory and minimally symptomatic (Hansen *et al.*, 1978).

In reviewing the plethora of available combination-chemotherapy studies, certain questions arise:

Does the choice of agents used in combination alter response? This question revolves particularly around the use of Adriamycin, VP-16, and the nitrosoureas. To date, no striking differences are apparent in complete-response rate, median or long-term survival, when studies using Adriamycin containing combinations are compared to those not employing Adriamycin. There are few, if any, direct comparative trials. Several studies have incorporated VP-16 into initial combination regimens, but the final results of these studies are currently not available. On the other hand, VP-16 does appear to be one of the most effective second-line agents after failure on initial combination chemotherapy (Hansen *et al.*, 1977). Although large studies employing the nitrosoureas (generally CCNU, 1-chloroethyl-3-cyclohexyl-1-nitrosourea) have yielded results comparable to studies not employing these agents, the disadvantage of their use is cumulative bone marrow toxicity, particularly with high-dose regimens. No consistent evidence exists that suggests that the use of nitrosoureas alters the central nervous system relapse rate.

What is the current role of radiotherapy, particularly in limited disease? For patients with limited disease, certain important points are being clarified by careful clinical investigations. Not unexpectedly, it appears that the use of radiation therapy followed by chemotherapy at relapse is inferior to the use of simultaneous chemotherapy plus irradiation (Kraus and Perez, 1979). Preliminary data from two studies have indicated that the objective response rate and survival associated with intensive combination chemotherapy alone are not significantly different from the same intensive chemotherapy plus radiotherapy (Stevens *et al.*, 1979; Hansen *et al.*, 1979). It must be emphasized that these data are preliminary and will only be conclusive when further evaluation shows that there are as many long-term, disease-free survivors in each treatment group.

There is a role for radiotherapy in the overall strategy for curing small cell anaplastic lung cancer which is well established. This is the use of elective cranial irradiation at the time of initial presentation to prevent central nervous system relapse. Most studies have employed 3000 rads in 10 fractions to the brain. The results of several nonrandomized, as well as randomized, studies have shown that the incidence of clinical brain relapse has been decreased from 22–28% to 6–8% with the use of elective brain irradiation as part of the initial treatment. These studies have been extensively reviewed by Bunn *et al.* (1978). Although an increase in survival has not been consistently demonstrated in these studies, the use of elective cranial irradiation must be considered as an integral part of the curative approach to small cell anaplastic lung cancer—particularly in patients with limited disease.

VII. CONCLUSION

In summary, it may seem somewhat paradoxical that the greatest strides in the therapy of lung cancer have been made in the most virulent histologic type—small cell anaplastic carcinoma. These developments have resulted from a better understanding of the clinical nature of the disease, and the advent of effective systemic therapy. Prior to the advent of combination chemotherapy, long-term disease-free survival occurred in only 0-5% of patients with limited disease. Currently, 15-30% of such patients can be expected to survive disease-free from 2 to 4 years. Extensive disease remains much less amenable to current therapies, with fewer than 10% of treated patients surviving disease-free at 2 years, and with a median survival in treated patients of approximately 6 months. It is hoped that further research will lead to an increased cure rate in limited-disease patients and to the development of the possibility for cure in those patients with extensive disease.

REFERENCES

Alberto, P., Brunner, K. W., Martz, C., Obrecht, J. P., and Sonntag, R. W. (1976). *Cancer* **38**, 2208-2216.
Bitran, J. D., Desser, R. K., De Messter, T. R., Coman, M., Evans, R., Billings, A., Griem, M., Rubenstein, L., Shapiro, C., and Golomb, H. (1976). *Cancer Treat. Rep.* **60**, 1225-1230.
Bodey, G. P., Lagokas, S., Guttierez, A. C., Wilson, H. E., and Selawry, O. S. (1977). *Cancer* **39**, 1026-1031.
Brittell, J. C., Eagan, R. T., Ingle, J. N., Creagan, E. T., Rabin, J., and Frytak, S. (1978). *Cancer Treat. Rep.* **62**, 1207-1210.
Broder, L., and Selawry, O. S. (1977). *Cancer Treat. Rev.* **4**, 219-259.
Bunn, P. A., Cohen, M. H., Ihde, D. C., Fossieck, B. E., Jr., Matthews, M. J., and Minna, J. D. (1977). *Cancer Treat. Rep.* **61**, 333-342.
Bunn, P. A., Nugent, J. L., and Matthews, M. J. (1978). *Semin. Oncol.* **5**, 314-322.
Chahinian, A. P., Arnold, D. J., Cohen, J. M., Purpora, D. P., Jaffrey, I. S., Teirstein, A. S., Kirschner, P. A., and Holland, J. F. (1977). *J. Am. Med. Assoc.* **237**, 2392-2396.
Choi, C. H., and Carey, R. W. (1976). *Cancer* **37**, 2651-2657.
Cohen, M. H. (1974). *Semin. Oncol.* **1**, 183.
Eagan, R. T., Ingle, J. N., Frytak, S., Rubin, J., Kuols, L. K., Carr, D. T., Coles, D. T., and O'Fallon, J. R. (1977). *Cancer Treat. Rep.* **61**, 1339-1345.
Edmonson, J. H., Lagakos, S., Stolbach, L., Perlia, C. P., Bennett, J. M., Mansour, E. G., Horton,

J., Regelson, W., Cummings, F. J., Israel, L., Brodsky, I., Snider, B. I., Creech, R., and Carbone, P. P. (1976a). *Cancer Treat. Rep.* **60**, 625–627.

Edmonson, J. H., Lagakos, S. W., Selawry, O. S., Perlia, C. P., Bennett, J. M., Muggia, F. M., Wampler, G., Brodovsky, H. S., Horton, J., Colsky, J., Mansour, E. G., Creech, R., Stolbach, L., Greenspan, E. M., Levitt, M., Israel, L., Ezdinli, E. Z., and Carbone, P. P. (1976b). *Cancer Treat. Rep.* **60**, 925–932.

Erozan, Y. S., and Frost, S. K. (1970). *Acta Cytol.* **14**, 565.

Fox, W., and Scadding, T. G. (1973). Lancet **2**, 616–617.

Ginsberg, S., Comis, R., King, R., Goldberg, J., Zamkoff, K., Gottlieb, A., Meyer, J., and Elbadawi, A. (1979). *Cancer Treat. Rep.* **63**, 1347–1349.

Goldberg, E. M., Shapiro, C. M., and Glicksman, A. (1974). *Semin. Oncol.* **1**, 205–215.

Greco, F. A., and Einhorn, L. H. (1978). *Semin. Oncol.* **5**, 233.

Hansen, H. H., Hirsch, F., and Dombernowsky, P. (1977). *Cancer* **40**, 633–637.

Hansen, H. H., Selawry, O. S., Simon, R., Carr, D. T., VanWyk, C. E., Tucker, R. D., and Sealy, R. (1976). *Cancer* **38**, 2201–2207.

Hansen, H. H., Dombernowsky, P., and Hirsch, F. R. (1978). *Semin. Oncol.* **5**, 280–287.

Hansen, H. H., Dombernowsky, P., Hansen, H. S., and Roth, M. (1979). *Proc. Am. Assoc. Cancer Res.* **20**, 277.

Harris, C. C. (1973). *Cancer Chemother. Rep., Part 3* **2**, 59–62.

Higgins, G. A., Shields, T. W., and Keehn, R. J. (1975) *Arch. Surg. (Chicago)* **110**, 570.

Hirsch, F., Hansen, H. H., Dombernowsky, P., and Hainau, B. (1977). *Cancer* **39**, 2563–2567.

Kraus, S., and Perez, C. (1979). *Proc. Am. Soc. Clin. Oncol.* **20**, 316.

Lee, R. E. (1974). *Semin. Oncol.* **1**, 245–252.

Legha, S., Muggia, F. M., and Carter, S. K. (1977). *Cancer* **39**, 1415–1424.

Livingston, R. B. (1977). *Cancer Treat. Rev.* **4**, 153–165.

Livingston, R. B. (1978). *Semin. Oncol.* **5**, 299–304.

Livingston, R. B., Moore, T. N., Heilbrun, L., Bottomley, R., Lehane, D., Rivkin, S. E., and Thigpen, T. (1978). *Ann. Intern. Med.* **88**, 194–199.

Lowenbraun, S., Krauss, S., Smalley, R., and Huguley, C. (1975). *Proc. Am. Assoc. Cancer Res.* **16**, 246.

Lukeman, J. M. (1973). *Cancer Chemother. Rep., Part 3* **4**, 79–94.

McKneally, M. F., Maver, C., and Kausel, H. W. (1976). *Lancet* **1**, 377–379.

Margolis, R., Hansen, H. H., Muggia, F. M., and Kanouwha, S. (1975). *Cancer* **34**, 1825–1829.

Matthews, M. J. (1974). *Semin. Oncol.* **1**, 175–182.

Matthews, M. J. (1976). *In* "Lung Cancer: Natural History, Prognosis and Therapy" (L. Israel and A. P. Chahinian, eds.), p. 23, Academic Press, New York.

Matthews, M. J. (1979). *In* "Proceedings of the Second National Cancer Institute Conference on Lung Cancer Treatment" (F. M. Muggia and M. Rozencweig, eds.), p. 134. Raven, New York.

Matthews, M. J., Gazdar, A. F., and Ihde, D. C. (1978). *Proc. Am. Assoc. Cancer Res.* **19**,

Morrison, R., Seeley, T. J., and Cleland, W. P. (1963). *Lancet* **1**, 683–687.

Mountain, C. F. (1976). *In* "Lung Cancer: Natural History, Prognosis and Therapy" (L. Israel and A. P. Chahinian, eds.), p. 108, Academic Press, New York.

Mountain, C. F. (1977). *In* "Lung Cancer, Clinical Diagnosis and Treatment" (M. J. Strauss, ed.), p. 185. Grune & Stratton, New York.

Mountain, C. F. (1978). *Semin. Oncol.* **5**, 272–279.

Mountain, C. F., Carr, D. T., and Anderson, W. A. (1974). *Am. J. Roentgenol., Radium. Ther. Nucl. Med.* **120**, 130–138.

Muggia, F. M., Kzezoski, S. K., and Hansen, H. H. (1974). *Cancer* **34**, 1683–1690.

Roswit, B., Patno, M. E., Rapp, R., Veinbergs, A., Feder, B., Stuhlbarg, J., and Reid, C. B. (1968). *Radiology* **90**, 668–697.

Ruckdeschel, J. C., Codish, S. D., Shanahan, A., and McKneally, M. F. (1972). *N. Engl. J. Med.* **287**, 1013–1017.
Silverberg, E. (1979). *Ca.* **29**, 6–21.
Stevens, E., Einhorn, L., and Rohn, R. (1979). *Proc. Am. Soc. Clin. Oncol.* **20**, 435.
Tischler, A. S. (1978). *Semin. Oncol.* **5**, 244–252.
Zelen, M. (1973). *Cancer Chemother. Rep., Part 3* **4**, 31–42.

10
CLINICAL CHARACTERISTICS OF CANCER IN THE BRAIN AND SPINAL CORD

Victor A. Levin and Charles B. Wilson

I.	Introduction	167
II.	Tumors of the Brain	168
	A. Incidence and Classification	168
	B. Neurology of Intracranial Tumors	171
	C. Neurology of Acute and Life-Threatening Syndromes Caused by Brain Tumors	177
	D. Diagnostic Tests	179
	E. Evaluation of Patients with Intracranial Tumors during Therapy	186
III.	Meningeal Carcinomatosis	190
	A. Leukemia	190
	B. Solid Tumors	191
IV.	Tumors of the Spinal Cord	192
	A. Incidence and Classification	192
	B. Neurology of Spinal Cord Tumors	194
	C. Diagnostic Tests	195
	References	197

I. INTRODUCTION

Malignant neoplasms are generally defined as aberrant growth of abnormal cells or tissues that grow at a rate independent of host tissue. Most malignant neoplasms are also capable of metastases to distant sites. Left unchecked, these neoplasms lead to death. This mechanism is somewhat different in the central nervous system (CNS). CNS tumors rarely metastasize outside of the CNS, and

CANCER AND CHEMOTHERAPY, VOL. II

167

even well-differentiated and histologically benign intracranial tumors can pursue a "malignant" course to death. Intracranial tumors produce signs and symptoms primarily through expansion, compressing and displacing vital neural tissue. This difference between CNS tumors and non-CNS tumors, with the former's complex signs and symptoms, requires prompt diagnosis and expeditious management to obtain optimal therapeutic results.

We will discuss the classification and incidence of CNS tumors, their basic neurology, and laboratory studies used in their diagnosis. In addition, because careful follow-up of patients undergoing radiation therapy and chemotherapy is critical, methods for assessing the results of therapy and following patients with CNS tumors will be presented.

II. TUMORS OF THE BRAIN

A. Incidence and Classification

The incidence of intracranial tumors is in excess of 16.7 per 100,000 population; most of these tumors are metastatic or astroglial in origin. The relative frequency of the seven most common families of intracranial tumors is given in Table I. Incidence figures for metastatic tumors compiled over the past several decades show a two- to fourfold increase in the number of patients with metastatic brain tumors. The explanation for this increase is either that diagnostic techniques today allow more precise diagnosis of intracranial tumors, or that sys-

TABLE I

Brain Tumors at All Ages[a]

Type	Percentage[b]
Metastatic	50
Glioblastoma	15
Astrocytoma	10
Other gliomas (ependymoma, oligoden-droglioma, medulloblastoma)	3.5
Meningioma	9
Nerve sheath (e.g., neurinomas)	4.5
Pituitary	2.5
Other (unspecified)	5.5

[a] Data taken from Tables 3-1C, 3-5, and 3-6A of Office of Biometry and Epidemiology (1977).

[b] These percentages for the incidences for the tumors listed above were extrapolated from the limited breakdown of tumor types cited.

TABLE II

Type of Tumor as a Function of Age at First Presentation[a]

Under age 15 (%)[b]	Age 15 to 45 (%)[b]	Over age 45 (%)[b]
Astrocytoma (20)	Metastatic (23.0)	Metastatic (59)
Medulloblastoma (26)	Glioblastoma (14.2)	Glioblastoma (8.8)
Ependymoma (4.8)	Astrocytoma (13.0)	Meningiomas (6.2)
Glioblastoma (2.4)	Pituitary (7.2)	Astrocytomas (4.0)
Metastatic carcinoma (9.8)	Other gliomas (6.5)[c]	Neurinomas (3.0)
Brain stem glioma (2.4)	Meningioma (5.9)	Pituitary (1.9)
Optic glioma (2.3)	Neurinomas (2.6)	Other gliomas (1.1)[c]
Papilloma of choroid plexus (2.3)	Angiomatas (0.7)	Angiomata (0.3)
Meningioma (1.0)		
Craniopharyngioma (2.4)		

[a] From Cuneo and Rand (1952); Office of Biometry and Epidemiology (1977).

[b] (%) = Percentage of tumors adjusted for the incidence of all tumors at each of the three ranges cited.

[c] Includes oligodendroglioma, ependymoma, medulloblastoma, neuroblastoma.

temic tumors are now better controlled, which results in greater life expectancy and, therefore, a longer period of risk during which primary tumors can metastasize.

Although CNS tumors are the second leading cancer-related cause of death in children under 15 years of age, and the third leading cancer-related cause of death in adolescents and adults between the ages of 15 and 34, the majority of intracranial tumors occur over the age of 45, with the peak incidence in the seventh decade. Table II lists the frequency of intracranial tumors by tumor type and age at first presentation. From this table it is evident that metastatic tumors are far more common after than before the age of 45. Similarly, glioblastoma, which is rare below the age of 15, increases in incidence to 8.8% of all tumors after the age of 45. Astrocytoma and other glial tumors less malignant than glioblastoma multiforme actually decrease in frequency with increasing age. Meningiomas increase from 1% of all tumors in patients under the age of 15 to 6.2% of tumors in patients over 45 years of age.

Secondary, or metastatic, tumors of the brain are slightly more common in males than in females, primarily because of the higher incidence of tumors of the lung, bronchus, and trachea in males. Table III summarizes the frequency with which extracranial tumors metastasize intracranially. Fully 24% of all intracranial tumors can be traced to tumors originated in the respiratory system and pharynx; modification of smoking habits could markedly reduce the incidence of these tumors.

TABLE III

Metastatic Tumors of the Brain

Site	Male (%)	Female (%)
Lung, bronchus, trachea	61	31
Other	16	17
Breast	1	28
Genitourinary	7	12
Skin	3	3
Intestine	3	4
Buccal cavity, pharynx	5	1
Stomach	2	1
Other GI	1	0.5
Uterus		3
Prostate	2	

Table IV lists the tremendous diversity in primary intracranial tumors that is clearly a function of the diversity of brain cells capable of transformation into tumors. Although the etiology of primary intracranial tumors is not known with certainty, experimentally a variety of carcinogens and viruses have been shown to produce glial and sarcomatous tumors. However, an association of specific etiological agents with human cancer has yet to be established.

TABLE IV

Classification of Primary Intracranial Tumors by Cell of Origin

Normal cell	Tumor
Astrocyte	Astrocytoma, astroblastoma, glioblastoma
Ependymocyte	Ependymoma, ependymoblastoma
Oligodendrocyte	Oligodendroglioma
Microgliocyte	Reticulum cell sarcoma or microglioma
Arachnoidal fibroblasts	Meningioma
Nerve cell or neuroblast	Ganglioneuroma, neuroblastoma, retino-blastoma
External granular cell or neuroblast	Medulloblastoma
Schwann cell	Schwannoma (neurinoma)
Melanocyte	Melanotic carcinoma
Choroid epithelial cell	Choroid plexus papilloma or carcinoma
Pituitary	Adenoma
Endothelial cell or "stromal" cell	Hemangioblastoma
Primitive germ cells	Germinoma, pinealoma, teratomas, cholesteatoma
Pineal parenchymal cells	Pinealcytoma
Notochordal remnants	Chordoma

B. Neurology of Intracranial Tumors

Unlike patients with stroke, patients with cerebral tumors rarely present with "classic" anatomically distinct neurological syndromes. The reason for this is that tumors produce symptoms primarily by two mechanisms: by mass effect, due either entirely to the tumor or to the tumor and surrounding edema; or by infiltration and destruction of normal tissue.

1. General Signs and Symptoms

Tumors of the cerebrum produce general signs and symptoms alone or in combination with focal signs and symptoms. Infiltrative tumors, such as the various grades of astrocytoma, oligodendroglioma, and some of the more primitive neuroectodermal tumors, can produce headache, gastrointestinal upset such as nausea and vomiting, personality changes, and slowing of psychomotor function.

Headache is a common nonspecific symptom in patients with brain tumors, and although it can vary in severity and quality, it most commonly occurs in the early morning hours or upon first awakening. Sometimes patients do not complain of headache per se, but rather of an uncomfortable feeling in the head. Because the brain does not have pain-sensitive structures, tumor headache has been attributed to local swelling and distortion of pain-sensitive nerve endings associated with blood vessels, primarily in the meninges. Once a tumor has achieved a critical volume, causing compression and displacement of brain, the onset and demise of headache seem to be correlated with changes in intracranial pressure.

Although there is not an exact relationship between the location of tumor headache and the location of the tumor, more often than not frontal and temporal tumors produce headache in frontal, retro-orbital, or temporal regions, whereas infratentorial tumors produce occipital and retroauricular headache. However, occasionally retro-orbital headaches are also associated with infratentorial tumors.

Patients also complain of nausea and occasionally vomit, but this symptom is more common with patients harboring infratentorial tumors than with patients harboring supratentorial tumors. Although textbooks discuss projectile vomiting as a not-infrequent generalized symptom of brain tumors, in our experience it is common in children but rare in adults. Reasons for a lower incidence of vomiting may be that patients with tumors are diagnosed earlier than in previous years, and receive glucocorticoids that can dramatically modify many of the generalized signs and symptoms of brain tumors.

Often it will be apparent to the family as well as the examiner that the patient is suffering from mental dysfunction. This may take the form of slowing of psychomotor activity. Characteristically, patients with brain tumors tend to sleep longer at night and tend to nap during the day.

Seizures, as a presenting symptom, occur in approximately 20% of patients with supratentorial brain tumors. They are likely to take the form of focal motor seizures for metastatic tumors and rapidly growing infiltrative malignant gliomas. In slowly growing astrocytomas, oligodendrogliomas, or meningiomas, generalized seizures may antedate the clinical diagnosis by weeks to years.

2. Focal Cerebral Syndromes

The *frontal lobe syndrome* varies greatly from patient to patient and can vary from a picture of headache and very mild slowing of contralateral hand movements to contralateral spastic hemiplegia, marked elevation in mood, or loss of initiative and dysphasia (dominant lobe). Strictly unilateral lesions of the right frontal lobe can cause left hemiplegia, slight elevation in mood, difficulty in adapting to new situations, loss of initiative, and even occasional primitive grasp and sucking reflexes. Left frontal lobe disease can cause right hemiplegia and a nonfluent dysphasia with or without some apraxia of lips, tongue, or hand movements.

Bifrontal disease, a condition usually associated with infiltrative gliomas, can cause variable degrees of bilateral hemiplegia, spastic bulbar palsy, severe impairment of intellect, lability of mood, dementia, and prominent primitive grasp, suck, and snout reflexes.

Temporal lobe syndromes, like frontal lobe syndromes, can range from mild symptoms, detectable only on very careful testing of perception and spatial judgment, to severe impairment of recent memory. Lesions of either temporal lobe can result in homonymous quadrantanopsia, auditory hallucinations, and even aggressive behavior. Involvement of the nondominant temporal lobe can, in addition, result in minor perceptual problems and spatial disorientation. Involvement of the dominant temporal lobe can result in dysnomia, impaired perception of verbal commands, and even a full-blown fluent Wernicke-like aphasia. Bilateral disease, involving both temporal lobes, is rare in comparison to the bilaterality of frontal lobe tumors.

Parietal lobe syndromes affect sensory more than motor modalities, although mild hemiparesis is sometimes seen with extensive parietal lobe tumors. Disease of either parietal lobe can produce a decrease in the perception of cortical sensory stimuli that may be mild and observed only by testing of sensory extinction, or it may be more severe with deep infiltrative tumors, leading to hemianesthesia and other hemisensory abnormalities. There also may be a homonymous hemianopsia or visual inattention. Involvement of the nondominant parietal lobe can lead to perceptual abnormalities and, in severe cases, to anosognosia and an apraxia for dressing oneself. Unilateral disease of the dominant parietal lobe can result in alexia, dysgraphia, and certain types of apraxia.

Involvement of *occipital lobes* can lead to a contralateral homonymous hemianopsia or visual aberrations that may take the form of imperception of color, object size, or object location. Bilateral occipital disease can lead to cortical blindness.

The classical disconnection syndromes associated with *corpus callosum lesions* are rarely seen in patients with brain tumors. The main reason for this is that even though infiltrative gliomas frequently cross the corpus callosum in the region of the genu or the splenium, there is normally involvement of additional structures that complicate neurological interpretation. Interruption of association fibers in the anterior part of the corpus callosum causes a failure of the left hand to carry out spoken commands. Lesions in the splenium of the corpus callosum result in an inability of patients to read or name colors because of the interruption of visual fibers connecting the right occipital lobe and left angular gyrus.

Frequently, tumors in the *thalamus* and, less commonly, in the *basal ganglia,* can reach 4 cm in diameter before the patient has symptoms severe enough to seek medical attention. These patients can present with headaches resulting from trapping of the lateral horn of one of the ventricles that produces hydrocephalus and increased intracranial pressure. Patients can present with a mild sensory abnormality on the contralateral side, which is only detected by testing of sensory extinction.

Some patients will complain of intermittent paresthesia on the contralateral side; because they are episodic and seizure-like, anticonvulsant drugs are sometimes successful. With more involvement of the basal ganglia, contralateral intention tremor and hemiballistic-like movement disorders can also be observed. It is uncommon for thalamic tumors to present in a manner typical of thalamic strokes unless bleeding into the tumor has occurred.

Involvement of the *brain stem* is due, in order of decreasing frequency, to astrocytoma, glioblastoma, and ependymoma. In 90% of patients, the initial manifestation of a brain stem glioma is a cranial nerve palsy involving the VIth and VIIth cranial nerves on one side. This is usually followed by involvement of long tracts resulting in hemiplegia, unilateral limb ataxia, ataxia of gait, paraplegia, hemisensory syndromes, gaze disorders, and occasionally hiccups. Less commonly, long-tract signs precede the cranial nerve abnormalities.

Astrocytoma is more likely to involve the midbrain and produce hydrocephalus, vomiting, drowsiness, and cerebellar signs, whereas glioblastoma more frequently involves the medulla. Children with glioblastoma characteristically have a more rapidly progressive course and are more likely to have VIIth, IXth, Xth, and VIth cranial nerve deficits along with dysarthria, personality change, and head tilt. Unlike the expansive posterior fossa tumors, headache, vomiting, and papilledema occur late.

Fourth ventricular tumors, by virtue of their location, tend to produce obstructive hydrocephalus early in their development. As a result, headache and vomiting may be prominent symptoms, usually associated with disturbances of gait and balance. With rapidly progressing lesions, a cerebellar herniation picture may develop (see below).

Tumors of the *cerebellum* produce, in general, different patterns. In slowly growing tumors, the first symptoms may be due to increased intracranial pressure (such as headache and nausea), and may include imbalance in gait or ataxia of a limb. In more rapidly growing cerebellar tumors, there may be quite prominent morning headache, vomiting, a stumbling gait with frequent falling, nystagmus and dizziness, and visual symptoms caused by papilledema. Bilateral VIth nerve palsies are uncommon. Abnormal posturing of the head is often seen in children; characteristically, the head is tilted back and away from the side of the tumor. Posturing of the head is curious in that it indicates unilateral cerebellar–foramen magnum herniation.

For the purposes of localization, midline lesions in and around the cerebellar vermis lead to truncal and gait ataxia, whereas lesions in a cerebellar hemisphere lead to unilateral appendicular ataxia, most readily observed in upper extremity movements.

Acoustic neurinomas (schwannoma, neurinoma) are so classic in their presentation that they warrant discussion as the main tumor responsible for the *cerebellopontine angle syndrome*. Almost all of these patients have involvement of the auditory or vestibular portions of the VIIIth nerve; over 50% have facial weakness, disturbance of taste, and sensory loss of the face; approximately 40% have ataxia of gait; and fewer than 25% have unilateral appendicular ataxia. By the use of audiological tests, the localization of the deafness and vestibular dysfunction to the auditory and vestibular nerve, rather than their end organs, is an important diagnostic characteristic of these tumors. These tumors are quite large at the time that they are first discovered. Currently, the majority of acoustic neurinomas are detected when unilateral sensorineural hearing is investigated, and consequently neurologic abnormalities are usually limited to impaired function of cochlear, vestibular, and facial nerves. Most of these patients also have an elevation of protein in the cerebrospinal fluid (CSF).

Table V summarizes the differential diagnostic features of cerebellopontine angle tumors and other, less common syndromes of *tumors at the base of the skull*.

The *optic chiasm syndromes* are usually caused by pituitary adenomas, and less commonly by craniopharyngiomas and meningiomas. Most patients (60%) present clinically with defects of the visual field; less commonly they present with blindness and optic atrophy. The visual field abnormality is usually a partial or complete bitemporal hemianopsia. With the lesion expanding from below the optic chiasm, the upper temporal quadrants are affected first. Patients can also present with scotomata in either eye. With long-standing, slowly progressive disease, unilateral or bilateral optic atrophy can be observed. Although only 20% of patients have headache as a symptom, expansion of tumor may involve the hypothalamus and compression of the IIIrd ventricle, leading to internal hydrocephalus.

Although included among brain tumors by tradition, tumors of the *pituitary gland* have distinct clinical features and little in common with other intracranial

TABLE V

Differential Diagnosis of Tumors at the Base of the Skull[a]

Site of lesion	Associated tumors	Clinical findings
Anterior parts	Carcinomas invasive from frontal and ethmoid sinuses; meningiomas	Unilateral anosmia, seizures, frontal lobe syndrome
Superior orbital fissure	Meningiomas, carcinoma of nasopharynx	IIIrd, IVth, V_1, VIth nerve lesions with ophthalmoplegia and pain and hypesthesia in V_1 distribution
Cavernous sinus	Chondromas, meningiomas, sellar and parasellar tumors	IIIrd, IVth, VIth, and sometimes Vth nerve involvement with ophthalmoplegia
Apex of the petrous temporal bone	Cholesteatoma, chondroma, meningioma, neurinoma, sarcoma	Vth and VIth nerve involvement with sensory and motor findings and diplopia
Sphenoid and petrous bones	Meningioma, chondroma, nasopharyngeal carcinoma, metastasis	IIIrd, IVth, VIth nerve lesions resulting in ophthalmoplegia; V may be associated with trigeminal neuralgia syndrome
Jugular foramen	Glomus jugular tumors, neurinomas, chondromas, cholesteatoma, meningioma, nasopharyngeal carcinoma	IXth, Xth, XIth nerves producing difficulty with swallowing, speaking, and weakness of strap muscles of neck
Cerebellopontine angle	Neurinoma, meningioma, cholesteatoma, metastasis, cerebellar tumors	VIIth nerve lesions causing loss of hearing, vertigo and nystagmus; cerebellar lesions producing ataxia of limbs and gait; Vth, VIIth, and occasionally IXth and XIIth nerve lesions; brain stem symptoms and signs of increased intracranial pressure

[a] Adapted from Bingas (1974).

tumors. The anterior pituitary (adenohypophysis) gives rise to a variety of tumors, the majority of which are endocrine-active, i.e., they produce hormones that create various syndromes of endocrine hyperactivity (Table VI). A small number of pituitary tumors produce no detectable hormones or produce hormones in quantities that assume no clinical significance. Although endocrine-active tumors may attain a large size, patients with endocrine-inactive tumors generally seek medical attention because of optic chiasmal compression–hypopituitarism as a consequence of a large mass.

Pituitary hormones are detectable by radioimmunoassay techniques, and prod-

TABLE VI

Clinical Syndromes Produced by Endocrine-Active Pituitary Adenomas

Hormone produced	Clinical syndrome
Growth hormone	Gigantism and acromegaly
Prolactin	Amenorrhea and galactorrhea, impotence
ACTH	Cushing's disease, Nelson's syndrome (following adrenalec-tomy)
TSH (rare)	Hyperthyroidism

ucts of the appropriate target organs can be measured—e.g., T3, T4, and cortisol. When a pituitary adenoma exceeds a diameter of 1 cm, compression of the normal anterior lobe causes pituitary hypofunction. Compression leads to detectable hyposecretion of specific cells, with production of growth hormone being most sensitive, followed closely by gonadotropins. Cells producing thyroid stimulating hormone (TSH) and adrenocorticotropic hormone (ACTH) are much more resistant, and their function is impaired only at a later stage of growth.

TABLE VII

Differential Diagnosis of Tumors by Location and Age at Onset of Symptoms

Location	Child	Adult
Supratentorial	Astrocytoma	Metastatic
	Glioblastoma	Glioblastoma
	Oligodendroglioma	Astrocytoma
	Sarcoma	Meningioma
	Neuroblastoma	Oligodendroglioma
	Mixed glioma	Mixed glioma
Infratentorial	Astrocytoma	Metastatic
	Medulloblastoma	Astrocytoma
	Ependymoma	Glioblastoma
	Brain stem glioma	Ependymoma
		Brain stem glioma
Sellar and parasellar	Craniopharyngioma	Pituitary, meningioma
	Optic glioma	Epidermoid
Base of the skull		Neurinoma
		Meningioma
		Chordoma
		Carcinoma
		Dermoid, epidermoid

Table VII summarizes the differential diagnosis of tumors by location in children and adults. It should serve as a guide and is not by any means an exhaustive enumeration of all the possible tumors that can occur in those locations. For a more extensive description of CNS tumor pathology, the reader is referred to Rubinstein and Russell's textbook on neuropathology (1977) or the Armed Forces Institute of Pathology Fasicile *Brain Tumors of the Central Nervous System* by Rubinstein (1972). For a more extensive description of the neurology of CNS tumors, a standard textbook of neurology, such as *Principles of Neurology* by Adams and Victor (1977), should be read.

C. Neurology of Acute and Life-Threatening Syndromes Caused by Brain Tumors

Because the brain and the spinal cord are surrounded by a rigid skull and dural membranes, lesions that are rapidly expanding within or abutting the brain or spinal cord can cause displacement of vital structures leading, in the brain, to respiratory arrest and death and, in the spinal cord, to paraplegia or quadriplegia.

In order to understand the sequence of events leading to temporal lobe–tentorial (uncal) herniation and cerebellar–foramen magnum herniation, one must have a good visual image of intracranial anatomy. The tentorium cerebelli forms a rigid tissue partition between the cerebral hemispheres above and the cerebellum and brain stem below. Through this opening passes the midbrain centrally and the IIIrd nerve anterolaterally. Immediately lateral to the IIIrd nerve lies the medial portion of the temporal lobe called the uncus. An expanding mass lesion situated supratentorially may displace the uncus medially and inferiorly beneath the tentorium. Table VIII summarizes the neurological findings and pathological cause for the events that make up the temporal lobe–tentorial herniation syndrome.

Mass lesions in the infratentorial compartment can displace brain tissue upward through the tentorial opening, but more commonly brain tissue is forced downward through the foramen magnum. In the latter syndrome, the cerebellar tonsils move caudally through the foramen magnum and in so doing wedge against the medulla, causing the findings summarized in Table IX.

These two herniation syndromes will invariably lead to death unless there is prompt intervention. The immediately intravenous administration of hyperosmotic agents (mannitol, urea) and large doses of glucocorticoids (methylprednisolone, dexamethasone) should be given as an emergency procedure.

Cerebellar–foramen magnum herniation frequently results from, or is contributed to by, obstructive hydrocephalus. In those cases, emergency removal of fluid from the more cephalad ventricular system may relieve symptoms and be life saving. Surgical intervention is indicated only if the reason for the herniation is treatable. In the case of cerebellar–foramen magnum herniation aggravated by acute obstructive hydrocephalus, ventricular–atrial or ventricular–peritoneal shunting is frequently necessary.

A rapid increase in the volume of the supratentorial compartment leading to herniation can be caused by a number of different factors. A very rapidly growing glioblastoma can produce this picture, although it is more usual for it to occur as a terminal or near-terminal event following ineffective therapy for the tumor. It can also occur when there is a dramatic increase in the amount of edema associated with metastasis to the brain or with hyponatremia and hypo-osmolar syndromes. Sometimes the injudicious use of parenteral 5% dextrose–water will be sufficient to produce hypo-osmolality, an increase in brain water, and temporal lobe herniation. We have also seen temporal lobe herniation follow a group of shortly spaced seizures. Presumably the seizures, which are associated with hypoventilation, produce a local hypoxia around the tumor with a resultant increase in brain edema.

Hemorrhage into a tumor is not as common as one would expect, although the

TABLE VIII

Temporal Lobe–Tentorial (Uncal) Herniation[a]

Neurological findings	Pathological cause
Pupillary dilatation and ptosis	Compression of ipsilateral oculomotor nerve between herniating tissue and petroclinoid ligament
Ipsilateral hemiplegia	Compression of contralateral cerebral peduncle against tentorium (Kernohan's notch)
Contralateral hemiplegia	Compression of ipsilateral cerebral peduncle; when associated with compression of contralateral peduncle, bilateral corticospinal-tract signs will be present.
Homonymous hemianopia	Compression of posterior cerebral artery against the tentorium can lead to occipital ischemia or infarction and contralateral homonymous hemianopia; occasionally bilateral field-cuts will occur.
Midbrain syndrome: Cheyne–Stokes respirations, stupor–coma, bipyramidal signs, decerebrate rigidity, dilated fixed pupils, gaze paresis, altered oculocephalic reflexes	Crushing of midbrain between herniating temporal lobe and opposite leaf of tentorium associated with vascular occlusion and perivascular hemorrhages
Coma, rising blood pressure, and bradycardia	These late signs occur from rising intracranial pressure and hydrocephalus as the aqueduct is compressed and the subarachnoid space becomes compromised.

[a] Adapted from Adams and Victor (1977).

TABLE IX

Cerebellar–Foramen Magnum Herniation[a]

Neurological findings	Pathological cause
Head tilt, stiff neck, arching of neck, pain or paresthesias over the neck	Downward displacement of inferior mesial cerebellar hemispheres through the foramen magnum; may be unilateral or bilateral
Tonic extensor spasms of limbs and body (cerebellar "fits") and later coma	Compressive effects of cerebellum or hydrocephalus on the upper brain stem
Respiratory arrest	Medullary compression

[a] Adapted from Adams and Victor (1977).

incidence of intratumor hemorrhage may increase somewhat because of iatrogenic thrombocytopenia associated with the current use of chemotherapy in the treatment of brain tumors. Tumors that most commonly bleed *de novo* are glioblastoma and metastases from the lung, melanoma, hypernephroma, and choriocarcinoma. Signs and symptoms of intratumoral hemorrhage may be temporized by the use of osmotic agents and glucocorticoids, but if extensive and life threatening, operation and decompression are indicated. Under no circumstances should a lumbar puncture be performed in any of the acute herniation syndromes. In fact, lumbar puncture should never be done indiscriminately. The indications for lumbar puncture will be covered in another section.

D. Diagnostic Tests

1. Neuroradiological and Nuclear Medicine Procedures

Clinical indications that a patient has a brain tumor require radiological confirmation. Radiodiagnostic methods are much more reliable today than they were in the past. The most significant recent advance in neuroradiology has been the development of computerized tomography (CT), which has permitted the diagnosis of benign as well as malignant intracranial tumors and, in many cases, has allowed the designation of these tumors as either benign or malignant. In addtion, the advent of CT scanning has given greater insight into the changes that tumors undergo during therapy, a subject covered in a later section.

Computerized tomography is based on the premise that summation of measured X rays transmitted through any given body from 360° polar space can define that body. X-Ray transmissions are reconstructed by a computer into a series of planes for visual imaging. CT scanning can precisely localize and distinguish meningiomas, metastatic tumors, and intratumoral cysts, and can suggest the malignancy of infiltrative gliomas. In the evaluation of suspected brain tumor patients, a CT scan should be obtained first without contrast enhancement and then after intravenous administration of a contrast agent.

Radionuclide (RN) brain scanning has to a great extent been superceded by CT scanning for the initial evaluation of patients with brain tumors. However, RN scans continue to be of value for following patients harboring primary and metastatic tumors. They are also quite helpful in following patients who develop subarachnoid spread of tumor; frequently, in these latter cases, they are more reliable than CT scans.

Whether surgery is being considered or not, patients initially presenting with signs and symptoms of brain tumor usually are evaluated with cerebral angiography. Over the years, techniques have been improved considerably, and angiography is now a step in the routine evaluation for many tumors. Magnification and subtraction techniques and improved interpretation of posterior fossa angiograms have increased the usefulness of this study. Angiography can localize most cerebral tumors, and the tumor type (i.e., degree and type of malignancy) may often be predicted by vascular patterns.

For infratentorial lesions, CT scanning still remains the screening procedure of choice, although diffuse lesions in the posterior fossa frequently may show better on RN brain scans. Extra-axial masses at the base of the brain and tumors adjacent to or within the ventricular and cisternal systems are best localized by air- or positive-contrast studies. Because the introduction of air contrast may alter intracranial pressure, surgical intervention must be anticipated immediately following these contrast studies.

Pneumoencephalography is the procedure of choice when air-contrast study is required. It allows visualization of basilar extra-axial masses more adequately than ventriculography, although ventriculography is preferred when access to the IVth ventricule may be limited from below by a posterior fossa mass, or when pneumoencephalography inadequately defines the ventricle or aqueduct of Sylvius. Polytomography in conjunction with pneumoencephalography has further enhanced the value of air-contrast studies in posterior fossa and parasellar tumors. The water-soluble iodinated contrast agent metrizamide is replacing air for most intracranial examinations that require visualization of the CSF-containing spaces.

Positive-contrast studies have their greatest value in the diagnosis of spinal cord tumors. Using electron-dense iodinated media, either water-soluble or oily, tumors that are extradural can be distinguished from those that are intradural, and commonly intradural extramedullary spinal cord tumors can be distinguished from intramedullary ones. In addition to identifying spinal cord tumors, positive-contrast studies are sometimes helpful in evaluating tumors at the base of the skull, particularly small acoustic neurinomas.

Although the purpose of this section is not to replace standard radiological textbooks, we believe that some radiographic examples may be of value to give a clearer picture of the comparative value of angiography, CT and RN scanning, and myelography. Figures 1A, 1B, and 1C show a typical subtracted cerebral angiogram, a CT scan, and an RN scan of a patient with a low-grade infiltrative astrocytoma. Characteristically, these tumors show a mass with displacement of cerebral vessels, but show no evidence of neovascularization that is typical of more malignant tumors. The CT scan shows no enhancement with contrast, and the radionuclide scan shows no permeability defect with leakage of isotope. Figures 2A, 2B, and 2C show the typical appearance of highly malignant glioblastomas. In comparison, the subtracted cerebral angiogram shows new vessel formation; the CT scan shows a rim of contrast enhancement, and the RN scan shows a large permeability defect with extravasation of isotope.

2. CSF Examination and Other Laboratory Tests

Lumbar puncture in a patient with headache, papilledema, and a presumed diagnosis of tumor is risky, because it increases the possibility of a fatal cerebellar–foramen magnum or temporal lobe–tentorial herniation. As a basic rule, lumbar puncture should follow rather than precede neurodiagnostic studies such as cerebral angiography and CT scanning. We have found the examination of CSF to be useful in following patients with intracranial tumors, particularly tumors such as medulloblastoma that have a propensity for seeding into the subarachnoid space. In these patients, an examination of the CSF for malignant cells (cytology), protein, and polyamines is of value because the appearance of malignant cells and an elevation of polyamines frequently precede clinical evidence of tumor progression and before progression becomes obvious by CT or RN scans or myelography. The examination of CSF is also of enormous importance in making the diagnosis of carcinomatosis of the meninges and CNS leukemia. In these cases, the appearance of malignant cells can be diagnostic; low glucose and high protein levels indicate the extent of the carcinomatosis or leukemic infiltration.

A high protein concentration with normal glucose and a normal cytology is seen in tumors of the base of the skull, such as acoustic neurinoma, and in spinal cord tumors. The appearance of xanthochromic CSF, due to high protein content, with an absence of red cells is quite characteristic of spinal cord tumors obstructing the subarachnoid space and producing stasis of the CSF in the caudal lumbar sac.

Sellar tumors can produce endocrinological abnormalities that, if not obvious on clinical examination, are measurable by the very sensitive radioimmunoassays that have been developed for pituitary hormones. Polycythemia developing with a presumed tumor of the posterior fossa (cerebellum) can be used as presumptive evidence for the diagnosis of hemangioblastoma. Aside from these examples, routine laboratory tests are of little value in the diagnosis of brain tumor.

The electroencephalogram (EEG) had a place, in past years, in the diagnosis of

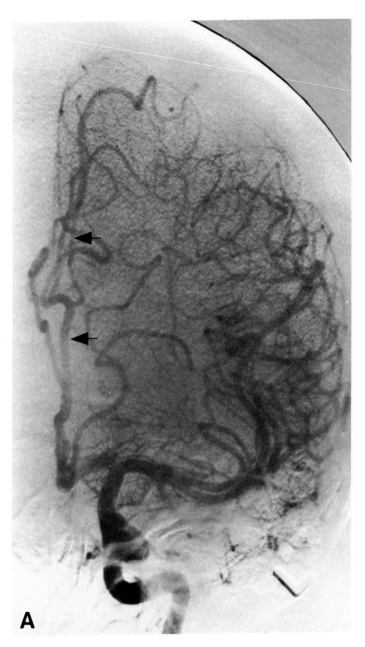

Fig. 1. A. Arteriogram; B, ^{99m}Tc-DPTA radionuclide brain scan; and C, computerized tomographic scan with contrast enhancement of patient with a well-differentiated (low-grade) astrocytoma. Arrows (A) show stretching and displacement of vessels but no new vessel formation. (Courtesy of Dr. David Norman.)

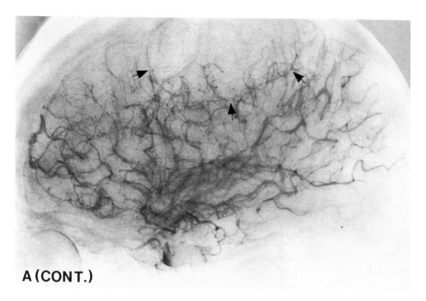

A (CONT.)

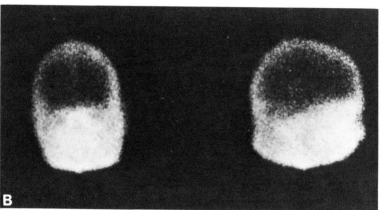

B

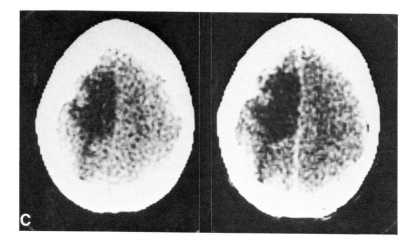

C

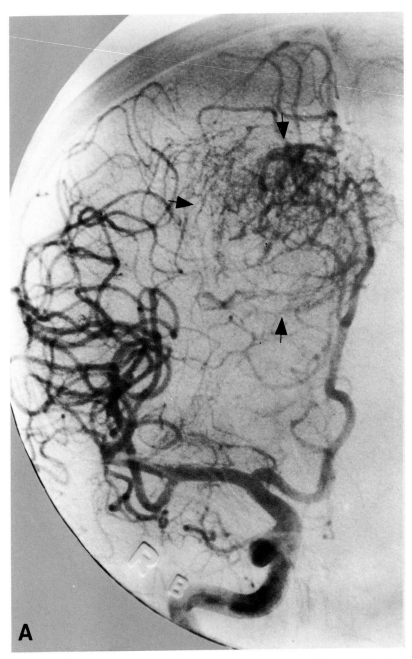

Fig. 2. A. Arteriogram; B, ⁹⁹ᵐ Tc-DPTA radionuclide brain scan; and C, computerized tomographic scan with contrast enhancement of patient with glioblastoma multiforme. The arrows (A) point to the new vessel formation characteristic of this tumor. (Courtesy of Dr. David Norman.)

184

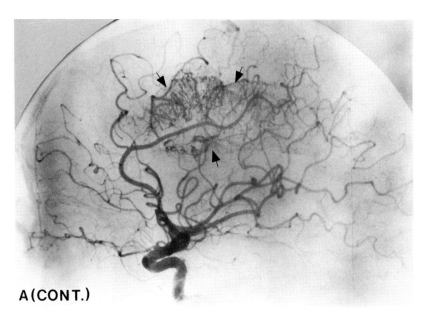

A(CONT.)

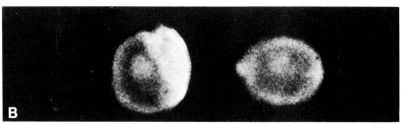

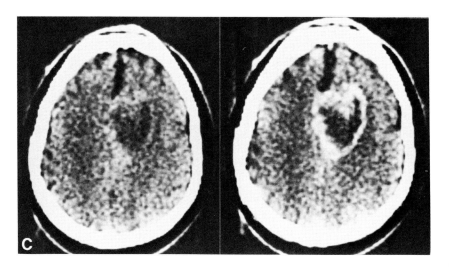

intracranial neoplasms. Characteristically, supratentorial tumors would produce polyphasic slow-wave (theta and delta waves) activity, which had some localizing value. Infratentorial lesions are sometimes associated with high-voltage slow waves seen particularly in anterior EEG leads. The lack of specificity in the EEG makes its value in the diagnosis of brain tumors quite limited. Its major value is in the diagnosis of seizure disorders and in following patients with brain tumors whose neurological deterioration may be related to subclinical seizures.

E. Evaluation of Patients with Intracranial Tumors during Therapy

Critical to the evaluation of the efficacy of any therapy for brain tumors is the reliability of the measurement of tumor growth (deterioration) or tumor regression (response). For years we have used sequential neurological examinations, CT scans, and RN scans to evaluate patients (Levin *et al.*, 1977); these methods will not be restated here. Instead, we will discuss factors other than cell growth that affect the clinical status of brain tumor patients.

1. Factors That May Produce Clinical Deterioration

The most common causes of neurological deterioration in brain tumor patients undergoing radiation therapy and/or chemotherapy are growth of the tumor and/or increased peritumoral edema. Both cause increased pressure in the cranial cavity and on adjacent functioning brain which causes impairment of cerebral blood flow. As a result, there is progressive impairment of functioning brain with resultant neurological deficits. These manifestations may include signs and symptoms of increased intracranial pressure and temporal lobe or cerebellar herniation (Tables VIII and IX).

The RN scan, CT scan, and cerebral angiogram can usually detect ineffective therapy by showing increased tumor size. Because tumor growth and clinical deterioration are end points for therapy, it is well to be aware of additional factors that can cause increased deficit without necessarily indicating treatment failure:

1. Hydrocephalus can occur as a result of obstruction of the ventricular system at the aqueduct of Sylvius, IVth ventricle, or foramen of Monro; except for obstruction of the foramen of Monro, obstructive hydrocephalus most often results from infratentorial tumors. Occasionally, hydrocephalus is caused by a cerebral subarachnoid convexity block due to infiltrative tumor (carcinomatosis, CNS leukemia, arachnoiditis). Hydrocephalus is usually treated with a ventricular shunting procedure, although sometimes the use of high-dose glucocorticoids will temporize the condition.

2. Hemorrhage into the tumor, although rare, can present as either an abrupt event or stepwise deterioration over hours. It is more likely to occur in a hypertensive patient. In addition, the incidence of intratumoral bleeding may increase

as more patients undergo myelotoxic chemotherapy and develop thrombocytopenia. The treatment for intratumoral hemorrhage is high-dose glucocorticoids initially, followed by surgery if necessary.

3. Fluid imbalance, particularly hyponatremia, can accentuate peritumoral edema. A common cause of hyponatremia is the use of excessive amounts of parenteral dextrose–water solutions. Salt-wasting syndromes, except in the immediate postoperative period, are not common in patients with brain tumors. The treatment in both cases is fluid restriction and, if herniation appears imminent, parenteral hyperosmotic therapy.

4. Hypertension can also accentuate intratumor and peritumor edema. The treatment should be directed to control of the hypertension. Sometimes high-dose glucocorticoids and hyperosmotic agents will be needed, but these may aggravate the hypertension or put an undue stress on the cardiovascular system, and they should be used with care.

5. Radiation therapy can cause deterioration in several ways. Early in the course of radiation therapy, edema or demyelination may cause progression of deficit, requiring an increase in glucocorticoid dosage. From 1 to 12 weeks (though usually from 6 to 12 weeks) following the completion of radiation therapy, a transient encephalopathy, with signs and symptoms of increased intracranial pressure, drowsiness, nausea, and exacerbation of preexisting neurological deficit, can occur (Hoffman *et al.*, 1979). This self-limited encephalopathy responds to steroids and resolves within several weeks without specific deficit. Steroids can then be discontinued. At times this delayed syndrome, observed in about 14% of patients completing a course of cranial irradiation, can be distinguished from tumor regrowth only by temporizing and finding that the patient's condition improves. This characteristic syndrome is not unique to brain tumors, but is also observed in leukemic children following prophylactic cranial irradiation.

From 4 months to 9 years following radiation therapy (but more often from 1 to 2 years), radiation necrosis can occur. Increased neurological deficit is noted that may or may not mimic tumor recurrence. There may be either atrophy or increased mass effect shown by CT. This complication is uncommon ($\simeq 5\%$) with proper dosimetry.

6. Seizures can complicate the evaluation of brain tumor progression. Their occurrence may suggest (rightly or wrongly) that the tumor is growing, and they may increase the deficit apart from any direct effect of the tumor. Recovery from increased weakness and mental dullness may take several hours to a week in postictal patients who are already brain injured. Even subclinical seizures can cause a similar deterioration, persisting for hours to days, which will resolve with control of the seizures. The EEG is usually diagnostic in these cases, and the treatment is better control of seizures. In this regard, we believe that patients receiving long-term chemotherapy frequently require higher doses of anticonvul-

sants because of deleterious drug interactions and increased degradation of the anticonvulsant drugs caused by drug-induced hepatic changes.

7.   Concurrent infection can produce neurological deterioration independent of tumor growth. Examples, although uncommon in brain tumor patients, are meningitis and cerebral abscess. The former can usually be distinguished by fever and meningismus; the latter, if in the same area as the tumor, is difficult to distinguish. In these situations, cerebral angiography and RN or CT scans can be helpful. More common infections are pneumonia and urinary tract infections. A debilitated patient with neurological damage is not only more susceptible to these infections, but may also have as a related complication increased lethargy and mental dullness for more than a week. During this period, an RN brain scan, CT scan, or angiogram will show no change; however, the EEG might show an increase in slow-wave activity.

Likewise, metabolic disorders, anemia, fatigue, or emotional depression can resemble clinical deterioration, including increase in focal deficit on testing. Again, brain scans (CT or RN) or other studies should be unchanged at these times.

Patients harboring responsive tumors may deteriorate after a course of chemotherapy. At least 10% of patients who eventually respond to therapy become significantly worse at the end of a first course of chemotherapy, and transient deterioration is occasionally observed even during the second year of continuous chemotherapy. Paradoxically, this clinical worsening early in therapy may result from an increase in tumor bulk resulting from "effective" therapy. Several factors contribute:

1.   The brain is surrounded by a rigid skull.
2.   Cell mass may increase when doomed cells either form giant cells or undergo one or more successful cell divisions before dying.
3.   The CNS has an inefficient mechanism for disposing of dead cells.
4.   Dead cells swell to occupy a larger volume than viable cells.
5.   Edema, probably caused by irritative products of cell lysis, may be present within the tumor mass and in adjacent brain.

Therefore, clinical deterioration and an enlarging abnormality as seen by RN (or CT) scan may not, after one course of chemotherapy, necessarily indicate an unresponsive tumor, and may in fact reflect the opposite. In about 20% of patients, a change in therapy at this point may lead to misinterpretation of response to both agents. We have avoided this pitfall by administering a second course regardless of the patient's response to the first course, using glucocorticoids as required. In this instance, improvement resulting from glucocorticoids must not be mistaken for oncolytic activity (see below).

2. *Factors That May Produce Clinical Improvement*

Theoretically, tumor regression should result in clinical improvement because of a reduction in the size of the tumor mass, i.e., killing of cells by chemotherapy and/or radiation therapy, followed by cell lysis and removal. However, if the neurological deficit is caused by infiltration with destruction of neural tissue rather than by compression and displacement of brain, clinical improvement may be negligible, despite oncolytic effectiveness.

Aside from the benefits of radiation and chemotherapeutic agents, clinical improvement is most likely to occur as a result of glucocorticoid administration. However, in order to assess accurately the effects of radiation therapy and chemotherapy in patients with intracranial tumors, glucocorticoid usage must be closely controlled. The following discussion highlights the circumstances where glucocorticoids are needed and how to limit their use.

Administration of glucocorticoids is usually begun before surgery for brain tumor. If a good surgical decompression has been achieved, steroid dose can be tapered off rapidly and discontinued within the first week or two following the operation. Some patients require steroid maintenance because a large volume of tumor remains, because tumor occupies the brain stem or spinal cord, or because of long-term prior usage.

Patients who no longer require glucocorticoids following the operation may later require them during or following radiation therapy, as discussed previously. Early in the course of radiation therapy, reactive edema is not uncommon, and occasionally there is a transient period of drowsiness and increased deficit at 6–12 weeks following the course of radiation therapy. The delayed radiation reaction usually resolves within 2 or 3 weeks, which is the only way to distinguish it with certainty from tumor progression.

Except for the provisions cited above, a patient's glucocorticoid requirement is most likely related to tumor growth or regression. The lowest dosage of glucocorticoid that will maintain a patient at his or her maximum level of comfort and function should be sought. Ordinarily this is discovered by decreasing the dosage until symptoms become more apparent, then increasing the dosage until symptoms subside; the dosage should then be kept constant. If the patient continues to do well, periodic attempts should be made to decrease the dosage. Keeping the dosage as low as the patient can tolerate minimizes the side effects of steroids and allows earlier recognition of tumor growth. If the patient becomes worse from physiological stress, such as a severe infection, glucocorticoid requirements generally increase, but should be returned to the original level when the stress resolves.

If deterioration is secondary to tumor growth, glucocorticoids may have to be increased indefinitely to keep the patient comfortable. For example, dexamethasone at 3 mg/day may have the desired effect for a patient with stabilized disease; a deteriorating patient may require dexamethasone increased to 64 mg/day or more.

Changes in glucocorticoid dosage affect the evaluation of the clinical state and response to cytotoxic treatment. A decrease in steroid requirement suggests improvement, assuming that the previous dosage was actually required. An increase in dosage suggests deterioration. Because increased steroid may (1) improve the neurologic status, (2) reduce the size of the lesion seen on RN brain scan and the mass effect seen on an angiogram, and (3) reduce the size of the tumor and the degree of contrast enhancement on CT scan, an attempt should be made to document tumor recurrence *before* increasing glucocorticoid dosage; this would rule out transient causes of deterioration, such as seizures or infection, so that a rational decision for change in treatment can be made.

III. MENINGEAL CARCINOMATOSIS

Leukemia and solid tumor cells can infiltrate the leptomeninges of the brain, spinal cord, and spinal nerve roots to produce neurological signs and symptoms. Leptomeningeal invasion begins in the pia-arachnoid and perivascular spaces of the CNS. Infiltration of the leptomeninges is usually diffuse, although nodular tumors occur. Hydrocephalus is a common complication of cancer-cell invasion of the arachnoid space.

Clinically, patients present with widespread multifocal signs and symptoms that fall into five categories: encephalopathy, increased intracranial pressure, meningeal irritation, cranial nerve palsies, and spinal nerve lesions (Hildebrand, 1978).

A. Leukemia

The effective management of leukemic infiltration of the cranial and spinal meninges and brain has been one of the major factors in the improved survival of children with acute leukemia. Before the use of prophylactic CNS irradiation and intrathecal methotrexate, 50–70% of children with acute lymphocytic leukemia (ALL) and acute myelocytic leukemia (AML) developed meningeal leukemia.

Meningeal leukemia is more likely to occur in ALL and AML, and up to 50% of children with leukemia may actually develop meningeal involvement during hematological remission. Over 70% of children present with manifestations of increased intracranial pressure such as headache, nausea and vomiting, and papilledema. Infiltration of the meninges also produces nuchal rigidity and cranial nerve (commonly VIth, VIIth, and VIIIth) findings. Depending on the extent and location of these infilrates, seizures, ataxia, and hypothalamic dysfunction can also be seen.

The diagnosis of increased intracranial pressure is usually obvious from radiographs of the skull showing splitting of the sutures (in children), and funduscopic examination that shows papilledema. Characteristically, the CSF shows an increased cell count, usually white cell blast forms, and in about two-thirds of these patients the glucose level is below normal; in about 50% of the patients, the protein level is elevated.

While meningeal leukemia is more common in ALL and AML, intracerebral (parenchymal) infiltrates are more common with AML. However, in comparison to meningeal infiltration, intracerebral leukemia is far less common. The onset of focal symptoms usually follows a spurt of leukemic cell proliferation that physically occludes small-caliber cerebral vessels. This occlusion commonly leads to vessel breakdown, intracerebral hemorrhage, and masslike spread of the leukemic cells.

B. Solid Tumors

Diffuse or multifocal seeding of the leptomeninges by carcinoma cells is an uncommon but by no means rare consequence of advanced systemic cancer. Although it has been reported most commonly with breast carcinoma, lymphomas, and lung carcinoma, it occurs secondarily to malignant melanoma and less commonly with pancreatic and gastric carcinoma.

Neurological signs are usually more prominent than symptoms. The most common symptoms are headache, altered mental state, and pain, and paresthesias in the distribution of spinal roots. On neurological examination the diagnosis is suggested by signs involving the neuraxis at more than one anatomical site. Mentation can be altered with dementia, lethargy, confusion, and poor attentiveness. Cranial nerves III, IV, VI, VII, and VIII are frequently involved. Neck

TABLE X

CSF in Leptomeningeal Carcinomatosis[a]

	Percentage abnormal	
Findings	Initial lumbar puncture	All lumbar punctures
Pressure > 150 mm H_2O	57	72
WBC $> 4/mm^3$	57	77
Positive cytology	45	79
Protein > 50 mg/dl	74	91
Glucose < 50 mg/dl	40	77

[a] Adapted from Olson et al. (1974).

pain, radiculopathy, motor weakness, sensory loss, and decreased deep tendon reflexes are also prominent features.

Although neurological signs and symptoms in a patient with systemic carcinoma may be suggestive of leptomeningeal carcinomatosis, the diagnosis requires confirmation to differentiate it from meningitis, intraparenchymal metastasis, and progressive multifocal leukoencephalopathy. Lumbar puncture has proved to be the most useful investigative test. Although a positive malignant CSF cytology is pathognomonic, it is not always observed. Olson *et al.* (1974) found positive cytology in 44% of patients in initial CSF examinations and in 78% of patients receiving multiple CSF examinations. Table X summarizes the CSF findings in 47 patients reported by Olson *et al.* In addition to the examination of CSF, myelography, CT scans, and RN scans can be helpful.

Treated or untreated, the clinical course is frequently progressive, with the development of signs and symptoms in multiple anatomical areas.

IV. TUMORS OF THE SPINAL CORD

A. Incidence and Classification

The overall incidence of spinal cord tumors is less than 15% of brain tumors. The same tumor types that occur in the brain also affect the spinal cord, although the frequency of specific tumors is strikingly different. Schwannomas and meningiomas account for approximately one-half of spinal tumors, with schwannomas being slightly more frequent; both types occur most exclusively in adult life. Gliomas constitute 20% of spinal tumors, and the majority are ependymomas with a predilection for the cauda equina. The usually cited frequency of metastatic tumors (20–25%) may be too low, especially with more successful palliation of systemic cancer. Furthermore, the incidence and frequency of metastatic tumors in any series of spinal tumors reflects the relative proportion of hospitalized patients with advanced cancer. A heterogenous group of uncommon tumors accounts for 10% of spinal tumors, with lipomas, dermoids, and hemangioblastomas predominating.

At our institution with its large brain tumor service, almost 10% of spinal tumors originate from an intracranial primary CNS tumor. The majority represent spinal subarachnoid seeding from medulloblastoma, with ependymoma, malignant astrocytoma, and germinoma following in that order.

In Table XI the distribution of various spinal tumors is expressed according to their frequency in a general hospital population.

Although different tumor types exhibit a predilection for certain spinal regions, taken altogether spinal tumors are distributed fairly evenly along the spinal axis. Approximately one-half of spinal tumors involve the thoracic spinal canal,

TABLE XI

Distribution of Spinal Tumors[a]

Tumor	Percentage
Schwannoma	25
Meningioma	20
Glioma	20
Metastatic	25
Other[b]	10

[a] From Sloof *et al.* (1964).

[b] Lipoma, dermoid, hemangioblastoma, subarachnoid seeding from primary intracranial tumor.

30% the lumbosacral spine, and the remainder the cervical spine including the foramen magnum. Schwannomas arise throughout the spine and often extend through an intervertebral foramen to acquire a dumbbell configuration. Meningiomas arise preferentially at the foramen magnum and in the thoracic spine; at both sites, they exhibit a striking dominance in females. The proximity of the mediastinum to the thoracic spine accounts for the frequency of extradural malignant pulmonary tumors in the thoracic spinal canal. Whereas astrocytomas are distributed throughout the spinal cord, the majority of ependymomas involve the conus medullarus and cauda equina. Spinal chordomas are characteristically sacral.

Further characterization of spinal tumors concerns their relationship to the spinal cord and dura mater (Table XII). The cranial dura is adhered firmly to the skull (with the exception of dural duplications of the falx and tentorium), and normally no extradural space exists between dura and skull. An entirely different anatomical relationship in the spinal canal accounts for a well-defined extradural

TABLE XII

Classification of Spinal Tumors by Their Location in Relation to the Spinal Cord and Dura Mater

Location	Usual tumor types
Extradural	Metastatic (carcinoma, lymphoma, myeloma, sarcoma), chordoma
Intradural	
Extramedullary	Schwannoma[a], meningioma
Intramedullary	Astrocytoma, ependymoma[b]

[a] May extend along nerve root into extradural and extraspinal spaces.

[b] Ependymomas originating from the filum terminale and involving the cauda equina, not intramedullary in the strictest sense, are included here by custom.

space containing epidural fat and blood vessels, and through the intervertebral foramina this extradural space communicates with adjacent extraspinal compartments, e.g., the mediastinum and retroperitoneal space. With rare exceptions, extradural tumors are metastatic, and the majority reach the extradural space through intervertebral foramina. The remaining metastatic extradural tumors represent extensions of bony metastases into the spinal canal, often in association with pathologic compression fractures and deformity of one or more vertebral bodies.

Tumors arising inside of the dural tube (intradural tumors) may originate within the spinal cord (intramedullary), or they may take origin outside the spinal cord (extramedullary). The two common extramedullary intradural tumors, schwannoma and meningioma, are attached respectively to sensory nerve roots and dura, and they involve the spinal cord by compression.

B. Neurology of Spinal Cord Tumors

A minority of cervical intramedullary tumors mimics syringomyelia, with dissociated sensory loss, weakness and wasting in the arms and hands, and variable long-tract involvement, but with this singular exception the clinical presentation of a spinal tumor does not indicate if it is extradural or intradural. The evaluation of symptoms usually reflects the tumor's rate of growth, with a history of days to a few weeks characterizing metastatic tumors, and a longer course, often many months, reflecting the slower growth of intradural tumors.

A spinal tumor produces two effects, local (focal), and distal (remote). Local effects indicate the tumor's location along the spinal axis, and distal effects reflect involvement of motor and sensory long tracts within the spinal cord.

Distal effects are common to all spinal tumors sooner or later, and symptoms and signs are confined to structures innervated below the spinal cord level of involvement. Although neurological manifestations commonly begin unilaterally, a full-blown Brown–Sequard syndrome of cord hemisection is rare. More characteristic is weakness—either spastic, if the tumor lies above the conus medullarus, or flaccid, if at or below the conus—and sensory impairment beginning in the feet. Impairment of bladder function occurs later in tumors above the conus, but may be an early manifestation of lower tumors. As a rule, the upper level of impaired long-tract function is several segments below the actual site of tumor involvement.

Local manifestation may reflect involvement of bone, pain constituting the cardinal symptom of tumors that are metastatic. Involvement of spinal roots produces pain, sensory impairment, and weakness with atrophy in the appropriate radicular distribution. Less often, involvement of spinal gray matter, either extensive pressure from extramedullary tumors or direct damage by intramedullary tumors, causes segmental sensory and motor changes.

Tumors at the foramen magnum are diagnosed incorrectly more often than spinal tumors at any other site. They can mimic multiple sclerosis, amyotrophic lateral sclerosis, and cervical disk disease, and the frequency of delayed diagnosis justifies the dictum that myelography and CT scans are indicated as diagnostic measures in any neurologic disease that can be accounted for by a lesion at or below the foramen magnum.

C. Diagnostic Tests

The diagnosis of a spinal tumor and its location along the spinal axis can be made with a high degree of accuracy on the basis of a detailed history and neurological examination. The clinical setting may provide a clue to the tumor type, e.g., a history of Hodgkin's disease or stigmata of neurofibromatasis. Plain radiographs have great diagnostic value: lytic or blastic lesions of the vertebral bodies are evident in 80% of metastatic spinal tumors; an enlarged intervertebral foramen can be associated with dumbbell-shaped schwannomas; erosion of the pedicles and vertebral bodies is common with slowly growing tumors, particularly in childhood.

The diagnostic study of greatest value is myelography. Spinal puncture below a tumor that has produced a total block of the subarachnoid space can, by suddenly changing pressure relationships, precipitate paraplegia. Consequently a spinal puncture should not be performed on any patient suspected of harboring a spinal tumor unless a neurosurgeon is available and myelography can be performed quickly in the event that there is a rapid change in neurological signs. The radiopaque contrast medium is injected by lumbar puncture unless the suspected tumor involves the cauda equina. In the majority of spinal tumors, myelography indicates not only its location within the spinal axis but also its relationship to the dura and spinal cord, e.g., intramedullary (Fig. 3). Air myelography, widely used abroad, has few advocates in this country. CT scans of the spine obtained on first generation scanners were disappointing, but the development of scanners with higher resolution and magnification has markedly increased their usefulness in the localization of spinal cord tumors. Spinal angiography may be used to supplement information obtained by myelography and CT scanning, but the indications for this procedure are limited.

Finally, what does examination of the CSF contribute to the diagnosis of spinal tumors? In practice, an isolated lumbar puncture is rarely indicated in a patient *suspected* of harboring a spinal tumor, and if the suspicion exists at all, myelography is preferable. If a lumbar puncture is performed, either alone or as a part of myelography, a Queckenstedt test is indicated if an intracranial mass has been excluded. When xanthochromic fluid is unexpectedly obtained from a spinal puncture performed on a patient suspected of non-neoplastic disease of the spinal

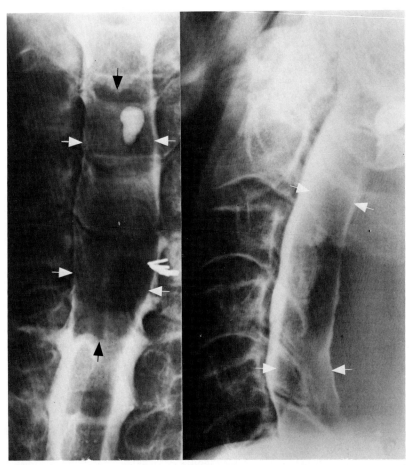

Fig. 3. Anteroposterior and lateral projections of cervical myelogram showing an expansive intramedullary tumor blocking the flow of contrast media in the subarachnoid space (arrows). (Courtesy of Dr. David Norman.)

cord, the needle should be left in place and arrangements made for emergency myelography, because the subarachnoid space collapses after CSF is removed below a spinal block, and subsequent spinal puncture may be impossible.

ACKNOWLEDGMENTS

This work was supported in part by NIH Center Grant CA-13525 and an American Cancer Society Faculty Research Award FRA-155 (VAL).

We thank Neil Buckley for editorial assistance.

REFERENCES

Adams, R. D., and Victor, M. (1977). "Principles of Neurology," pp. 586–617. McGraw-Hill, New York.

Bingas, B. (1974). *Handb. Clin. Neurol.* **17**, 136–233.

Cuneo, H. M., and Rand, C. W. (1952). "Brain Tumors of Childhood." Thomas, Springfield, Illinois.

Hildebrand, J. (1978). "Lesions of the Nervous System in Cancer Patients," EORTC Monogr. Ser., Vol. 5. Raven, New York.

Hoffman, W. F., Levin, V. A., and Wilson, C. B. (1979). *J. Neurosurg.* **50**, 624–628.

Levin, V. A., Crafts, D. C., Norman, D. M., Hoffer, P. B., Spire, J.-P., and Wilson, C. B. (1977). *J. Neurosurg.* **47**, 329–335.

Office of Biometry and Epidemiology (1977). "Survey of Intracranial Neoplasms." NINCDS, Bethesda, Maryland.

Olson, M. E., Chernik, N. L., and Posner, J. B. (1974). *Arch. Neurol. (Chicago)* **30**, 122–137.

Rubinstein, L. J. (1972). "Brain Tumors of the Central Nervous System," Fasc. 6, Atlas of Tumor Pathology, 2nd Ser. Armed Forces Inst. Pathol., Washington, D.C.

Rubinstein, L. J., and Russell, D. J. (1977). "Pathology of Tumors of the Nervous System," 4th ed. Williams & Wilkins, Baltimore, Maryland.

Sloof, J. L., Kernohan, J. W., and MacCarty, C. S. (1964). "Primary Intramedullary Tumors of the Spinal Cord and Filum Terminale." Saunders, Philadelphia, Pennsylvania.

11

GENITOURINARY CANCER
R. Bruce Bracken

I.	Introduction	200
II.	Renal Carcinoma	201
	A. Etiology	201
	B. Pathology	201
	C. Clinical Manifestations	203
	D. Diagnosis	203
	E. Staging	203
	F. Treatment	205
III.	Carcinoma of the Renal Pelvis	206
	A. Etiology	206
	B. Pathology	207
	C. Clinical Manifestations	207
	D. Diagnosis	207
	E. Staging	209
	F. Treatment	210
IV.	Carcinoma of the Ureter	210
	A. Etiology	210
	B. Treatment	210
V.	Female Urethral Carcinoma	212
	A. Etiology	212
	B. Pathology	213
	C. Clinical Manifestations	214
	D. Diagnosis	214
	E. Staging	214
	F. Treatment	214
VI.	Male Urethral Carcinoma	216
	A. Etiology	216
	B. Pathology	216
	C. Clinical Manifestations	216
	D. Diagnosis	217
	E. Staging	217
	F. Treatment	218
VII.	Penile Carcinoma	218
	A. Etiology	218
	B. Pathology	219
	C. Clinical Manifestations	219
	D. Diagnosis	221

CANCER AND CHEMOTHERAPY, VOL. II
199
ISBN 0-12-197802-8

	E.	Staging	221
	F.	Treatment	221
VIII.		Testicular Tumors	222
	A.	Etiology	222
	B.	Pathology	222
	C.	Histological Types	223
	D.	Clinical Manifestations	226
	E.	Diagnosis	227
	F.	Staging	227
	G.	Treatment	227
IX.		Bladder Cancer	231
	A.	Etiology	231
	B.	Pathology	232
	C.	Diagnosis	233
	D.	Staging	233
	E.	Treatment	234
X.		Prostate Cancer	237
	A.	Etiology	237
	B.	Pathology	237
	C.	Diagnosis	238
	D.	Staging	238
	E.	Treatment	239
		References	241

I. INTRODUCTION

Each year, almost 110,000 Americans develop urological neoplasms. In the past, results of single-modality therapy had seemingly reached a plateau. The introduction in 1970 of active combination chemotherapy for patients with germinal testicular cancer revolutionized the field of urological oncology. The success of mutlimodal therapy for patients with testis tumors has become a model on which to pattern therapy for other genitourinary (GU) malignancies. At present, in addition to testicular tumors, effective chemotherapy is successfully combined with surgery and irradiation only in bladder cancer. Prostatic, adult renal, penile, and urethral tumors have not yielded to chemotherapy yet, so that treatment of these neoplasms still depends on surgery and irradiation.

Refinement in the treatment of all GU tumors during the 1970s was made with a firm basis in the pathology of these malignancies, augmented by improved clinical staging afforded by improved lymphangiography and angiography, and by the addition of sonography and CT scanning.

The treatment of most stages of most urologic neoplasms impairs sexual function. True rehabilitation of the GU-cancer patient will require methods to assess, preserve, and restore this important function.

At present, we are in an exciting period and can approach the patient who has GU cancer and offer the combined expertise of the GU pathologist, radiologist, chemotherapist, radiologist, and urologist.

II. RENAL CARCINOMA

A. Etiology

Renal carcinoma strikes approximately 15,000 Americans per year, and over 6000 die from this malignancy. These tumors account for 86–89% of all renal malignancies. Etiologic factors include a possible increased incidence in male smokers. There is an increased incidence in the Scandinavian countries and in countries whose people ingest diets high in fats, oils, milk, and sugar. There is a low incidence in Japan, South America, and Eastern Europe.

B. Pathology

Electron-microscope studies have demonstrated that renal carcinomas arise from the epithelium of the proximal renal tubule (Bennington and Beckwith, 1975). The histological, electron-microscopic, and gross similarities between adenomas and carcinomas suggest that adenomas are merely small cancers. Renal parenchymal tumors are rarely recognized until they reach a size sufficient either to distort the renal outline or to impinge upon the collecting system (Fig. 1). Generally speaking, these lesions must reach a diameter of at least 5 cm before they can be consistently demonstrated on intravenous pyelogram. When a tumor has reached this size prior to its recognition, a high rate of metastases is hardly surprising at the time of diagnosis. Histologically, both adenoma and carcinoma are comprised of epithelial cells that have either clear or granular cytoplasm. Histological evidence of vascular invasion occurs in up to 75% of renal carcinomas, accounting for the high incidence of hematogenous metastases (55% pulmonary, 35% liver, and 33% osseous) once tumor dissemination occurs.

Lymphatic metastases, which occur in 35% of patients, are most characteristically noted to occur in the periaortic lymph nodes from the level of the renal vessels superiorly, to the bifurcation of the common iliac artery inferiorly. However, both mediastinal and supraclavicular lymph nodes may be the first site of lymphatic metastases in some patients.

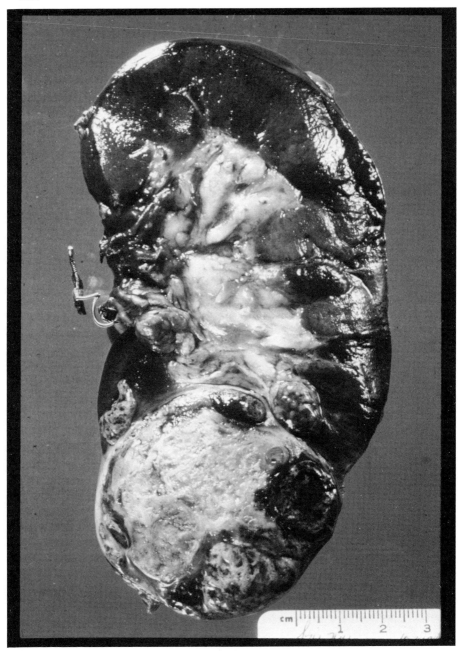

Fig. 1. Typical renal carcinoma.

C. Clinical Manifestations

Although most patients have symptoms, diagnosis may be made in 30–45% of patients when a renal mass is encountered in an individual who is asymptomatic. (Medellin, 1973). Anemia, weight loss, and weakness all occur in about one-third of patients; 61% have abdominal pain or gastrointestinal complaints, 60% have hematuria, 50% have flank pain, 33% complain of a mass, 17% have fever, 4% have erythrocytosis, and 2–4% of patients present with fever of unknown origin. Acute varicocele, hepatopathy, amyloidosis, neuromyopathy, hypertension, hypercalcemia, gonadotropin production, or an unusual cutaneous or subcutaneous lesion all herald the tumor occasionally. The classic triad of hematuria, mass, and flank pain occurs in 15% of patients, and one-half of these patients will already have metastatic disease. Distant metastases, which are present at diagnosis in 30% of patients, may cause the initial symptoms.

D. Diagnosis

A typical angiographic appearance is all that is necessary to establish a diagnosis of renal carcinoma (Fig. 2), and when this is present a tissue diagnosis is not required prior to starting treatment (Medellin, 1973). When the radiographic appearance is atypical, diagnosis is more uncertain, but in these cases a decision for definitive therapy should still be made on clinical grounds alone. We are unclear how "exploration" of the kidney can increase the accuracy of a thorough preoperative evaluation, and feel that an incisional biopsy reduces the likelihood of achieving local control with surgery when a malignancy is present. Occasionally, the diagnosis is first suspected when the biopsy of a metastatic deposit is more hemorrhagic than usual, histologically consistent with renal carcinoma, and special stains demonstrate the presence of glycogen.

E. Staging

Pathological staging is all that we have available for use at present to evaluate the status of the primary tumor. Unfortunately, angiographic staging is accurate in only 36% of cases (Bracken and Jonsson, 1979), and computerized tomography and ultrasonography are still inadequately evaluated as staging procedures. We prefer a 1-to-4 staging system (Johnson *et al.*, 1976a): Stage I tumors are confined within the renal capsule; stage II extend into perinephric fat but are contained with Gerota's fascia; in stage III there is gross evidence of venous or lyphatic invasion; and in stage IV there is local extension into adjacent organs, exclusive of the adrenal gland or distant metastases.

Patients should be assessed after taking a careful history by physical examination. The metastatic evaluation includes a complete blood count, urinalysis,

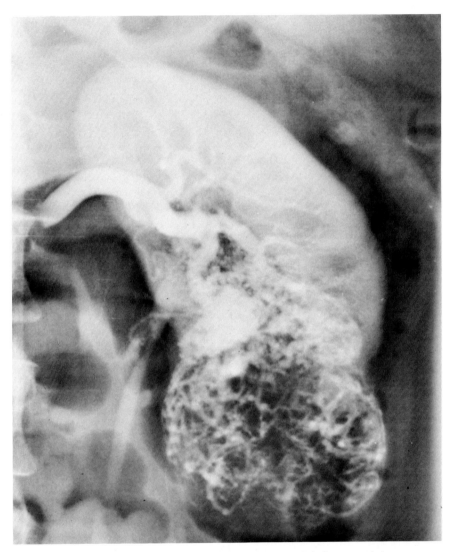

Fig. 2. Angiogram of a renal carcinoma with characteristic hypervascularity.

SMA-12, chest X ray, and bone scan (Fig. 3). An intravenous pyelogram, aorto-gram, bilateral selective renal arteriorgram, coeliac axis angiogram, and inferior vena cavogram with ipsilateral renal venogram (Medellin, 1973) are essential to make the diagnosis and estimate the extent of the primary tumor. Occasionally angiography defines distant metastases (Fig. 3). Both CT scan and ultrasonog-raphy are helpful adjuncts to these more established examinations, and perhaps with experience may reduce the need for angiography in selected patients.

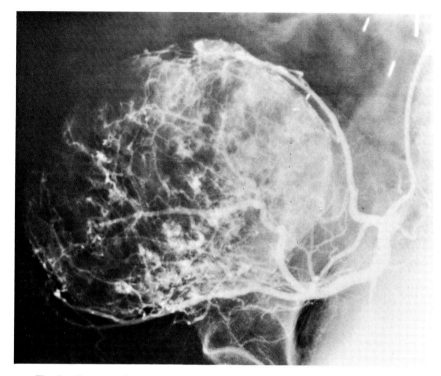

Fig. 3. Hypervascular angiographic appearance of a large metastatis to the right ilium.

F. Treatment

1. Localized Disease

Treatment for stage I, II, and III is radical nephrectomy, an operation that consists of early ligation of the renal pedicle and excision of the kidney and perinephric fat inside an intact capsule of Gerota's fascia (Johnson *et al.*, 1976a). Although paraaortic lymphadenectomy has been included along with radical nephrectomy, we have abandoned the procedure and feel that the added surgery has not improved survival in these patients. Heroic surgery to remove tumors that extend into the renal vein or inferior vena cava enjoys much popularity today, probably because there is no other effective form of treatment. However, the development of adjuvant therapy will be required to make this an attractive mainstay in our therapeutic armamentarium.

The disappointing impact that radiation therapy has had upon treatment results may be due in part to the lack of an accurate clinical staging system upon which to base preoperative therapy. It is our policy to restrict radiation therapy to patients who have either microscopic or gross tumor remaining after nephrectomy in either the renal fossa or periaortic lymph nodes. At present, there are no chemotherapeutic agents active enough to justify their use as an adjunct to therapy (Johnson *et al.*, 1976a).

2. *Metastatic Disease*

Treatment of metastatic disease remains truly frustrating. A variety of chemotherapeutic agents have been tried singly and in combination without success, and at present chemotherapy can be considered purely investigational (Johnson *et al.*, 1976a). Some authors have concluded that medroxyprogesterone acetate yields up to a 16% partial response rate, with duration of response varying between 3 and 36 months. However, recent prospective randomized clinical trials have failed to substantiate this beneficial effect. Nephrectomy alone cannot be justified in the face of pulmonary, liver, cerebral, or multiple osseous metastases because it has not improved survival in these patients (Johnson *et al.*, 1975). When nephrectomy was used in patients who have solitary osseous metastases, median survival was extended from 10.1 to 23 months (D. A. Swanson, personal communication).

The only significant therapy at present for patients with metastatic disease is available solely when the primary tumor remains *in situ*. Treatment consists of the combination of percutaneous renal artery embolization followed 4 to 7 days later by nephrectomy and Depo-Provera (400 mg I.M. twice weekly) (Bracken *et al.*, 1975). This has resulted in a 61% response rate (20% complete, 16% partial, 3% mixed, 23% stable), in patients with pulmonary or subcutaneous metastases. The responses frequently require 8–12 weeks to become evident, and perhaps this delay explains why patients with a shorter life expectancy (e.g., those with CNS, hepatic, multiple osseous, and extensive pulmonary metastases) fail to respond to therapy. The explanation for response is presumed to be an alteration in the host–tumor interaction. Whatever the mechanism, none of the components of the combination used alone—namely, infarction, nephrectomy, or Provera—induces consistent responses.

III. CARCINOMA OF THE RENAL PELVIS

A. Etiology

Carcinoma of the renal pelvis comprises 8–9% of renal tumors. In general, the etiology is similar to that described in the section on bladder cancer, except that Johansson *et al.* (1976) have noted an 8% incidence of upper-tract tumors in a series of patients with phenacetin nephritis. Squamous carcinomas are frequently associated with a long history of upper-tract calculus disease. Most interesting is the high incidence of upper-tract transitional tumors in patients who have a form of interstitial nephritis called endemic nephropathy (Petkovic, 1972). This association occurs in the Balkan countries, in rural villagers who reside in river valleys. These patients have a high incidence of low-grade, noninvasive papillary tumors that have a long stalk, and are therefore frequently suited to local excision. The benign histological features, the 10% incidence of bilaterality, and the associated nephritis that usually leads to death from renal failure after a long illness, dictate that surgery be conservative whenever feasible. It is the lack of these features in most other series that generally compels us to be more aggressive surgically in this country (Johnson *et al.*, 1974).

B. Pathology

Eighty-five percent of renal pelvic tumors are transitional-cell carcinomas, 14% squamous carcinomas, and 1% are adenocarcinomas. A history of previous bladder cancer may be present but if not, it may be anticipated to occur in 30–40% of individuals, and most frequently within a 2-year period following diagnosis (Johnson *et al.*, 1974). The risk of bladder cancer necessitates regular cystoscopic follow-up. Low-grade superficial tumors rarely spread, whereas high-grade invasive lesions invade the kidney (Fig. 4), perirenal tissues and great vessels, and metastasize most frequently to the lung, liver, and bone (Johnson *et al.*, 1974).

C. Clinical Manifestations

Most renal pelvic tumors occur in patients between ages 40 and 70, and there is a 3:1 male-to-female ratio. Hematuria occurs in 95%, pain in 40%, abdominal or flank mass in 2–15%, and vesical irritative symptoms occur in 15%.

D. Diagnosis

Renal pelvic tumors may present a diagnostic problem that cannot be resolved until the gross specimen has been pathologically assessed. However, these tumors may be clinically anticipated because they usually produce some type of radiographic abnormality such that a good-quality normal intravenous pyelogram and retrograde pyelogram effectively rule out the neoplasm. Failure to visualize a portion or all of the renal pelvis on intravenous pyelogram occurs in 75% of cases, and a filling defect as defined by retrograde pyelography in a similar percentage.

During retrograde pyelography, if the urologist obtains urine and washings from the renal pelvis, a cytologic diagnosis of carcinoma may be made in up to 61% of cases, whereas the diagnostic accuracy of cytology from voided urine is much less, ranging from 33–78%. The Gill brush technique (Gill *et al.*, 1973) has increased the accuracy of preoperative diagnosis to almost 100%. In this

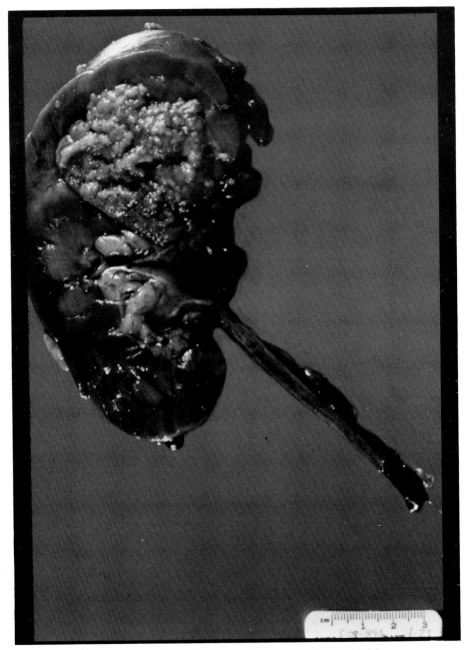

Fig. 4. Gross specimen of a transitional-cell tumor of the renal pelvis.

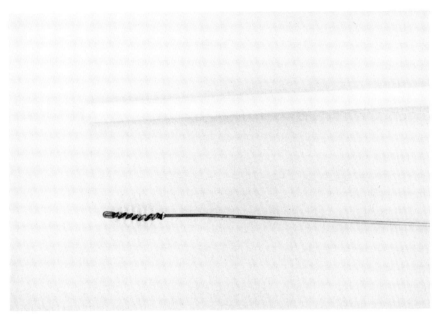

Fig. 5. Brush that is passed through a ureteral catheter that has an end hole, for obtaining a cytologic specimen from upper tract abnormalities that are suggestive of urothelial neoplasm.

technique (which combines retrograde pyelography and cytology), a small brush (Fig. 5) is advanced to the renal pelvic lesion through a retrograde catheter under radiographic monitoring, the suspicious area is brushed, and the renal pelvis is irrigated with saline. Both the irrigating fluid and the brush (which may have entrapped tissue fragments) are then examined by the cytologist.

E. Staging

The staging system used for both renal pelvic and ureteral tumors is similar, and both suffer from being pathological rather than clinical systems (Grabstald *et al.*, 1971). Group I are histologically benign papillomas; group II are low-stage carcinomas that are noninvasive; group III are high-stage tumors confined to the kidney (or for ureteral tumors, extension locally into periureteric fat); and group IV are high-stage tumors with distant metastases. If there is a concomitant bladder tumor, the subgroup A is designated and if there is not, this tumor falls into subgroup B.

Patients with either renal pelvic or ureteral tumors should have a careful history taken and be given a thorough physical examination. Metastatic evalua- tion consists of a complete blood count, SMA-12/60, urinalysis, urine cytology, chest X ray, and bone scan. The renal lesion is evaluated by intravenous pyelogram, retrograde pyelography, renal pelvic cytology and, when necessary, by cytology obtained via the Gill brush technique.

F. Treatment

Treatment consists of nephroureterectomy with excision of a cuff of juxtaureteral vesical mucosa. This is most readily accomplished if after nephrectomy the distal ureter is removed as described by Howerton *et al.* (1970). In this procedure, a ureteral catheter is passed through the remaining ureter until it coils up in the bladder. The end of the catheter is tied to the cut end of the distal ureter. A small anterior cystotomy is made and the coiled ureteral catheter is brought out of the bladder through it. Next, the catheter is gently pulled, and in so doing the remaining ureter is turned inside out upon itself and the entire structure is delivered into the bladder lumen. Finally, the ureter and adjacent vesical mucosa are excised and the mucosal defect sutured is closed.

Prognosis is related to tumor stage and grade with 5-year survival rates as follows: 83% with noninvasive tumors; 33% with high-stage lesions; 100% with grade I tumors; 66% with grade II tumors; and 31% with grade III tumors (Johnson *et al.*, 1974). When lymphatic, vascular, or renal parenchymal invasion occur, survival is reduced to approximately 1 year.

Neither the incidence of lymphatic metastases nor the value of lymphadenectomy is known for these tumors, and our current practice is to omit lymphadenectomy. Postoperative radiation therapy should be considered in non-metastatic high-stage or high-grade tumors, in hopes of improving local control rates. Chemotherapy for metastatic disease consists of combination, cyclophosphamide, Adriamycin , and *cis*-platinum, as discussed in the section on bladder cancer.

IV. CARCINOMA OF THE URETER

A. Etiology

Primary ureteral tumors make up 1% of upper-tract tumors, with 85% occuring in patients between 50 and 70 years of age. There is a 2:1 male-to-female predominance. Seventy-five percent occur in the lower one-third of the ureter. Pathology (Fig. 6), symptoms and signs, staging, and diagnostic evaluation (Fig. 7) are similar to those described under the section on tumors of the renal pelvis.

B. Treatment

The treatment of choice consists of nephroureterectomy including a cuff of normal bladder mucosa adjacent to the ureteral meatus. A distal ureterectomy

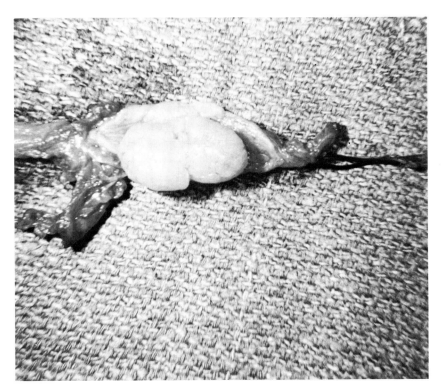

Fig. 6. Gross specimen of ureteral carcinoma.

and ureteral reimplantation should be considered (a) whenever a lower one-third ureteral tumor has a papillary appearance on intravenous pyelogram or retrograde pyelography and there is no significant hydronephrosis; or (b) when a grade I, stage A lesion protrudes from the lower ureter into the bladder lumen. The lower ureter should be exposed extraperitoneally, and if palpation discloses no evidence of ureteral muscle invasion or regional metastases, distal ureterectomy and excision of bladder cuff is performed. Provided frozen-section examination confirms that the ureteral tumor is low grade and noninvasive, reimplantation should proceed. Mobilization of both the distal ureter and bladder, with fixation of the bladder to the psoas muscle (psoas hitch), should be performed whenever necessary to eliminate tension across the ureteroneocystostomy suture line. Unfortunately, in most cases the favorable pathological and anatomical circumstances required for distal ureterectomy and reimplantation are not encountered; then nephroureterectomy including the bladder cuff should be the standard procedure (Fig. 8). Prognosis depends on the tumor stage, and 5-year survival rates range between 46 and 91% in stage A, 10 and 43% in stage B, and 0% in stages C and D.

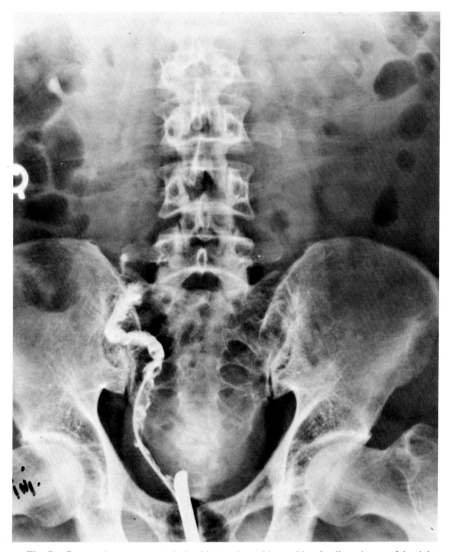

Fig. 7. Retrograde ureterogram obtained in a patient with transitional-cell carcinoma of the right ureter.

V. FEMALE URETHRAL CARCINOMA

A. Etiology

Urethral carcinoma in the female represents 0.02% of all malignant disease in women. No specific etiological factors have been determined; urethral diver-

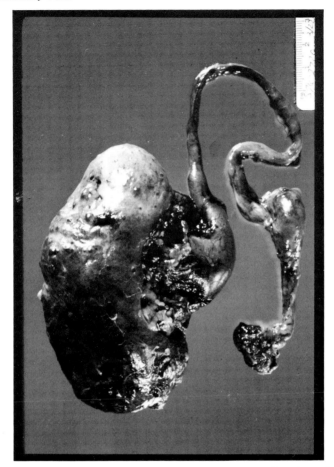

Fig. 8.   Nephroureterectomy specimen in a patient with transitional-cell carcinoma in the lower third of the ureter.

ticula, urethral caruncles, chronic urinary tract infection, urethritis, prior childbirth, and primary tumors of the bladder, vulva, cervix, or vagina all appear to be unrelated. A review of 81 patients treated at the M.D. Anderson Hospital and Tumor Institute will form the basis of this section (Bracken *et al.*, 1976).

B. Pathology

Squamous carcinoma accounts for 41% of these tumors, transitional carcinomas 30%, adenocarcinomas 23%, undifferentiated tumors 4%, and melanomas 2%. We feel that these tumors, with the exception of melanoma, are very similar in their natural history and radiosensitivity, and so should be considered identical for treatment purposes. The neoplasm originates from the epithclial or glandular structures of the urethra, then grows into the lamina propria and urethral muscle. With further growth, tumor extends into the vagina, bladder base, labia, and clitoris. At diagnosis, regional lymphatic metastases to the inguinal, external iliac, and obturator lymph nodes were present in 19% of patients in our study, and a similar percentage developed evidence of nodal metastases during the treatment and follow-up periods. Distant metastases occur late in the course of the disease and are most frequently noted in the lung, liver, and bone.

C. Clinical Manifestations

Symptoms of urethral carcinoma consisted of urethral bleeding in 56%, symptoms of urethral obstruction in 38%, dysuria in 30%, frequency in 25%, mass at the introitus 21%, perineal pain in 10%, vaginal discharge in 4.8%, incontinence in 3.6%, and dyspareunia in 1%. Physical findings consisted of the visible and palpatory evidence of the primary tumor or its metastases (Fig. 9).

D. Diagnosis

Diagnosis is preferably made by transurethral biopsy, unless a particular anterior urethral lesion lends itself to easy local excision.

E. Staging

The staging system proposed by Grabstald *et al.* (1966) both parallels the pathogenesis of urethral tumors and provides a guide to treatment and prognosis. In stage O, tumor is confined to the mucosa; in stage A, there is infiltration of the lamina propria; in stage B, there is infiltration of the urethral muscle; in stage C, there is periurethral extension to the bladder base, vagina, labia, and clitoris; in stage D, there is regional lymphatic or distant metastatic disease.

Clinical staging requires a thorough history and physical examination, and the metastatic evaluation consists of a complete blood count, SMA-12, bone scan, chest X ray, intravenous pyelogram, and bilateral pedal lymphangiogram. Urethroscopy and examination of the urethra under anesthesia are mandatory to best assess the local extent of tumor growth.

F. Treatment

In our experience, single-modality treatment had a prohibitively high incidence of local failure, which ranged from 22% in small tumors treated with radiation and surgery, through 46% in patients treated with radiation therapy

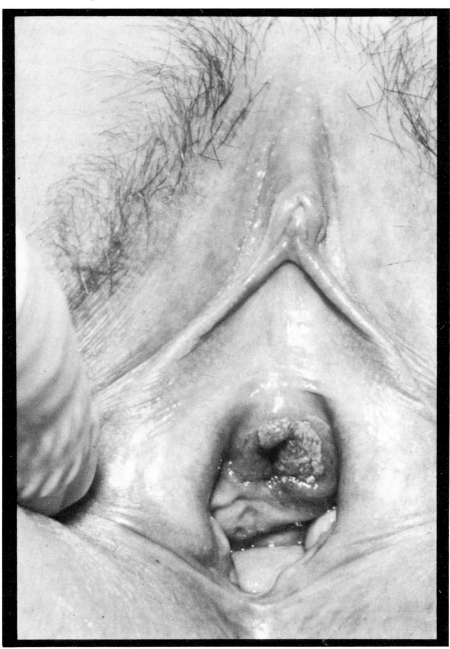

Fig. 9. Carcinoma of the female urethra.

alone, to 64% in patients treated with surgery alone (Bracken *et al.*, 1976). Once local failure was recognized, only 3 of 33 patients were salvaged by secondary forms of treatment. In attempting to improve local control, we have changed our treatment and now combine radiation and surgery as follows: In all stage O, A, and some small B lesions, local resection with 5000 rad interstitial radiation therapy; in B and C lesions, 5000 rad external radiation therapy through a four-field-box technique, followed in 6 weeks by cystectomy and limited vulvectomy; when inguinal lymph node metastases are present, bilateral staged therapeutic groin dissections are added; when pelvic lymph node metastases are present, patients receive definitive radiation therapy. It is too early to assess the results of this change in treatment policy.

When distant metastases occur, no specific type of chemotherapy has had an adequate trial. Our current recommendation would be the combination of cyclophosphamide, Adriamycin, and *cis*-platinum as described under the section on bladder cancer.

VI. MALE URETHRAL CARCINOMA

A. Etiology

Although the male urethra is a common site of benign disorders, it is rare to encounter a neoplasm of this structure, and fewer than 400 primary tumors have been described. The etiology is poorly understood, except to note that one-third of patients have had a past history of gonoccal urethritis, and many patients have had chronic urethral strictures. A review of patients at the M.D. Anderson Hospital and Tumor Institute will provide the basis for the opinions expressed in this section (Johnson *et al.*, 1976a).

B. Pathology

Squamous carcinoma is the most common tumor and is present in 67% of cases, with transitional cell carcinoma noted in 16%, adenocarcinoma and undifferentiated carcinoma each 7%, and melanomas reported occasionally. In spite of the adjacent vascular corpus spongiosum, local growth and regional lymphatic metastases to inguinal, external iliac, and obturator nodes are usually well established before hematogenous metastases manifest.

C. Clinical Manifestations

Clinical symptoms are mostly related to urethral obstruction and consist of slowing or spraying of the urinary stream, urinary tract infection, urethral or

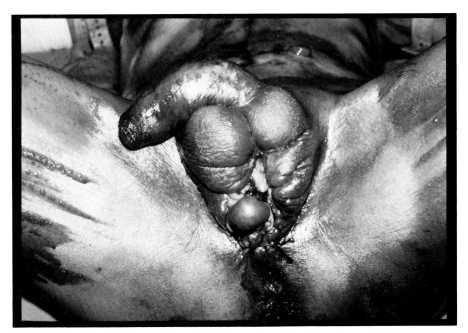

Fig. 10.   Carcinoma of the male bulbous urethra with urethrocutaneous fistula.

periurethral mass, hematuria, and urethral discharge or bleeding. Local signs consist of a urethral mass (Fig. 10), single or multiple urethrocutaneous fistulae (watering-pot perineum), periurethral abscess, or signs of malignant inguinal lymphadenopathy.

D. Diagnosis

Diagnosis is established by transurethral biopsy (preferred) or open biopsy of the primary tumor.

E. Staging

We have divided our cases into (a) those confined within the corpus spongiosum; (b) those extending locally into the adjacent structures of the penis, perineal musculature, and inferior pubic rami; (c) those with regional lymphatic metastases; and (d) those with distant metastatic disease.

Clinical evaluation consists of careful history-taking and physical examination, and metastatic evaluation consists of a complete blood count, SMA-12/60, chest X ray, bone scan, intravenous pyelogram, and bilateral pedal lymphangiogram. Endoscopic evaluation and bimanual examination under anesthesia are essential to assess the extent of the local lesion.

F. Treatment

1. Anterior Tumors

Treatment is dependent upon the location of the tumor. Anterior lesions (distal to the penoscrotal junction) are treated by either partial penectomy or total penectomy and perineal urethrostomy—the decision dependent upon the length of the remaining penis after the lesion is excised with a 2-cm margin. When the remaining penil length is sufficient to direct the urinary stream with the patient standing, a partial penectomy is indicated, but when the remaining urethra is too short for satisfactory voiding, a total penectomy with perineal urethrostomy is recommended. With either operation, local tumor control should approach 90%. Staged therapeutic inguinal lymphadenectomies are performed whenever lymph nodes metastases are present, but prophylactic dissections should be avoided.

2. Posterior Tumors

Posterior urethral tumors often invade beyond the urethra into the perineal musculature, and one-third invade the inferior pubic rami. Another one-third are so extensive locally and have so much associated inflammation and infection that they are not amenable to definitive treatment. Our initial experience showed that single-modality therapy failed to control any posterior tumors, and this caused us to change our treatment recommendations to a combination of radiation and surgery whenever feasible. At present, we recommend careful staging, and if no evidence of distant metastases is found, an ileal-conduit urine diversion is performed. During the postoperative convalescent period, a 2000-rad tumor dose is delievered to the perineum, and this should be followed immediately by anterior exenteration with *en bloc* resection of the symphysis pubis, both inferior pubic rami, and the entire urethra and phallus. Four patients have been managed satisfactorily by this technique, and all are free of disease for a minimum of 2 years postoperatively.

3. Palliation

For the one-third of patients whose posterior tumors are not suited to definitive therapy, palliative measures such as incision and drainage of abscesses, suprapubic cystostomy, and neurosurgical measures to control pain may be of palliative benefit to the patient and ease nursing care.

VII. PENILE CARCINOMA

A. Etiology

Cancer of the penis accounts for 2% of all malignancies of the genitourinary tract, but represents less than 0.1% of all male malignancies (Johnson, 1973).

TABLE I

Geographic Incidence of Penile Cancer

Indonesia	37.8%	India	10.0%
China	27.9%	Europe	4.9%
Mainland	24.5%	Puerto Rico	3.4%
Taiwan	3.5%	Venezuela	2.8%
Burma	24.2%	Great Britain	1.3%
Ceylon	13.7%	Uganda	1-2%
		United States	1-2%

This tumor's geographic incidence is truly fascinating, because although the incidence in the United States is 1 new case per 500,000 in the male population annually, this tumor is extremely common in many relatively undeveloped countries in which circumcision is not practiced and poor hygiene abounds (Table I). Although no specific etiological factors are obvious, smegma is carcinogenic, and the association of phymosis with 75-90% of cases suggests this to be a good etiological possibility. Inflammation and a history of veneral disease (27%) are common in the background of patients with cancer of the penis. The disease virtually does not strike Jews or Muhammadans, presumably because they practice circumcision shortly after birth. If the current stand against routine circumcision taken by the American Academy of Pediatrics and other groups is followed, one wonders how this will affect the future incidence of penile cancer in this country.

B. Pathology

Most penile cancers are squamous carcinomas and grossly they may be nodular, exophytic (Fig. 11), ulcerative, or fungating. By decreasing order of frequency, the common sites of occurrence are the glans, coronal sulcus, prepuce, and shaft. Bowen's disease and erythroplasia of Queyrat are forms of carcinoma *in situ* and therefore are malignant, not premalignant, lesions. Tumors directly invade the adjacent tissues of the penis and urethra, or they metastasize by emboli to the inguinal or external iliac lymph nodes. Associated infection of the primary tumor may cause reactive hyperplasia or frank suppuration of regional lymph nodes, and so all lymphadenopathy need not be malignant.

C. Clinical Manifestations

The age of onset ranges from 2.5 to 91 years, with a median of 65 years. Symptoms consist of the penile lesion alone in 41% of patients, penile discharge in 37%, pain in 27%, bleeding in 16%, and dysuria in 11% (Johnson, 1973). Physical findings are related to the primary tumor (nodular, ulcerative, fungat-

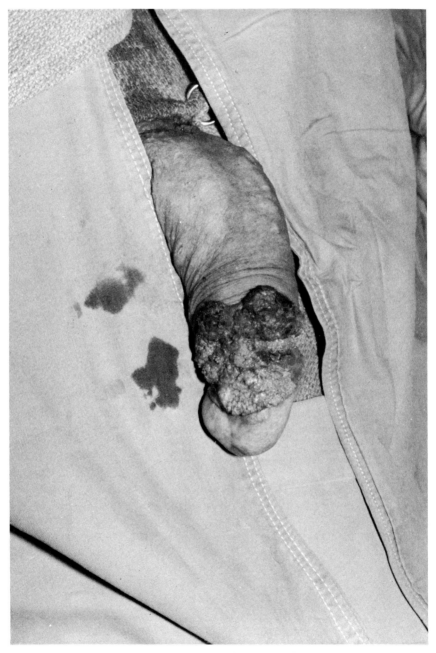

Fig. 11. Gross appearance of carcinoma of the penis.

ing, autoamputating), and in addition, almost 80% of these patients will have clinical inguinal lymphadenopathy. In 50% of patients this lymphadenopathy will resolve 4–6 weeks after the inflamed, infected primary lesion has been excised, because it is a reaction to the local infection.

D. Diagnosis

Diagnosis is proved by biopsy and frozen section. Prior to biopsy a patient should be informed and consent to whatever definitive surgery is required should the biopsy demonstrate carcinoma. Prior to biopsy, a tourniquet should be placed at the base of the penis to minimize chances for tumor-cell dissemination by the procedure. After biopsy, the instruments, gloves, and surgical drapes should be changed and the tumor covered with a sterile condom to prevent implantation of tumor cells into the open wound during penectomy.

E. Staging

We prefer a 1–3 staging system: Stage I is tumor confined to the penis; stage II is clinical suspicion of regional lymph node metastases; stage III is disseminated disease.

A careful history should be taken, a thorough physical examination should be given, and patients should have a complete blood count, SMA-12/60, chest X ray, intravenous pyelogram, and pedal lymphangiogram. The status of the inguinal lymph nodes is determined solely by palpation, and this part of the physical examination is obviously most important in staging.

F. Treatment

1. Stage I

For stage I patients, partial penectomy—excising at least a 2-cm margin of normal penis proximal to the tumor—is the treatment of choice when the remaining penis is long enough to direct the urinary stream while the patient is standing. If adequate excision would set the urethra too close to the symphysis pubis or scrotum so that clean urination would be impossible from a standing position, total penectomy should be recommended. The 5-year survival rate from surgery is 65% and local tumor control is 90%. Definitive radiation has been plagued by a 30–50% incidence of local recurrence and by painful radiation ulcers that may require biopsy to differentiate them from recurrent disease.

Clinical experience suggests that examination of the groin will diagnose 90% of patients who have inguinal lymph node metastases present at the time of examination. We feel the potential morbidity of groin dissection hardly justifies prophylactic inguinal lymphadenectomy in all patients to pick up the 10% of patients whose positive nodes are missed at the original examination. Furthermore, it is suggested by literature that survival potential is not reduced if lymphadenectomy is delayed until malignant inguinal nodes become clinically evident.

2. Stage II

Patients with stage II lesions should undergo the same treatment for the primary tumor as described for stage I. Following this, staged inguinal lymphadenectomies are performed because lymphatic drainage from the penis is bilateral. The 5-year survival in stage II is 20%.

3. Stage III

The experience with chemotherapy for metastatic penile cancer has been limited and so remains both individualized and investigational. Bleomycin has shown good responses in localized cases but has been unsatisfactory for the treatment of metastatic disease. (Ichikawa et al., 1969). A combination of bleomycin, vincristine, cyclophosphamide, methotrexate, and 5-fluorouracil has produced some partial but no complete responses (M. L. Samuels, personal communication). A. Yagoda (personal communication) reported partial responses in 6 of 10 with the use of cis-platinum.

VIII. TESTICULAR TUMORS

A. Etiology

For most physicians, testicular tumors are an interesting but rarely encountered malignancy (Mostofi and Price, 1973). The etiology is not understood. Factors such as trauma, heredity, and atrophy, although suggested, have not been substantiated. Six to eleven percent of testicular tumors occur in cryptorchid individuals (80% in the maldescended testis, 20% in the normally descended member) who have between a 20 and 40% greater chance than a normal individual to develop a testis tumor—a risk that may be reduced by orchidopexy prior to age 7.

B. Pathology

1. General

The current U.S. classification of testicular tumors is shown in Table II (Mostofi and Price, 1973). Because combinations of different tumors occur in at

TABLE II

Pathological Classification of Testicular Tumors

Tumors showing one histological pattern
Seminoma
  Typical seminoma
  Anaplastic seminoma
  Spermatocytic seminoma
Embryonal carcinoma
  Embryonal carcinoma—adult
  Polyembryoma
  Embryonal carcinoma—infantile
Choriocarcinoma
Teratoma
  Mature
  Immature
Tumors showing more than one histological pattern
Embryonal carcinoma and teratoma (teratocarcinoma)
Others

---

least 40% of cases, clinicians prefer the grouping system shown in Table III
(Dixon and Moore, 1952) as a more practical guide to staging and treatment.
Because of the high percentage of mixed elements, each tumor must be step-
sectioned to ensure recognition of all existing components.

C. Histological Types

1. Seminomas

These are the most common pure lesion (Fig. 12) and occur in a slightly older
patient population. They have not been reported in prepubertal patients. Since
seminomas are radiosensitive, they are generally treated by radiation therapy.
There are three separate histological varieties of seminoma—classic, anaplastic,
and spermatocytic.

TABLE III

Classification of Germinal Testicular Tumors[a]

Group I	Seminoma, pure
Group II	Embryonal carcinoma, pure or with seminoma
Group III	Teratoma, pure or with seminoma
Group IV	Teratoma with embryonal carcinoma, choriocarcinoma, or seminoma
Group V	Choriocarcinoma, pure or with seminoma and/or embryonal carcinoma

[a] After Dixon and Moore (1952).

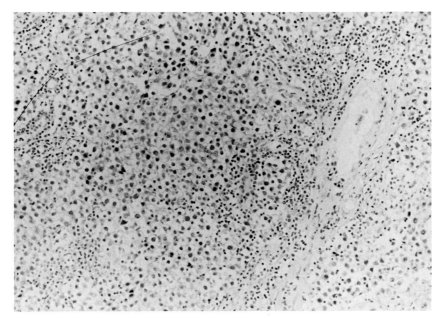

Fig. 12. Histological section of seminoma.

2. Embryonal Carcinomas

These are classically separated into infant and adult types. The infantile form (Fig. 13), also known as the clear cell adenocarcinoma, endodermal sinus tumor, and yolk sac tumor, produces alpha-fetoprotein in both adults and children. This lesion makes up 60% of testis tumors in childhood, in whom the overall incidence of metastases is about 25%. However, when metastases occur the hematogenous route is more common (60%) than the lymphatic (40%). Adult embryonal carcinomas are more likely to metastasize than the infantile form, but do so generally by way of the lymphatics, with only about 25% having initial hematogenous dissemination.

3. Mature Teratomas

These make up 1–9% of adult series (Fig. 14), in whom the malignant tumor spreading predominantly via the lymphatics. This lesion constitutes 40% of testis tumors in children less than 10 years of age, in whom it is benign.

4. Pure Choriocarcinoma

This makes up 1–4% of adult series. Both syncytiotrophoblastic and cyto-trophoblastic elements are required for diagnosis. The syncytiotrophoblastic cell is responsible for the elaboration of human chorionic gonadotropin. The characteristic mechanism of tumor dissemination is hematogenous, although regional

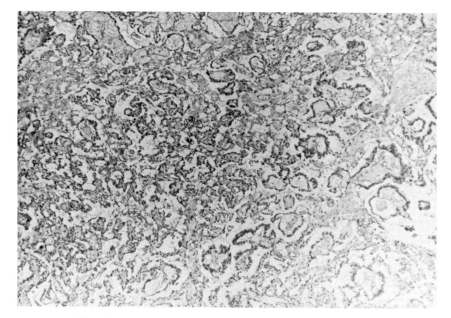

Fig. 13. Histological section of embryonal carcinoma, infantile type.

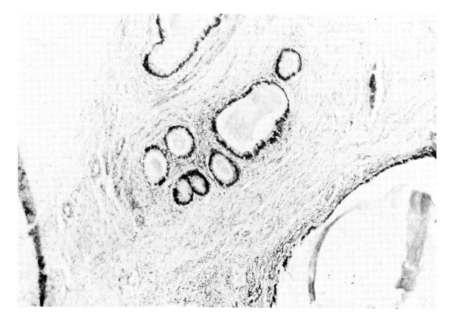

Fig. 14. Histological section of teratoma.

lymphatic metastases occur in virtually all patients. These tumors do not occur in childhood (Fig. 15).

5. Mixed Tumors

Forty percent of primary germinal testicular tumors are mixed lesions, with the most common combination being teratocarcinoma. This occurs in from 9 to 32% of all series and spread is most commonly via the lymphatics, with only 7% having initial hematogenous metastases.

D. Clinical Manifestations

Testicular tumors occur with an incidence of 2 to 3 per 100,000 males annually, and are the second most common neoplasm and neoplastic cause of death in men between the ages of 20 and 34. These tumors are even more uncommon in blacks. Symptoms consist of scrotal swelling present in 74–91% of cases, testicular pain in 13–49%, a history of testicular trauma in 6–21%, and a history of maldescent in 6–11%. One to eight percent are asymptomatic. Symptoms of metastatic disease herald the tumor in 4–14% of cases. Physical signs include increased testicular weight, firmness and nodularity, with an associated hydrocele present in 5–10% of patients. Symptoms of metastatic disease include supraclavicular adenopathy, gynecomastia, abdominal mass, backache, and con-

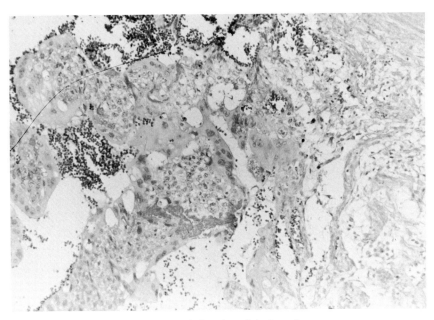

Fig. 15.   Histological section of choriocarcinoma.

stitutional symptoms such as weight loss, anorexia, or shortness of breath
(Johnson *et al.*, 1976b).

E. Diagnosis

If the diagnosis is clinically certain, it may be proved by an inguinal orchiectomy performed after ligation and incision of the spermatic cord at the internal
inguinal ring prior to manipulation of the testis (Fig. 16). If the diagnosis is less
obvious clinically, the testis should be explored or biopsied in a fashion identical
to that described except that the veins and lymphatics of the spermatic cord are
first occluded by means of an atraumatic clamp or tourniquet to prevent tumor
dissemination during manipulation of the testis. After a positive biopsy, gloves,
sterile drapes, and all instruments used in the biopsy are discarded and the
operation proceeds with clean supplies, thereby lessening the risk of wound
implantation (Guinn, 1976).

F. Staging

The treatment-oriented staging systems we use in both seminoma and non-
seminomatous testicular tumors are based upon the 1–3 system originally proposed by Boden and Gibb (1951). Stage I is tumor confined within the tunica
albuginea; stage II is regional lymphatic metastatic disease; and stage III is
distant metastases.

Clinical stage is assigned after careful evaluation of the orchiectomy specimen, a history and physical examination, complete blood count, SMA-12/60,
alpha fetoprotein, HCG titer, chest X ray, intravenous pyelogram, and bilateral
pedal lymphangiogram. In selected instances, other studies augment the information obtained in the above; these include an inferior vena cavogram, whole lung
tomograms, abdominal CT scan, and abdominal ultrasonography.

Stage in seminoma is assigned clinically after all indicated tests have been
completed. In non-seminomatous tumors, when the clinical evaluation is negative, clinical stage cannot be assigned until a complete retroperitoneal lymphadenectomy has been performed and all excised nodes have been examined by
the pathologist (Fig. 17).

G. Treatment

1. Seminomas

Treatment of stage 1 seminoma consists of 2500 rads to the ipsilateral ilioin-
guinal and periaortic areas up to T12, and results in a 95% 3-year survival.

Stage II is divided into patients who have retroperitoneal metastatic deposits

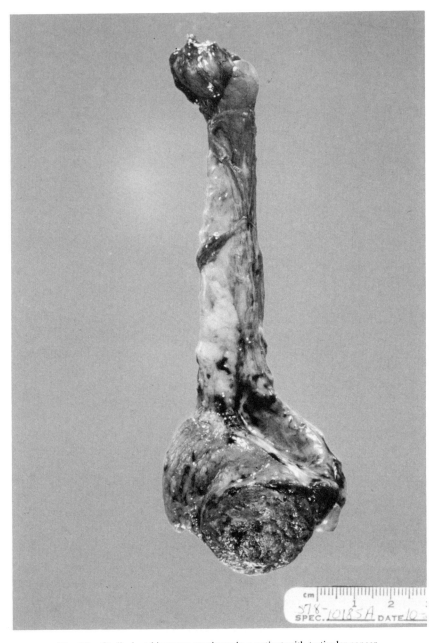

Fig. 16. Radical orchiectomy specimen in a patient with testicular cancer.

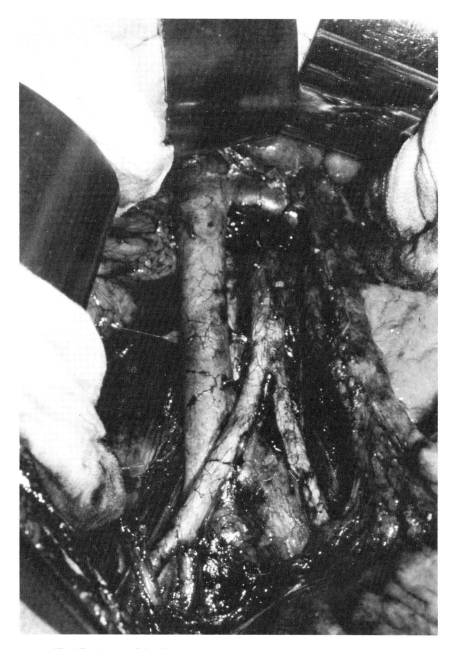

Fig. 17. Extent of the dissection in a staging retroperitoneal lymphadenectomy.

either smaller (A) or larger (B) than 10 cm in diameter. In the former instance, treatment is as in stage I except for a 500- to 1500-rad boost to the site of metastatic disease and, after a 3-week rest, by a "prophylactic" 2500-rad tumor dose to the mediastinal and appropriate supraclavicular areas. In stage IIB, patients receive 2000-rad whole abdominal radiation followed by a 500- to 1500-rad boost to the tumor mass. Mediastinal and supraclavicular radiation is delivered as in stage IIA. Three-year survival in stage II is 78%.

Patients with stage IIIA have mediastinal and/or supraclavicular adenopathy. The retroperitoneum and mediastinum are treated as in stage II, depending upon extent of disease present, but in addition, a 500- to 1500-rad boost is delivered to the supradiaphragmatic tumor deposit(s). The 3-year survival rate in IIIA is 60%. Patients with disseminated disease (IIIB) require individualized treatment consisting of chemotherapy with or without radiation therapy. Until recently, response to chemotherapy has been less dramatic than that noted with non-seminomatous tumors. *cis*-Platinum employed in doses of 120 mg/m² each week for a total of five to six treatments has resulted in the best complete response rate achieved in disseminated seminoma.

2. Non-Seminomatous Testicular Tumors

Stage I patients have an anticipated 5- and 10-year survival rate of 100% for teratoma, 93% for teratocarcinoma, and 74% for embryonal carcinoma. We do not routinely employ adjuvant chemotherapy for any stage I patient, although a case may be made for its use in embryonal carcinoma.

Patients with stage IIA have lymph node metastases removed surgically in spite of a negative lymphangiogram. In the past, a 48% 5-year survival rate was achieved by using 4500-rad postoperative radiation therapy. At present, we have discontinued postoperative radiation therapy in hopes that adjuvant chemotherapy using four courses of Velban and bleomycin may improve these results. Patients with stage 11B all had positive lymphangiograms, and then received a 2500-rad tumor dose to the regional paraaortic lymph nodes prior to retroperitoneal lymphadenectomy. In stage 11B₁, lymphatic metastases were sterilized by radiation therapy and 95% of these patients remain without evidence of disease, whether or not they received an additional 2000-rad postoperative tumor dose. Currently, these patients are given no postoperative radiation therapy. In stage IIB₂, viable lymphatic metastases are completely excised. In the past, 73% of these patients survived 5 years when treatment was completed by an additional 2000-rad treatment postoperatively. For the present, we have discontinued the postoperative portion of "sandwich" radiation therapy and have substituted four courses of adjuvant chemotherapy in hopes of improving survival further.

Patients with stage III disease must be subdivided on the basis of tumor burden in order to compare treatment results between different centers (Samuels *et al.*,

1976). Stage IIIA comprises supraclavicular lymph node metastases; stage $IIIB_1$ is gynecomastia with no other disease evident; $IIIB_2$ is minimal lung involvement defined as five or fewer metastases in each lung, all less than 2 cm in diameter; stage $IIIB_3$ is advanced lung disease in which there is a mediastinal mass, a malignant pleural effusion, or an intrapulmonary lesion greater than 2 cm in diameter; stage $IIIB_4$ is advanced abdominal disease in which there is a palpable retroperitoneal mass or major ureteral deviation by a large extranodal mass; stage $IIIB_5$ comprises nonpulmonary visceral metastases in the liver, brain, or gut.

A tremendous improvement in chemotherapy for metastatic disease has resulted from the discovery of the effectiveness of combination vincoleukoblastine and bleomycin on germinal tumors. Samuels and others (1976) have modified the original drug doses and means of administration so that present complete response rates are 57% in stage IIIA, almost 100% in stage $IIIB_1$, 81% in stage $IIIB_2$, 57% in stage $IIIB_3$, 17% in stage $IIIB_4$, but virtually nil in stage $IIIB_5$. Other authors have added *cis*-platinum, Adriamycin, thereby modifying the original and/or drug combination, and all report good results (Cvitkovic *et al.*, 1977; Einhorn and Donohue, 1977). The question of the optimum treatment regimen, duration of therapy, and the need for long-term maintenance therapy will need to be answered by measuring treatment results against a scale of tumor burden as outlined above. The role for surgery in these patients is yet to be established, but two approaches are presently available. In the first, debulking both pulmonary and retroperitoneal metastases is undertaken after initial courses of chemotherapy have demonstrated that the tumor responds to chemotherapy (Skinner, 1977; Merrin *et al.*, 1976). In the second, surgery is used to provide histological evidence of response in clinically unevaluable areas such as the retroperitoneum in patients who have either no evidence of disease or in whom abnormalities persist in spite of otherwise complete response to therapy. After surgery, continued chemotherapy can be logically based on the presence or absence of histologically malignant tissue (Johnson *et al.*, 1976c).

IX. BLADDER CANCER

A. Etiology

Approximately 30,000 new cases of bladder cancer occur each year in the United States, and almost 10,000 deaths can be attributed to this malignancy annually. Bladder neoplasia is unusual prior to age 40, with the median age ranging between 60 and 70 years. The usual male-to-female ratio is 2:1. In spite of the much-publicized association between exposure to both identified and suspected industrial carcinogens and the subsequent development of bladder cancer, in the majority of patients the causative factor(s) remains obscure. 4-Amino-diphenyl, benzidine, 4-nitrodiphenyl, and betanapthylamine are four

carcinogens in the work place known to cause bladder cancer after a latent period
of up to 40 years after exposure. A history of phenacetin intake and/or cigarette
smoking are more prevalent among patients with bladder cancer. There is also a
well-known association between *Schistosoma hematobium* and the development
of squamous carcinoma in the bladder noted in countries such as Egypt, where
infestation with this parasite abounds (Johnson *et al.*, 1976a).

B. Pathology

Ninety-seven percent of bladder cancer is epithelial in origin, and of these 90%
are transitional-cell carcinomas, 6–7% squamous carcinomas, 3–4% undifferentiated carcinomas, and 0.5–2% are adenocarcinomas. Transitional-cell carcinomas are frequently multifocal in both place and time, either within the
bladder or throughout the urothelium (Fig. 18). This multifocal potential necessitates regular endoscopic evaluation of the bladder and urethra in affected individuals, and regular intravenous pyelograms to assess the upper tracts. Squamous, undifferentiated, and adenocarcinomas differ from transitional cell tumors
because they are usually solitary within the bladder, and the risk of their occurrence elsewhere in the urothelium is remote (Koss, 1975).

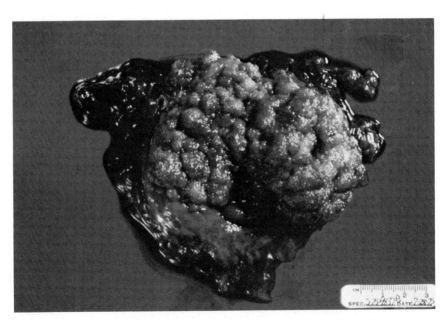

Fig. 18.   Cystectomy specimen in a female with extensive multifocal transitional carcinoma of
the bladder.

The available natural-history information suggests that untreated bladder cancer usually kills the host within 2 years after first symptoms occur, frequently from ureteral obstruction with the tumor still confined to the pelvis. Lymphatic invasion occurs in only 5% of tumors superficial to the muscle, but either lymphatic or vascular invasion occurs in 40% of individuals once muscle invasion has developed. Bladder tumors may grow by direct extension into the adjacent organs (prostate and seminal vesicle in the male; vagina, uterus, and adenexa in the female); and they may metastasize by lymphatic emboli to the regional pelvic lymph nodes and hematogenously, most commonly to the lungs, bone, and liver.

C. Diagnosis

Hematuria is the initial symptom of bladder cancer in 75–80% of patients, and in 50% the duration of this symptom is less than 1 month. Twenty-five percent of patients have so-called irritative bladder symptoms (frequency, dysuria, and painful urination). Twenty percent of patients will be asymptomatic, and the diagnosis is made from an investigation of microscopic hematuria or pyuria.

In the absence of metastatic disease there are no specific findings to aid the physician in making a diagnosis of bladder cancer unless the primary tumor mass is large enough to be palpable on rectal or vaginal examination. Diagnosis is made at cystoscopy and proved by transurethral biopsy.

D. Staging

The staging systems popularized in this country are all based on the observations by Jewett and Strong (1946). These authors demonstrated that the depth that a bladder tumor had invaded the bladder wall was directly related to its potential for metastases. Refinements by Marshall (1956) have resulted in the staging system in vogue today. In stage O, either papillary or *in situ* carcinoma is confined to the mucosa; stage A refers to tumor invasion of the lamina propria; stage B is superficial muscle invasion with B_2 reserved for deep muscle invasion; in stage C there is invasion through the bladder muscle into perivesical fat; stage D_1 refers to direct invasion into the substance of adjacent organs, pelvic lymph node metastases, or postsurgical would implantation into the abdominal wall; D_2 refers to extrapelvic metastases.

The primary tumor should be evaluated cystoscopically and biopsied transurethrally. Following transurethral resection, bimanual examination is carefully performed. When the bimanual examination is normal, the tumor stage is assigned according to the histological evidence of invasion derived from the biopsies. When there is thickening of the bladder wall, stage B_2 is assigned; a palpable mass in three dimensions indicates a stage C tumor; and palpable evidence of invasion of adjacent organs, fixation to the pelvic side wall, or extension into the substance of the lower abdominal wall indicates stage D_1. The presence of metastatic disease is assessed initially by a history and physical examination, complete blood count, SMA-12/60, chest X ray, bone scan, and bilateral pedal lymphangiogram (Fig. 19). In addition to these examinations, an intravenous pyelogram is mandatory to assess the status of the upper tracts.

E. Treatment

Treatment is based upon the stage of disease. In patients with papillary stage O or A tumors, treatment consists of transurethral resection, which results in a 63–81% 5-year survival but is associated with a 60–70% local recurrence rate (Johnson *et al.*, 1976a). The latter necessitates cystoscopy at intervals of 3 months for 3 years after resection of the last tumor, then at less frequent intervals for life. Contraindications to definitive transurethral resection are inaccessability of the lesion to the resectoscope, poorly differentiated tumors, rapid recurrence of multiple tumors with an increasingly high grade, or invasion of the stroma of the prostate gland. When superficial tumors are so extensive that transurethral resection cannot eradicate all the disease, intravesical chemotherapy may assist the resectionist. We feel that thiotepa and bleomycin are helpful only for patients with a small tumor burden (Bracken *et al.*, 1977). Mitomycin C appears to be the most effective agent available to date, with a response rate of 76–81%; this drug can eradicate multiple small-volume superficial tumors (Mishina *et al.*, 1975). When transurethral resection and intravesical chemotherapy fails, cystectomy is the only definitive therapy that can control the malignant process, since external and intracavitary radiation therapy have failed to control the disease in the past, partial cystectomy has a high local recurrence rate, and mucosal denudation has caused a prohibitively high incidence of bladder contracture.

When tumors infiltrate superfical muscle (B_1), transurethral resection, partial cystectomy, or preoperative radiation and cystectomy may be used satisfactorily, but the treatment decision must be individualized. The 5-year survival rate approximates 60%. With B_2 and C tumors, cystectomy (Fig. 20) or definitive radiation produced 5-year survivals ranging from 11–20%. The combination of preoperative radiation followed by cystectomy has improved 5-year survival rates to the 50% level, largely by reducing the incidence of pelvic recurrence to less than 10% (Chan and Johnson, 1978). However, survival rates have reached a plateau, and neither varying the type of cystectomy nor the delivery of radiation therapy seems to have improved the prospects for these patients. Adjuvant

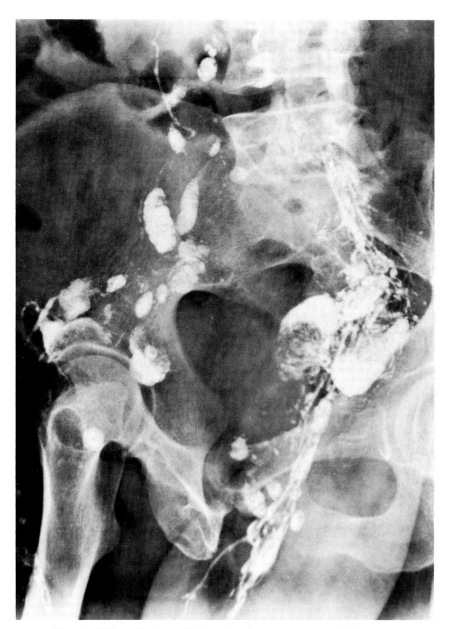

Fig. 19.   Filling defect in a pelvic lymph node due to metastatic bladder cancer.

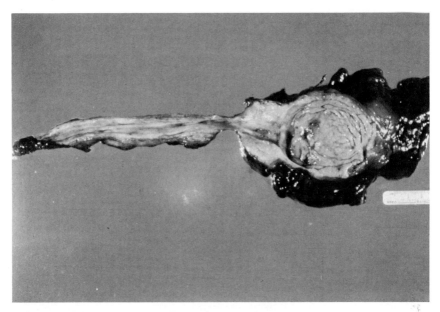

Fig. 20. Radical cystectomy specimen includes perivesical peritoneum and fat, prostate, seminal vesicles, ampullae of the vasa, and the entire urethra.

chemotherapy is the next logical extension of therapy, and a number of centers are planning this treatment at present.

The 5-year survival results in D_1 tumors treated by cystectomy is virtually zero when the tumor has invaded adjacent pelvic organs, metastasized to more than two pelvic lymph nodes, or when the tumor has been implanted in the abdominal incision during open bladder surgery (LaPlante and Brice, 1973; Dretler *et al.*, 1973). If only one or two pelvic lymph node metastases are present, 13–33% of patients have been reported to survive 5 years after radical surgery. On the other hand, 6500- 7000-rad definitive radiation therapy with 25-MEV X rays results in a 10–19% 5-year survival rate in all patients with any of the D_1 presentations, except those patients who have tumor implantation into the abdominal wall (Miller and Johnson, 1973).

Chemotherapy for stage D_2 tumors has been encouraging only since the introduction of *cis*-platinum alone or in combination. Response rates between 50 and 89% have been reported, with complete responses obtained in about 25% of patients. Responses have been noted in the primary tumor as well as in lymphatic, pulmonary, hepatic, and osseous metastases. At present it is too early to define either the duration or the completeness of response, and at present the management of the apparent complete responder is undetermined (Sternberg *et al.*, 1977).

X. PROSTATE CANCER

A. Etiology

In the United States, adenocarcinoma of the prostate is the second commonest malignancy that occurs in males, the commonest neoplasm in black males, and the commonest malignancy in men over age 75. Approximately 60,000 prostate tumors will be recognized annually, and almost 20,000 deaths in the United States are attributed to this malignancy each year.

The etiology remains undetermined; age, life in the United States, sexual habits, prior veneral disease, hormonal imbalance, and a viral origin are among potential possibilities. The incidence of latent carcinoma (clinically undetectable but recognized pathologically) seems similar throughout the world, but the development of clinical cancer is more common in the developed western nations than in areas such as Japan and the Orient. Considering the incidence of latent prostatic cancer and the number of men over age 50, it is estimated that there is a pool of between 4 and 12 million men in the United States with the latent form of disease, from which the 60,000 clinical cases are derived each year. Increased longevity in the western cultures compared to that experienced in underdeveloped nations, and the advanced median age of men with prostatic tumors may explain the higher incidence of the clinical cancer in our culture, because it has been estimated that 20 years are required for the latent tumor to become clinically manifest.

B. Pathology

Ninety-seven percent of prostatic tumors are adenocarcinomas. These tumors have evaded a simple and easily accepted grading system. At present no system is universally accepted, in spite of the fact that most urologists and pathologists realize that patients with well-defined tumors generally have a good prognosis, whereas those who have undifferentiated tumors fare poorly.

With increasing age the prostate is commonly subject to two pathological processes—benign prostatic hyperplasia and adenocarcinoma. Benign prostatic hyperplasia originates from the periurethral portion of the gland, whereas cancer usually originates in the outer compressed portion of the lateral and posterior lobes in the region of the so-called surgical capsule. Mostofi and Price (1973) have shown that prostatic carcinoma is a multifocal process in 85% of patients in whom the organ was totally excised as treatment for clinically localized disease. With further growth the tumor penetrates through the prostatic capsule and invades the adjacent seminal vesicles, bladder base, urethra, and periprostatic skeletal muscle. Direct invasion of the rectum is unusual. and is apparently restricted by Denonvillier's fascia. Lymphatic metastases occur in most patients who have metastatic disease, with primary lymph drainage to the obturator, external iliac, hypogastric, common iliac, presacral, and periaortic nodes. Blood-borne metastases enter the periprostatic valveless venous plexus of Battson, which accounts for the common distribution of osseous metastases to the pelvis, the lumbosacral, thoracic, and cervical spine, the base of the skull, and the proximal humeri, femora, and ribs. Pulmonary (usually lymphatic in type) and hepatic metastases are recognized uncommonly during life, and when they occur they are generally accompanied by clinically evident osseous metastases. The common sites of metastases at postmortem include bones, lymph nodes, bone marrow, lung, liver, and adrenal gland.

C. Diagnosis

Prostatic cancer is usually asymptomatic while the malignancy is confined within the prostate. Once local extension occurs, urinary obstruction and/or irritative symptoms, hematuria, or perineal pain commonly occur. Symptoms of metastatic disease include bone pain, anorexia, weight loss, loss of energy, and symptoms of anemia.

The only consistent way to detect prostatic carcinoma is by digital rectal examination. Suspicion is aroused by unusal induration or hardness in the gland, which is produced by the prostatic stromal reaction to the tumor. Obviously, if the tumor does not incite this response, clinical diagnosis is more difficult. Diagnosis is proved most commonly by transrectal or transperineal biopsy (Fig. 21), and less commonly by transurethral resection.

D. Staging

The staging system used for prostatic carcinoma at M.D. Anderson Hospital is modified from that described by Delregado (Johnson *et al.*, 1976a). Stage A is two or fewer microscopic foci of tumor; stage B is any tumor confined within the prostatic capsule that consists of three or more microscopic foci; In stage C the tumor extends through the prostatic capsule, and in stage D there is disseminated disease.

Digital rectal examination alone is used to stage the extent of the local disease. There is a great need for a more reproducible and possibly accurate method to quantitate the local extent of these tumors, but unfortunately none exists today.

Metastatic disease in assessed by a complete blood count, SMA-12/60, prostatic acid phosphatase, bone scan, chest X ray, and bilateral pedal lymphangiogram. Occasionally, moderate elevation of the prostatic acid phosphatase may be noted in stage C lesions but in general, gross elevations are associated with metastases. Bone scans may provide an earlier estimate of osseous metastases,

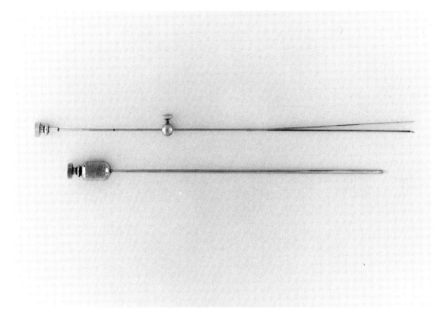

Fig. 21. Hutchins needle for transperineal or transrectal needle biopsy of the prostate.

but the evaluation of the skeleton provided by skeletal radiographs is important in the overall management of patients with this malignancy (Fig. 22).

E. Treatment

1. Stage A

When a patient undergoes subtotal prostatectomy for the relief of obstructive voiding symptoms and has one or two microscopic foci of well-differentiated adenocarcinoma, he should be returned to the operating room for a repeat transurethral resection. If there is no further cancer in the resected tissue, additional therapy is not indicated. If there is more cancer, the patient has a B lesion (Johnson *et al.*, 1974).

2. Stage B

For well-differentiated stage B lesions, the best results of therapy that have been published were obtained from total prostatectomy, confirming a 5-year survival rate ranging between 54 and 92%, with a 15-year survival rate with no evidence of disease of 33%. Complications consist of a 95%-plus chance for erectile impotence, a 15–20% chance for incontinence, and the potential for

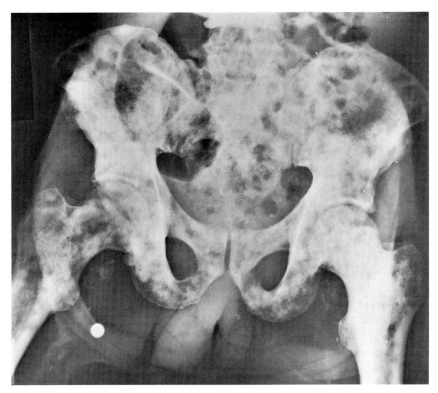

Fig. 22. Osteoblastic metastases.

stricture at the vesicourethral anastomosis. Definitive radiation should be offered
for patients who refuse surgery, with the expectation of no evidence of disease at
5 years of 72%, and at 10 years of 48%. Patients over 75 years of age should be
treated with endocrine therapy, because their 5-year survival rates equal those
achieved with surgery or irradiation and their reduced life expectancy does not
justify the potential risks of definitive treatment. Poorly differentiated B lesions
should be treated by irradiation therapy.

3. Stage C

Radiotherapy has recently become the dominant form of definitive therapy for
patients with this stage of disease. External radiation, interstitial radiation using
I^{125} seeds, and the combination of interstitial gold and external radiation therapy
are the current accepted ways to deliver the radiation. Unfortunately, the patient
populations treated by each form of therapy are different enough to preclude
comparison of these various types of therapy. Bagshaw reports results for external radiation therapy of a 5-year survival rate of 46% with no evidence of

disease, and a 10-year rate of 30% with no evidence of disease. Less popular treatment alternatives include total prostatectomy for resectable lesions and endocrine therapy, which may confirm a 5-year survival rate of 40–50% with disease.

4. Stage D

Details of treatment for this stage vary considerably throughout the world, but initial therapy is based upon the androgen-dependency of most prostatic tumors. We prefer to treat all patients with 5 mg of diethylstilbestrol and bilateral scrotal orchiectomy, and anticipate a 70–80% response rate, a 2.5-year median survival rate, and a 20% 5-year survival rate for this group of patients. Other authors initiate endocrine therapy with either estrogens or orchiectomy and add the therapy initially withheld when and if endocrine failure occurs. When this is done, a 17–36% chance to reinduce a response is possible. When relapse after endocrine therapy occurs, the median survival is 6–9 months. A variety of therapies to reinduce a lost endocrine response has resulted in the use of adrenal suppression with steroids or aminoglutethimide, adrenalectomy, hypophysectomy, or the use of high-dose intravenous Stilphostrol®.

Local radiation frequently palliates isolated symptomatic osseous metastases, whereas intravenous[32] P may palliate diffuse bone pain. Since 1973, patients failing endocrine therapy have been treated with experimental chemotherapy by institutions participating in the National Prostatic Cancer Group. For chemotherapy purposes, patients are divided into those having a history of prior pelvic radiation and those without, since bone marrow reserve may be depleted by radiation. In the non-irradiated group, cyclophosphamide and 5-fluorouracil have emerged with an established palliative role in the improvement of pain and performance status while achieving few objective responses. Palliation was achieved less consistently in the previously radiated group of patients; estracyt is currently the best drug tested in this group to date. At present, chemotherapy for prostatic cancer is in its infancy, and one must await future developments to see if this form of treatment will become an established therapy for elderly men with advanced disease.

REFERENCES

Bennington, J. L., and Beckwith, J. B. (1975). Tumors of the kidney, renal pelvis and ureter. In "Atlas of Tumor Pathology," Vol. XII. Armed Forces Inst. Pathol., Washington, D.C.
Boden, G., and Gibb, R. (1951). Lancet 2, 1195–1197.
Bracken, R. B., and Jonsson, K. (1979). Urology 14, 96–99.
Bracken, R. B., Johnson, D. E., Goldstein, H. M., Wallace, S., and Ayala, A. G. (1975). Urology 6, 6–10.
Bracken, R. B., Johnson, D. E., Miller, L. S., Ayala, A. G., and Rutledge, F. (1976). J. Urol. 116, 118–192.

Bracken, R. B., Johnson, D. E., Rodriguez, L., Samuels, M. L., and Ayala, A. G. (1977). *Urology* **9**, 161-163.

Chan, R. C., and Johnson, D. E. (1978). *Urology* **12**, 549-552.

Cvitkovic, E., Cheng, E., and Whitmore, W. F. (1977). *Proc. Am. Assoc. Cancer Res.* **18**, 324.

Dixon, F. J., and Moore, R. A. (1952). Tumors of the male genital system. *In* "Atlas of Tumor Pathology," Vol. XII. Armed Forces Inst. Pathol., Washington, D.C.

Dretler, S. P., Ragsdale, B. D., and Leadbetter, W. F. (1973). *J. Urol.* **109**, 414-416.

Einhorn, L. H., and Donohue, J. P. (1977). *In* "Urologic Clinics of North America" (E. Fraley, ed.), p. 407. Saunders, Philadelphia, Pennsylvania.

Gill, W. B., Lu, C. T., and Thomsen, D. (1973). *J. Urol.* **109**, 573-578.

Grabstald, H., Hillaris, B., Henschke, U., and Whitmore, W. F. (1966). *J. Am. Med. Assoc.* **197**, 835-842.

Grabstald, H., Whitmore, W. F., and Melamed, M. R. (1971). *J. Am. Med. Assoc.* **216**, 845.

Guinn, G. A. (1976). *In* "Testicular Tumors" (D. E. Johnson, ed.). Medical Examination Publishing Co., Inc., Flushing, New York.

Howerton, L. W., Lich, R., Goode, L. S., and Amin, M. (1970). *J. Urol.* **104**, 817-820.

Ichikawa, T., Nakano, I., and Hirokawa, I. (1969). *J. Urol.* **102**, 699-707.

Jewett, H. J., and Strong, G. H. (1946). *J. Urol.* **55**, 366-372.

Johansson, S., Angervall, L., Bengtsson, U., and Wahlqvist, L. (1976). *Cancer* **37**, 1376-1383.

Johnson, D. E. (1973). *Cancer Bull.* **25**, 50.

Johnson, D. E., de Berardinis, M., and Ayala, A. G. (1974). *South. Med. J.* **67**, 1183-1186.

Johnson, D. E., Kaesler, K. E., and Samuels, M. L. (1975). *J. Urol.* **114**, 27-29.

Johnson, D. E., Bracken, R. B., Wallace, S., Ayala, A. G., Samuels, M. L., Hussey, D. H., and Miller, L. S. (1976a). *In* "Cancer Patient Care at M.D. Anderson Hospital and Tumor Institute" (R. L. Clark and C. D. Howe, eds.), pp. 361-414. Yearbook Publ. Chicago, Illinois.

Johnson, D. E., Bracken, R. B., and Blight, E. M. (1976b). *J. Urol.* **116**, 63-65.

Johnson, D. E., Bracken, R. B., Ayala, A. G., and Samuels, M. L. (1976c). *J. Urol.* **116**, 66-68.

Koss, L. G. (1975). Tumors of the urinary bladder. *In* "Atlas of Tumor Pathology," Vol. XI. Armed Forces Inst. Pathol., Washington, D.C.

LaPlante, M., and Brice, M. (1973). *J. Urol.* **109**, 261-264.

Marshall, V. F. (1956). *Cancer* **9**, 543-550.

Medellin, H. (1973). *Cancer Bull.* **25**, 42-47.

Merrin, C., Takito, H., and Weber, R., Wajsman, Z., Baumgartner, G., and Murphy, G. (1976). *Cancer* **37**, 20-29.

Miller, L. S., and Johnson, D. E. (1973). *Proc. Nat. Cancer Conf., 7th, 1972*, pp. 771-782.

Mishina, T., Oda, K., Murata, S., Mou, Y., and Takohask, T. (1975). *J. Urol.* **114**, 217-219.

Mostofi, F. K., and Price, E. B. (1973). Tumors of the male genital system. *In* "Atlas of Tumor Pathology," Vol. VIII. Armed Forces Inst. Pathol., Washington, D.C.

Petkovic, S. D. (1972). *J. Urol.* **107**, 220-223.

Samuels, M. L., Lanzotti, V. S., Holoye, P. Y., Boyle, L. E., Smith, T. L., and Johnson, D. E. (1976). *Cancer Treat. Rev.* **3**, 185-204.

Skinner, D. G. (1977). *In Surg. Clin. North Am.* **4**, 465.

Sternberg, J. J., Bracken, R. B., Handel, P. B., and Johnson, D. E. (1977). *J. Am. Med. Assoc.* **238**, 2282-2287.

12

GYNECOLOGICAL CANCERS
Laurence H. Baker

I.   Introduction 243
II.   Ovarian Cancer 245
III.   Cancer of the Cervix 250
IV.   Endometrial Carcinoma 254
    References 255

I. INTRODUCTION

Malignant neoplasms of the female genital tract account for almost one-fifth of all cancers occurring in women. Data compiled by the American Cancer Society (1979) indicates that in 1980, 75,500 new cases of cancer involving the uterine cervix, uterine corpus, ovary, vagina, and accessory structures will be discovered. Additionally, it is projected that over 45,000 new cases of *in situ* carcinomas of the cervix will be detected and treated. An estimated 22,800 deaths will occur as a result of these malignancies.

In general, although it appears that the incidence of ovarian cancer increases with age, carcinomas of both the uterine cervix and corpus decrease with age, reaching their peak rate of occurrence at around age 50 (Fig. 1) (Hreshchyshyn, 1973). Data from the Cancer Survival and End Results of the National Cancer Institute reveals that the overall 5-year survival rate for women with cervical cancer of all stages is approximately 55%, compared to 74% in women with endometrial carcinoma and only 30% in those with ovarian cancer (Table I) (DeVita *et al.,* 1976). Explaining in large part the survival differences among these diseases, the same survey shows that although nearly half the patients with cervical cancer and 80% of those with endometrial carcinoma have localized disease, less than a third with ovarian cancer have localized malignancy. Hence, far-advanced disease is found in nearly two-thirds of the patients with ovarian cancer, compared to slightly more than 10% in patients with endometrial and

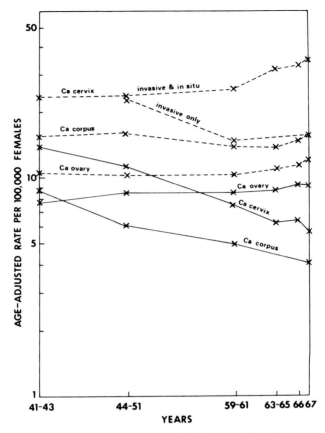

Fig. 1.   Trends in morbidity associated with gynecological cancer. (From Hreshchyshyn, 1973.)

cervical cancers (Table II) (De Vita *et. al.,* 1976). Additionally, because carcinomas of the uterus or cervix are far more detectable on physical examination
than are carcinomas of the ovary, significant delays between onset of disease and
diagnosis occur more frequently in ovarian cancer.

Modern advances in both gynecological cancer diagnosis and management
have been described by Gusberg (1976). The decade of the 1940s witnessed the
development and refinement of radiotherapeutic and surgical techniques. In the
1950s, the importance of early diagnosis of precancerous lesions was recognized
with the concept of hyperplasia leading to dysplasia, leading to carcinoma *in situ*
and, finally, to microinvasion. The 1960s brought the establishment of a firm
biological base with the development of the fields of (a) cell kinetics and
physiology (in relation to chemotherapy); (b) radiobiology; (c) tumor immunology; (d) steroid endocrinology; and (e) epidemiology (which provided definitions

TABLE I

Gynecological Cancer Survival End Results[a]

Disease site	Time period	Follow-up period (yr)	Percentage alive[b]			
			All stages	Local disease	Regional disease	Distant metastasis
Cervix	1965–1969	5	56	78	44	10
	1960–1964	5	57	77	43	9
	1950–1959	10	54	72	41	NA[c]
Ovary	1965–1969	5	32	76	32	12
	1960–1964	5	33	75	32	10
	1950–1959	10	26	64	25	NA
Endometrium	1965–1969	5	74	85	45	21
	1960–1964	5	73	83	46	14
	1950–1959	10	68	80	48	NA

[a] From DeVita et al. (1976).

[b] Relative survival, not necessarily disease-free, after all therapies.

[c] NA, data not available.

of high risk). During the 1970s, the findings of the previous 3 decades were translated into therapeutic action. Thus, the factors contributing to the decline in mortality from gynecological cancers include emphasis on early diagnosis, widespread use of cytological screening, advancements in radical surgery, improvement of radiotherapy, and the introduction of chemotherapy. Based on these modes of detection and therapy, a sequential order of treatment in cancer of the uterine cervix was described by DeVita et al. (1976), and is illustrated in Fig. 2.

II. OVARIAN CANCER

The peak incidence of ovarian cancer occurs in women between 50 and 60 years of age. In the past several decades, the mortality rate for ovarian cancer has increased to the point where 1 out of every 100 female deaths can be attributed to this malignancy (Griffiths, 1973).

The effective management of ovarian cancer is based on a thorough understanding of its natural history in terms of both signs and symptoms, as well as accurate staging. It is readily apparent from Table III (Young and DeVita, 1975) that these signs and symptoms represent late manifestations of the disease; nearly three-quarters of the patients have disease disseminated beyond the ovary at the time of diagnosis. As previously stated, this is chiefly because the ovary does not easily lend itself to

TABLE II

Treatment Modalities for Gynecological Cancer[a]

Disease site	No. of cases	Percentage classified[b]				Percentage treated[c]				
		Local-ized	Re-gional	Dis-tant	Un-known	Sur-gery[c]	Radia-tion	Sur-gery + radia-tion	Drug or hormone therapy + other therapies	Un-treated
Cervix	4599	45	43	11	1	7	73	4	11	5
Ovary	2977	28	7	61	4	15	6	17	52	8
Endometrium	3944	79	8	11	2	7	14	6	69[d]	3

[a] From DeVita et al. (1976). Period of 1965–1969.
[b] Initial classification at diagnosis.
[c] Initial course of therapy or that given within 4 months of diagnosis.
[d] Monthly hormonal therapy.

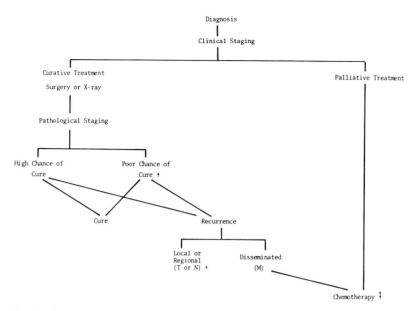

Fig. 2.   Treatment flow in cancer of the uterus (cervix and endometrium). (From DeVita *et al.*, 1976.)

TABLE III

Symptoms and Signs of Ovarian Carcinoma[a]

Symptoms and signs	Patients (%)
Symptoms	
Low abdominal pain	54
Abdominal enlargement	53
Gastrointestinal complaints	21
Genitourinary complaints	20
Abdominal vaginal bleed- ing	18
Pelvic pressure	17
Backache	13
Signs	
Pelvic mass	87
Abdominal mass	77
Ascites	31
Weight loss	28

[a] From Young and DeVita (1975).

physical examination. The staging of ovarian cancer, then, can be divided into two parts—both a clinical and surgical staging.

Clinical staging is based on physical examination, which specifically includes careful attention to pelvic exam and proctoscopy. Occasionally, X rays are of assistance, including X rays of the thorax and abdomen, intravenous pyelogram, barium enema, upper GI series, and a lymphangiogram to assess the status of the para-aortic nodes. Cytological examination of ascitic or pleural fluid is important in the staging of ovarian cancer. Increasingly more popular in the assessment of this disease is evaluation by peritoneoscopy. However, because of the difficulty in clinically assessing ovarian cancer, further attempts to delineate specific features are investigated at the time of laparotomy. These include (a) unilateral or bilateral disease; (b) fixation; (c) presence or absence of peritoneal implants; and (d) sites of peritoneal implants in the pelvis, in the cul-de-sac, on the peritoneal surface, in the lateral paracolic spaces, on the surface of the liver, and under the diaphragm. These procedures permit an accurate staging system ranging from stage IA, describing growth limited to one ovary with no ascites, to stage IV, which represents growth in one or both ovaries but with distant metastases outside of the peritoneal cavity (Table IV) (Kottmeier, 1969).

The prognosis of patients with ovarian cancer is not only related to the extent of disease; histological features of the disease process appear to be of importance as well. Eighty-five to ninety percent of all ovarian cancers are epithelial in origin. Pathologically, they are classified as serous or mucinous cystadenocarcinomas, solid and endometrioid carcinomas, differentiated adenocarcinomas, undifferentiated carcinomas, malignant germ cell tumors, and malignant mesen-

TABLE IV

IFGO[a] Staging of Carcinoma of Ovary

Stage	Involvement
IA	Growth limited to one ovary; no ascites
IB	Growth limited to one or both ovaries; no ascites
IC	Growth limited to one or both ovaries; ascites present, with malignant cells in the fluid
IIA	Growth involving one or both ovaries with extension and/or metastasis to uterus and/or tubes only
IIB	Growth involving one or both ovaries with extension and/or metastasis to other pelvic tissues
III	Growth involving one or both ovaries with widespread intraperitoneal metastasis to the abdomen (including omentum, intestine, mesentery, liver, retroperitoneal lymph glands, and other abdominal organs)
IV	Growth involving one or both ovaries, with distant metastasis outside the peritoneal cavity

[a] International Federation of Gynecology and Obstetrics.

TABLE V

Histological Classification and Frequency of Malignant Ovarian Tumors

Tumor type	Percentage
Serous cystadenocarcinoma (with or without papillary changes)	48
Undifferentiated adenocarcinoma	16
Endometrioid adenocarcinoma	14
Mucinous cystadenocarcinoma	11
Mesonephroid adenocarcinoma	5
Malignant germinal cell tumors (dysgerminomas, granulosa cell, arrheno-blastoma, malignant teratomas)	6

chymal tumors (Table V). Within these cell types, survival is dependent upon the degree of differentiation of the tumor that is represented by a histological grade. Figure 3 (Malkasian *et al.*, 1975) illustrates the difference in survival within each stage as a result of the grading of the malignancy.

The treatment of ovarian cancer includes the major modalities of surgery, radiotherapy, and chemotherapy. Table VI (Bagley *et al.*, 1972) summarizes the results of various therapies utilizing these modalities. Because many patients have stage III and IV disease upon presentation, chemotherapy has assumed an increasingly important role in management. It has been shown that a combination

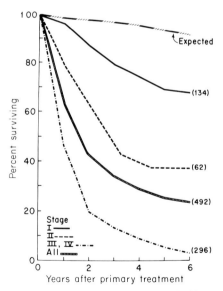

Fig. 3. Serous cystadenocarcinoma (492 graded cases): survival by stage. Number of cases in each subgroup is shown at right of survival curve. (From Malakasian *et al.*, 1975.)

TABLE VI

Ovarian Carcinoma: Five-Year Survival Rate Following Various Therapies; Summary of Multiple Series[a]

IFGO[b] stage	Five-year survival (%)		
	Surgery only	Surgery and radiotherapy	Surgery and chemotherapy
I	67 (32–78)	60 (40–71)	94[c]
IA	63	65	—
IB	70	52	—
IC	—	43	—
II	24 (0–33)	37 (27–69)	—
IIA	—	62[b]	—
IIB		39	—
III–IV	1 (0–3)	7 (6–16)	7(0–9)
III	—	6	—

[a] Bagley et al. (1972).

[b] International Federation of Gynecology and Obstetrics.

[c] Data from only one series.

of drugs appears to be more effective than single-agent therapy, which was the previously accepted standard (Young and Anderson, 1977). Many combinations appear to be active in the management of ovarian cancer, including various combinations using an alkylating agent such as cyclophosphamide, melphalan, cis-diamine dichloroplatinum, Adriamycin™, hexamethylmelamine or mitomycin-C. Other drugs known to have activity in this disease include 5-fluorouracil and methotrexate.

Of equal importance in the use of combination drug strategies has been the observation that "second look" surgical operations seem to enhance survival of patients with advanced disease. This allows for the removal of tumor not otherwise clinically suspected because of the difficulties inherent in the examination of the abdomen. Of particular concern are the previously described regions examined during laparotomy for sites of peritoneal implants. The use of combination chemotherapy together with "second look" surgery is an example of the multidisciplinary approach which has gained currency in the treatment of gynecological cancers.

III. CANCER OF THE CERVIX

Invasive carcinoma of the uterine cervix is now the second most common malignant neoplasm of the female genital tract, and the fifth most common cancer in women. At one time, it was one of the predominant causes of cancer death in women, but has now been surpassed in rate of mortality by ovarian cancer (American Cancer Society, 1979). Whether or not earlier detection of cervical cancer has led to improved survival, however, remains a subject of some dispute.

The etiology of cervical cancer, like all other cancers, remains unclear at this time. A relationship between herpes virus type 2 infections and invasive carcinomas of the uterine cervix has been described (Josey *et al.*, 1976; Simon, 1976). The basis for this statement is the observation that type 2 antibodies are present in a far higher percentage of patients with carcinoma of the cervix than in a comparable control group of women. Cervical cancer has also often been correlated to race, with the rate of invasive cancer of the cervix found to be twice as great in black females (American Cancer Society, 1979). This, however, is probably best explained by the fact that this disease tends to occur more frequently in educationally and socioeconomically underprivileged women and is not due to inherent biological factors (Christopherson and Parker, 1960). Much speculation has existed regarding the relationship between early and frequent sexual activity and the incidence of cervical cancer, though supporting evidence is by no means conclusive.

Approximately 95% of all cervical carcinomas are of the squamous cell variety and nearly all of the rest are adenocarcinomas. Despite the fact that 1 in 20 carcinomas of the cervix are adenocarcinomas in origin, there appears to be very little difference in the behavior when compared to squamous cell carcinomas, either in terms of natural history or response to treatment. Like ovarian cancer, the prognosis and treatment strategy of carcinomas of the uterine cervix also depend on a precise staging system that is essentially based on clinical findings (Table VII) (Kottmeier, 1971).

Stage I lesions are defined as those clearly confined to the uterine cervix, whereas stage IV lesions denote those that have extended beyond the true pelvis or have invaded the mucosa of the urinary bladder or rectum. One of the major difficulties in planning treatment for patients with cervical carcinoma is the assessment of para-aortic nodes. The importance of para-aortic node involvement in prognosis and therapy is becoming increasingly recognized. Table VIII (Lewis, 1975) outlines five series, showing the incidence of para-aortic node involvement by stage. Para-aortic node involvement obviously constitutes stage IV advanced disease and, therefore, requires aggressive therapy. Failure to determine para-aortic node involvement may result in a treatment plan that may not include this disease site.

One of the reasons for the improved prognosis of this disease has been the introduction of the Papanicolaou (Pap) smear. Examination by cytology of the cervical mucosa is easily accomplished and has lead to recognition of precancerous lesions as well as early nonvisible cancer. Table IX shows the Papanicolaou

TABLE VII

Clinical Stages in Carcinoma of the Uterine Cervix[a]

Pre-invasive carcinoma
Stage 0   Carcinoma in situ, intraepithelial carcinoma. Stage 0 cases should not be included in any
          therapeutic statistics.
Invasive carcinoma
Stage I   Carcinoma strictly confined to the cervix (extension to the corpus should be disregarded).
   Stage IA   The cancer cannot be diagnosed by clinical examination: (1) early stromal invasion,
              (2) occult cancer.
   Stage IB   All other stage I cases
Stage II   The carcinoma extends beyond the cervix but does not extend onto the pelvic wall. The
           carcinoma involves the vagina but not the lower third.
   Stage IIA   No obvious parametrial involvement
   Stage IIB   Obvious parametrial involvement
Stage III   The carcinoma extends onto the pelvic wall. On rectal examination there is no cancer-
            free space between the tumor and the pelvic wall. The tumor involves the lower third of
            the vagina. There is hydronephrosis or a nonfunctioning kidney.
   Stage IIIA   No extension onto the pelvic wall
   Stage IIIB   Extension onto the pelvic wall
Stage IV   The carcinoma extends beyond the true pelvis or involves the mucosa of the bladder or
           rectum. (The presence of a bullous edema does not permit assignment to stage IV).

[a] From Kottmeier (1971).

classification of cervical cytologic specimens; it ranges from Class 1, or normal, to Class 5, which represents clearly defined areas of malignant cells (Papanicolaou, 1954). Early lesions, then, are usually detected by a Pap smear done in a routine fashion. However, in more advanced lesions, patients usually

TABLE VIII

Incidence of Metastases to Para-Aortic Nodes Determined at the Time of Pretreatment Laparotomy[a]

Stage	Averette et al. (1972)		Buchsbaum (1972)		Nelson et al. (1974)		Piver et al. (1974)		Rutledge	
	No.	%	No.	%	No.	%	No.	%	No.	%
I	3/40	8	0/27	0	—	—	—	—	0/21	0
II	4/18	22	1/12	8	5/31	17	1/19	5	7/50	14
III	2/10	20	7/20	35	13/28	46	12/32	38	14/41	34
IV	1/2	50	1/2	50	—	—	2/5	40	0/1	0
Total	10/70	14	9/61	15	18/51	31	15/56	27	21/113	18

[a] From Lewis (1975).

TABLE IX

Papanicolaou Classification of Cervical Cytologic Specimens

Class 1	Smear containing only normal cells
Class 2	Smear containing cells having some atypical features, such as vacuolization, cytoplasmic granules, double nuclei, and nuclear enlargement, but none suggestive of a malignant cell
Class 3	Smear containing cells having abnormal features suggestive of, but not definite for, malignant cells
Class 4	Smear containing malignant cells
Class 5	Smear containing malignant cells more bizarre than Class 4

have a visible lesion and frequently have vaginal bleeding, vaginal discharge, or signs and symptoms compatible with extension of the disease outside of the uterine cervix.

Several treatment modalities are effective in the management of cervical carcinomas. In the United States, most patients are treated with radiotherapy. Carcinoma of the cervix is one of the most curable of all internal cancers. Nearly 60% of patients with invasive carcinoma of the cervix that are treated in a major radiotherapy center will survive more than 5 years. Younger patients with early invasive carcinoma of the cervix are frequently treated by radical hysterectomy, often called the Wertheim hysterectomy. Reasons for this form of surgical treatment are detailed in Table X (DeVita *et al.*, 1976). There has also been an attempt to define the role of chemotherapy in the treatment of cervical cancer (Table XI) (DeVita *et al.*, 1976). A vigorous systematic and rational search continues in an attempt to discover effective therapies for this disease.

TABLE X

Reasons for Radical Hysterectomy as the Treatment of Choice for Carcinoma of the Cervix (Stages IB and IIA)[a]

1. Survival equal to that after irradiation
2. Mortality and fistula complication < 1% in skilled hands
3. Permanent morbidity less than with irradiation
4. Vagina, rectum, bladder, and ureter damaged to some degree by irradiation
5. Preservation of good vaginal function
6. More accurate assessment of stage of malignancy and more accurate application of therapy
7. Survival rate of 50-60%, with pelvic lymph node metastases
8. Relief from patient anxiety due to removal of tumor
9. Less time and expense for patient than irradiation

[a] From DeVita *et al.* (1976).

TABLE XI

Role of Chemotherapy in Cervical Cancer[a]

1. Patients untreatable by local modalities: stage IV (approximately 4% of all patients initially) and patients unable to tolerate surgery and/or radiotherapy
   Goals: palliation and cure
2. Patients with recurrent disease post surgery and/or post radiotherapy
   Goals: palliation and cure
3. Patients treatable by local modalities (surgery and/or radiotherapy), but with low potential of cure: stages IIB, III
   Goal: cure

[a] From DeVita *et al.* (1976).

IV. ENDOMETRIAL CARCINOMA

Increased interest has focused on endometrial carcinomas, as a result of a relative and actual increase in the incidence of the disease, which is possibly related to the discovery of its relationship to the use of exogenous hormone (estrogen) (Hertz, 1976).

Nearly 90% of all carcinomas of the body of the uterus are adenocarcinoma in origin. The remaining 10% comprise unusual tumors, predominantly of sarcomatous origin. A general body habitus is associated with this disease and consists of women who are obese, hypertensive, and adult-onset diabetics. These women also tend to have long-standing histories of menstrual dysfunction. Additionally, there appears to be a correlation between the presence of benign adenomatous hyperplasia and increased risk of developing endometrial carcinoma (Gusberg and Kaplan, 1963).

Carcinoma of the uterine corpus grows slowly and remains within the endometrium for long periods of time. When invasion occurs, it is usually to the myometrium first and then to the cervix. Once a tumor is present in the myometrium, it can then spread either by the myometrium lymphatics or through the extensive vascular supply of the myometrium, or both.

The staging system of endometrial cancer is clinical. Stage I cancer is divided into two groups, IA and IB, based upon the size of the uterus, which offers a good index of the invasiveness of the malignancy. Approximately 85% of patients will present with a symptom of abnormal uterine bleeding. Later signs of invasive carcinoma, such as pain and constant constitutional symptomology, may develop. Diagnosis is made by endometrial and endocervical biopsies or fractional curettage, which determines both spread of the tumor to the endocervix and the size of the uterus.

In stage IA (grades I and II) carcinomas of the endometrium, abdominal hysterectomy is viewed as the optimal treatment, whereas preoperative radiotherapy is indicated for stage IA (grade III) and IIB carcinomas. External radiation and/or intracavitary irradiation, followed by hysterectomy, appears to provide the best prognosis for long-term survival. Because endometrial carcinomas appear to exhibit hormonal dependence, approximately 30% of these patients will experience clinical remission as a result of the administration of progesterone. Chemotherapy of endometrial carcinoma is less well defined. Although agents such as 5-fluorouracil, cyclophosphamide, Adriamycin, and various combinations of chemotherapeutic agents have shown activity against this disease, meaningful response rates and prolongation of survival have yet to be demonstrated.

ACKNOWLEDGMENT

The author is indebted to Dr. V. K. Vaitkevicius, M.D., F.A.C.P., Professor and Chairman of Oncology, Wayne State University School of Medicine, and Dr. Julian P. Smith, M.D., F.A.C.O.G., Professor, Department of Gynecology and Obstetrics, Director of the Division of Gynecologic Oncology, Wayne State University School of Medicine, for their guidance and critical review of this manuscript.

REFERENCES

American Cancer Society (1979). "1980 Cancer Facts and Figures." Am. Cancer Soc., New York.
Bagley, C. M., Jr., Young, R. C., Canellos, G. P., and DeVita, V. T. (1972). N. Engl. J. Med. **287**, 856–862.
Christopherson, W. M., and Parker, J. E. (1960). Cancer **13**, 711–713.
DeVita, V. T., Wasserman, T. H., Young, R. C., and Carter, S. K. (1976). Cancer **38**, 509–525.
Griffiths, C. T. (1973). In "Cancer Medicine" (J. Holland and E. Frei, eds.), p. 1710. Lea & Febiger, Philadelphia, Pennsylvania.
Gusberg, S. B. (1976). Cancer **38**, 409–410.
Gusberg, S. B., and Kaplan, A. L. (1963). Am. J. Obstet. Gynecol. **87**, 662.
Hertz, R. (1976). Cancer **38**, 534–537.
Hreshchyshyn, M. M. (1973). In "Cancer Medicine" (J. Holland and E. Frei, eds.), p. 1709. Lea & Febiger, Philadelphia, Pennsylvania.
Josey, W. E., Nahmias, A. J., and Zuher, N. M. (1976). Cancer **38**, 529–530.
Kottmeier, H. L. (1969). In "Cancer of the Uterus and Ovary," pp. 17–32. Yearbook Publ., Chicago, Illinois.
Kottmeier, H. L. (1971). Int. J. Gynecol. Obstet. **9**, 172–179.
Lewis, J. L., Jr. (1975). In "Cancer Therapy" (M. J. Staquet, ed.), p. 342. Raven, New York.
Malkasian, G. D., Decker, D. G., and Webb, M. J. (1975). Semin. Oncol. **2**, 191–201.
Papanicolaou, G. N. (1954). "Atlas of Exfoliative Cytology." Harvard Univ. Press, Cambridge, Massachusetts.
Simon, J. W. (1976). Gynecol. Oncol. **4**, 108–116.
Young, R. C., and Anderson, A. (1977). Recent Adv. Cancer Treat. **3**, 325–342.
Young, R. C., and DeVita, V. T. (1975). In "Prognostic Factors and Criteria of Response" (M. J. Staquet, ed.), p. 320. Raven, New York.

13

MALIGNANT MELANOMA
Frank E. Smith

I.	Introduction	257
II.	Epidemiology	258
III.	Pathology	259
	A. Gross Pathology	260
	B. Microscopic Pathology	263
IV.	Clinical Findings	265
V.	Diagnosis	268
VI.	Prognosis	269
VII.	Treatment	270
VIII.	Conclusion	272
	References	272

I. INTRODUCTION

Malignant melanoma is an uncommon tumor, usually arising in the skin, and represents 1.4% of all malignancies reported annually in the United States. This tumor arises from melanocytes, and most commonly pigment is demonstrable intracellularly. In a minority of instances such pigment is not demonstrable within individual cells and hence gross examination of such tumors will not reveal the external coloration that characterizes the majority of melanomas. Since melanocytes are by proportion much more frequent in skin, melanoma is most frequently primary in that tissue (Table I). Malignant transformation in melanocytes may occur in cells present in anatomical sites beyond the skin, so that primary tumors have occured in the gastrointestinal tract, meninges, adrenals, retina, nasal cavities, bronchus, and vagina. It is estimated that approximately two-thirds of melanomas arise in preexisting benign nevi or "moles" of the skin. Since moles are exceedingly common in most individuals, it is all the more remarkable that malignant melanoma represents such a small component of all malignancy in man.

CANCER AND CHEMOTHERAPY, VOL. II

TABLE I

Patients with Melanoma of Skin (M.D. Anderson Hospital, 1944–1971)[a]

Location of primary	Percentage	Males	Females
Head and neck	21	359	209
Trunk	22	374	239
Upper extremity	21	271	297
Lower extremity	25	199	492
Unknown primaries	4.5	87	33
Others	6.5	70	105
Total		1360	1375

[a] From McBride (1973).

II. EPIDEMIOLOGY

The mechanism of malignant change in melanoma is unknown, but several observations have been made that have identified factors which have some influence on the occurrence and course of the disease.

There has been a great deal of controversy regarding sunlight in the pathogenesis of melanoma. In this regard, a variety of melanoma, lentigo maligna, occurs almost exclusively on sun-exposed areas, whereas the other two common types of melanoma, superficial and nodular, may occur on exposed or unexposed skin surfaces. A counter argument has been that native Africans and blacks who live in other geographic areas have a much lower incidence of melanoma than whites, despite their heavy exposure to ultraviolet radiation from the sun and larger number of melanocytes in the skin compared to Caucasians.

Familial influences on the incidence of melanoma are well described in both the animal kingdom and man (Smith *et al.,* 1966). Hereditary influences in fish, flies, salamanders, mice, swine, and horses have been well documented, and in some species the propensity for developing malignant melanoma can even be transmitted as a dominant trait. The fact that all gray horses, if they live long enough, will eventually develop melanoma was well known in the sixteenth century. Familial melanoma in humans does not appear to follow Mendelian law, but should be included in that category of neoplasm that may occasionally occur in close relatives. Familial melanoma has been known in siblings and offspring, occurring in approximately one-half of the cases within 2 years of recognition of the marker tumor. This observation has prompted some to speculate that a common carcinogenic influence may have been present in the afflicted subjects, possibly an oncogenic virus. In this manner, for example, a mother and son or sister and brother who develop melanoma at approximately similar times raise suspicion of a common pathogenesis.

Hormonal influences have also been implicated in the appearance and course of melanoma. For example, melanoma is an unusual tumor in the pediatric age group, but at puberty, preexisting nevi may undergo malignant change. The influences responsible for this change, at a time when major hormonal adjustments are occurring, are unknown, but clinical observations regarding this phenomenon have been known for many years. The clinical danger in this observation is that individual patients in the prepubertal age group may in truth be harboring a malignant melanoma that may be overlooked and consequently may be inadequately treated or not treated at all. The juvenile nevus may closely resemble malignant melanoma grossly, but is usually well demarcated and smooth and does not metastasize. Because of similarities in appearance of "benign juvenile nevus" and malignant melanoma, pathologists pay close attention to the age of patients whose biopsies appear before them for interpretation, despite the fact that pediatric "melanoma" can be treated initially in a less aggressive manner than suspect lesions in adults. If a patient is approaching puberty and the pathologic picture is suspicious, the prudent judgment would be to approach treatment as if the lesion were malignant. A prospective "error" in this situation can prevent a retrospective realization of melanoma in the rare individual instances when young patients present themselves to the clinicians.

In a similar fashion, pigmentary changes in the skin and nipples occur not only at puberty but also during pregnancy. Transformation of benign nevi to malignant melanomas during pregnancy has been noted, and the risk for a pregnant woman's mole to become malignant may be as high as three times that of the nonpregnant female. Regional nodal metastases in similarly staged melanoma patients who are pregnant occur twice as commonly as expected. Transmission of melanoma to the fetus from the mother is rare, but has been reported (Reynolds, 1955).

The fact that as many as 40% of melanomas are estrogen-receptor-positive is an interesting finding, the significance of which is unknown (Nathanson *et al.*, 1978).

III. PATHOLOGY

An exact diagnosis of melanoma by its gross appearance can be very difficult, and in questionable situations a biopsy is mandatory. The traditional opinion that suspected melanomas must be excised to minimize the possibility of hematogenous dissemination has been overstated. Needle biopsy or incisional biopsy are now considered reasonable practice by most clinicians when the question of possible malignant melanoma arises. Differences in prognosis have not been demonstrated when biopsies other than wide excision have been employed.

Classification of melanoma by depth of invasion is extremely important in prognosis. Three systems are depicted in Fig. 1.

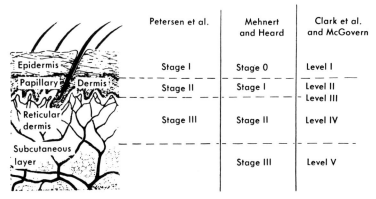

Fig. 1. Classification of melanoma by depth of invasion. From Dellonand Ketcham (1973).

A. Gross Pathology

Malignant melanomas have grossly observable characteristics that should be considered:

1. Over 80% of melanomas have an irregular border. Three-quarters of melanomas are the superfisial spreading variety. About 7% of melanomas are classified as lentigo maligna, a superficial melanoma with an irregular border; it has an extremely long natural course (Fig. 2, color plate). Nodular melanoma is a well-demarcated lesion and represents 15–20% of primary melanomas (Fig. 3).

2. Pigmentation may be highly suggestive of melanoma. Various combinations of red, white, blue, and brown may be present alone or, more commonly, in combination (Fig. 4, color plate). Reddish discoloration is representative of a superficial inflammatory response to the presence of the lesion. Blue or brown pigmentation denotes pigmentary deposition within the tumor. White areas around the lesion denote scarring, or "healing," in that the local immunologic battle between tumor and host may be resolved in this zone with the formation of cicatricial tissue (Fig. 5 and 6). Spontaneous resolution of a nevus or melanoma may be seen, and in this situation a depigmented, whitish area in the skin remains.

Nonpigmented melanomas also occur and may be as frequent as one-sixth of all such tumors. Such a lesion is seen in Fig. 7. Because of the lack of the usual bluish or brown color on external examination, the diagnosis must be made histologically. Not infrequently, experienced pathologists express difficulty in microscopic interpretation of this lesion.

3. The occurrence of "satellite" lesions around a primary melanoma is a very distinctive circumstance (Fig. 8). These lesions represent intracutaneous lymphangitic metastases and are somewhat unique observable evidences of melanoma.

So called "in-transit" metastases in melanoma are characterized as nodules in the skin proximal to a primary lesion. Their significance is that of more distant

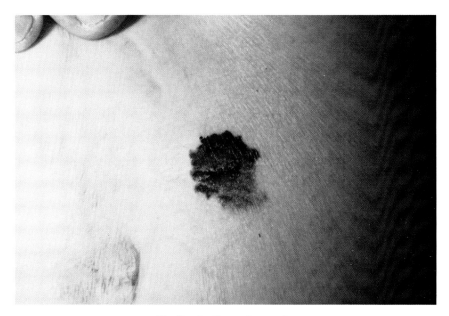

Fig. 2. Lentigo maligna melanoma.

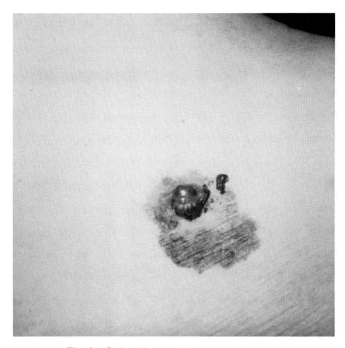

Fig. 4. Red, white, and blue coloration in melanoma.

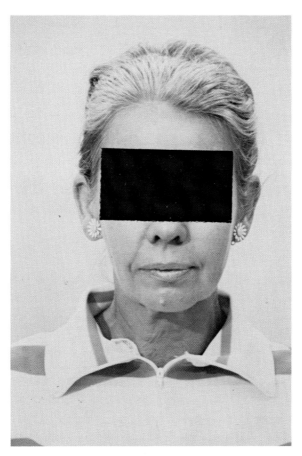

Fig. 15. Melanosis: The pigmentary deposition of widespread melanoma accounts for the abnormal skin hue in this patient with advanced disease.

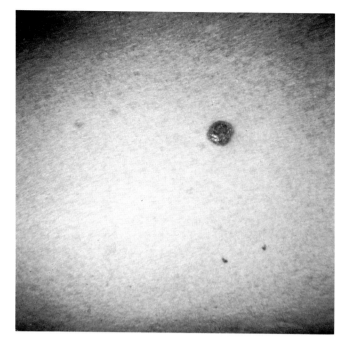

Fig. 3. Nodular melanoma.

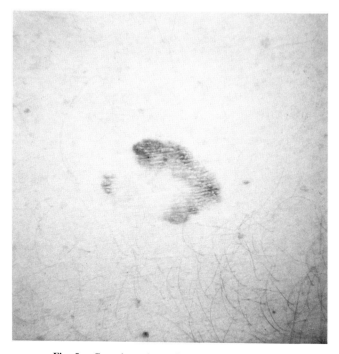

Fig. 5. Central scarring and "clearing" in melanoma.

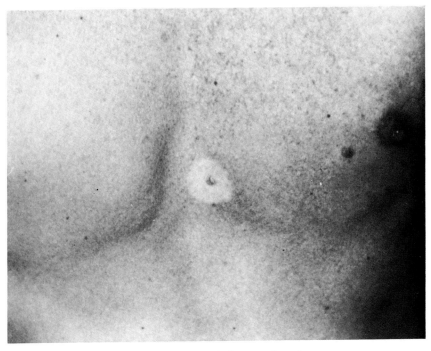

Fig. 6. Spontaneous resolution around a melanoma.

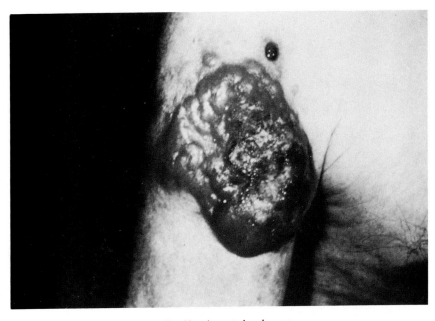

Fig. 7. Nonpigmented melanoma.

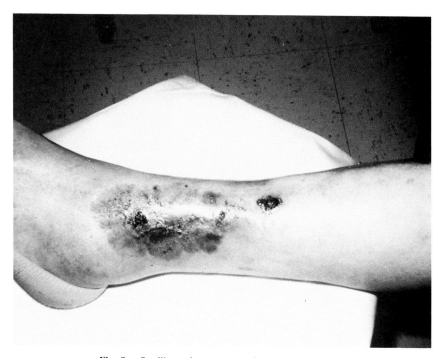

Fig. 8. Satellite melanomas around a primary lesion.

intracutaneous lymphatic metastases. These lesions may be benefited by intra-arterial chemotherapy when located on an extremity, as described below.

B. Microscopic Pathology

When malignant change occurs in a junctional nevus, very "active" cells are seen in the dermis and epidermis. Increased cellular activity is seen at the dermal–epidermal junction (Fig. 9). The microscopic histology is variable, and individual cells or cellular patterns may resemble carcinoma, sarcoma, or cells of nerve cell origin (Fig. 10). The most important microscopic feature is that of dermal invasion. If this is present along with other elements of malignancy—e.g., frequent mitoses, increased nucleolar size—the diagnosis is established. The stromal reaction adjacent to melanoma cells may include macrophages, lymphocytes, and plasma cells (del Regato and Spjut, 1977).

Early in the course of metastatic disease, regional lymphatics contain tumor, and regional nodes are frequently involved. Hematogenous dissemination is the other principle mode of spread and accounts for the frequency of involvement of multiple organ systems with metastatic disease.

Postmortem examination has shown that of patients with advanced disease,

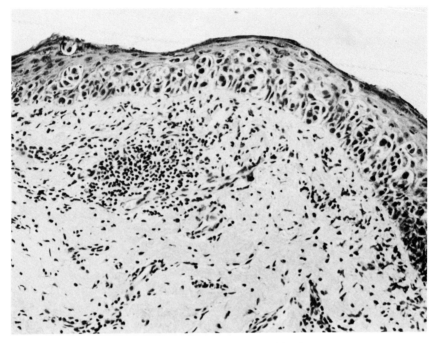

Fig. 9. Melanoma cells below the epidermis.

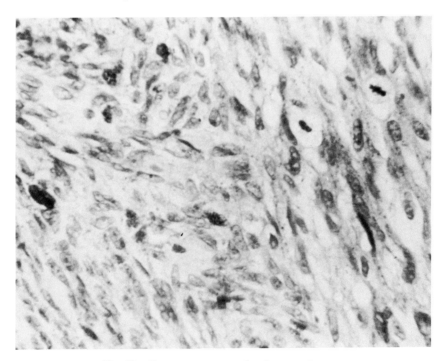

Fig. 10. Sarcometous pattern of malignant melanoma.

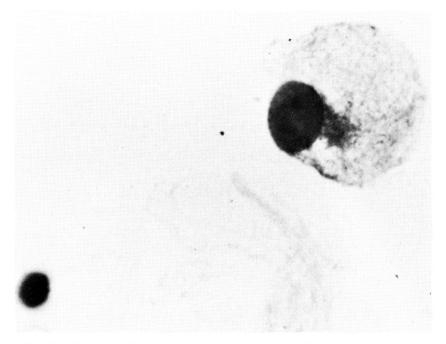

Fig. 11. Melanoma cell in cerebrospinal fluid from a patient with meningeal involvement.

approximately one-half have involvement of the central nervous system (CNS), heart (pericardium and myocardium), and bone (Fig. 11). Liver metastases are present in 60% of cases, and the lung is involved 70% of the time. When the tumor load is very high and hematogenous dissemination is ongoing, cytologic examination may reveal malignant cells in the peripheral blood, a most unusual finding for an epithelial neoplasm.

IV. CLINICAL FINDINGS

As noted previously, the majority of melanomas arise in preexisting nevi. The external features that may portend malignancy include growth, itching, increased pigmentation, ulceration, and bleeding.

Melanoma in Caucasians characteristically occurs in fair, red or sandy haired, blue-eyed or hazel-eyed persons. Approximately one-tenth of the population in the United States has these colorations, yet eight of ten melanomas occur in persons with these general features. The lesion is relatively uncommon in blacks in the United States, but is more frequent in African natives. When melanoma effects blacks, the sites most frequently involved include the soles of the feet, nail beds, and oral mucosa (Fig. 12). These anatomical areas are not pigmented in the black race. Melanoma is also infrequent in Asians.

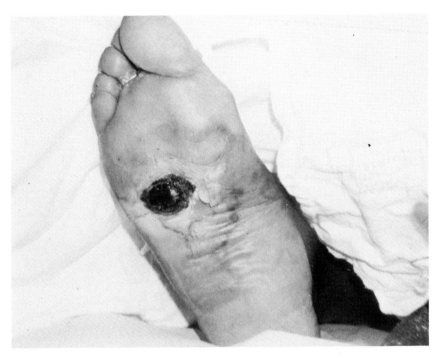

Fig. 12. Plantar melanoma.

Most commonly, the tumor occurs on the lower extremities, face, and neck. The trunk is quite commonly involved; genital melanoma is unusual. However, pigmented moles on the soles and in the genital area have a much increased risk of malignancy. Persistent moles on the plantar skin, whether pigmented or not, must be considered malignant until pathological proof discounts this possibility.

Although multiple primary melanomas have been described, such instances are happily very uncommon. Cutaneous metastases from malignant melanoma can be distinguished from multiple primary melanomas by histological examination: Metastatic lesions disrupt the epidermis, whereas primary tumors are found to have continuity with the stratum germinatum.

An unusual variant of pigmented tumor is the congenital "bathing trunk" nevus (Fig. 13). These lesions are large and suspiscious in appearance and their ominous characteristics suggest their malignant potential. Malignant transformation often occurs by puberty, and other forms of neoplasm may also be seen in these patients.

When metastases from a primary melanoma appear they do so by local extension and lymphatic and hematogenous dissemination. Late in the course of disease, blood-borne metastases predominate and are the most frequent cause of death. It is for these reasons that CNS metastases are very common in malignant

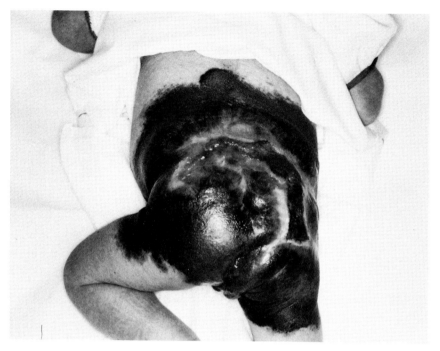

Fig. 13. The ''bathing trunk'' nevus. This patient required multiple surgical excisions of the estensive lesion.

melanoma compared to any other form of malignancy, including lung and breast primary tumors. Brain involvement is seen at postmortem in from 38 to 90% of patients in reported series. Other sites of common involvement include lung (70%), heart (55%), liver (65%), and bone (50%).

It must also be noted that melanoma frequently spreads to the stomach, lower gastrointestinal tract, kidneys, spleen, and skin (Fig. 14). The other epithelial tumors that involve the gastrointestinal tract, spleen, heart, and skin with any degree of regularity are carcinoma of the lung and breast. Lymphoproliferative neoplasms, lymphoma and leukemia, also commonly involve these sites. These neoplasms must be considered when differential diagnosis in an unknown primary situation occurs or when late recurrence or multiple primary malignancies are at issue. These patterns of spread of melanoma can also be of major importance (1) when biopsy of an unknown primary lesion is performed and the lesion itself is nonpigmented, or (2) when a nonmelanomatous, poorly differentiated epithelial neoplasm or non-Hodgkin's lymphoma presents to the physician, since the patterns of spread within this group of neoplasm can be so similar.

The predisposition to vascular metastases accounts for many failures of treatment, which is frequently aimed at the lymphatic surgical anatomy of the pri-

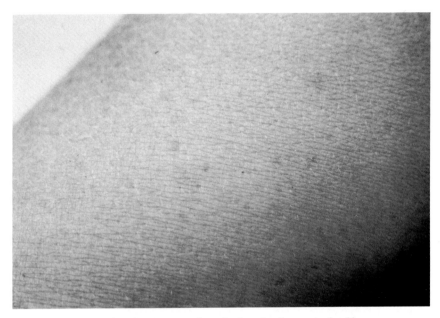

Fig. 14.   Hematogenous dissemination of melanoma to the skin.

mary, and probably has led to a general diminution of enthusiasm for radical initial surgery requiring extensive regional nodal dissection. This is particularly so when lesions may be quite distant from the regional nodes—e.g., an ankle melanoma that is treated locally in conjunction with a groin dissection. It is also evident from general patterns of hematogenous dissemination that modern approaches to treatment of widespread disease, which may include hepatic artery perfusion and prophylactic brain irradiation, have a reasonable clinical pathological basis.

When widespread disease activity is seen, deposition of melanin in the skin can be extensive. This is referred to as melanosis, a situation in which the hue of the skin may be blue or brownish. In this condition the urine often turns black or very dark, and the ferric chloride test on urine demonstrates the characteristic black discoloration, indicating the large amount of melanin present in the urine (Fig. 15, color plate). With this finding, the prognosis is limited because of the extensive tumor burden present.

V. DIAGNOSIS

Classically, a suspicious lesion is widely excised and is submitted for pathologic examination. The past dictum of wide local excision is currently less important since no evidence exists that other biopsy procedures—e.g., needle or incisional biopsy—decrease survival via hypothetical enhancement of vascular metastases. The realization of this situation removes much of the concern that previously surrounded the evaluation of potential melanomatous lesions.

Evaluation of melanoma, grossly and microscopically, has been described previously and is a critical feature of diagnosis. In this respect, pigmented tumors of several types may mimic melanoma grossly and microscopically, making diagnosis difficult. The juvenile nevus, senile keratosis, basal cell carcinoma, hemangioma, histiocytoma, and blue nevus are important differential considerations. Nonpigmented melanomas may be suspected by careful evaluation of the natural course of disease and a critical microscopic review.

Poorly differentiated melanoma may be confused microscopically with carcinoma of epithelial origin, sarcoma, and histiocytic lymphoma. In patients with widely disseminated tumor, the urine may be very dark in color and react positively with ferric chloride, as mentioned above. When diffuse cutaneous melanosis is present, the pigment released by the tumor is deposited in the skin. The external features of melanoma have been discussed previously.

VI. PROGNOSIS

As in all neoplasms, survival is related to the stage of disease at the time of diagnosis. The overall 5-year survival rate of all patients (i.e., patients presenting themselves to the physicians in all stages) is about 45%, or essentially the same as for patients with carcinoma of the breast. This survival rate emphasizes the fact that the ''lethal'' reputation attributed to malignant melanoma is perhaps not always deserved.

The most widely accepted staging system in melanoma is that of Clark and Mihm (1969) shown in Fig. 1. In essence, this system correlates survival with depth of penetration of the malignancy into the skin at the time of diagnosis. This staging method has largely replaced previous prognostic modes and now enjoys the support of most clinicians. In this classification, a level I lesion is depicted by atypical melanocytic hyperplasia confined to the epidermis. This is a premalignant lesion. Level II melanoma shows neoplastic cells penetrating the epidermal basement membrance and extending into the papillary dermis. Level III lesions show neoplastic cell accumulation at the interface between papillary and reticular dermis. Level IV consists of the extension of tumor cells between the bundles of collagen in the reticular dermis. In level V melanoma, the subdermal fat is invaded by tumor.

The information on overall survival must be balanced with individual variations in behavior of disease, which can fall well outside the norm. For example, late recurrences are not unusual in melanoma, as is the case in other malignancies—notably, carcinoma of the breast, renal cell carcinoma, and lymphomas. Thirteen percent of first recurrences or metastases in melanoma may be found more than 5 years after primary surgery. In this respect the patient should be forewarned that a 5-year survival free of disease is most encouraging but does not guarantee "cure."

If distant metastases are present at the time of diagnosis, survival is usually 1.5–3 years. In the instance of palpable regional nodes, the survival rate is diminished to 10% for 5 years. If regional nodes at diagnosis are palpably negative but show tumor on microscopic examination, the survival rate improves to 15–25% for 5 years. If regional nodes are palpable and microscropic examination is negative for tumor, the 5-year survival rate increases to 60%.

VII. TREATMENT

The primary treatment of melanoma remains wide local excision. Cautery of melanoma should not be performed inasmuch as pathological specimens are not obtained during this procedure. Recurrence following cauterization may be difficult to evaluate, in addition to the fact that adequate primary treatment has been denied to the patient. The surgical margins around a melanoma, or what constitutes a "wide local excision," is not easily defined, but many clinicians accept 3 cm around small lesions and 5 cm around large tumors. Skin grafting is a necessary concomitant procedure for closure of the surgical site.

Prophylactic node dissection at the time of, or following, the primary excision historically was considered mandatory. Aside from the fact that considerable morbidity may accompany radical nodal dissections, there is no convincing data that verify the proposal that prophylactic nodal dissection increases the survival of patients. The prevailing view now is that prophylactic nodal dissection is not an absolutely indicated procedure (Goldsmith et al., 1970). It must be stated, however, that such surgery allows more complete staging and can add prognostic information, as stated above, for the use of a clinician on behalf of a given patient.

Therapeutic nodal dissection is usually restricted to those patients whose melanoma lies in close anatomical proximity to the area of nodal drainage (Das Gupta and McNeer, 1964). This procedure has been most useful in the management of scalp lesions. Iliac and inguinal node dissections are currently seldom performed.

Amputations for limb lesions are also rarely performed now (Turnbull et al., 1973). The indications for amputation have fortunately become quite restricted since the advent of techniques of arterial perfusion with chemotherapeutic agents. Perfusional treatment has been advocated by Stehlin et al. (1975), and has several advantages. First, amputation of limbs may be avoided. Second, in-transit metastases can be successfully controlled by limb perfusion. Third, enhancement of antitumor effects may result if concomitant hyperthermia is employed. Fourth, doses of chemotherapy given in the vascular system isolated from the systemic circulation may allow much higher amounts of chemotherapy to be delivered to the tumor site than is tolerated in conventional systemic chemotherapy. Lastly, perfusion may also be employed for liver metastases, since this organ is frequently a major site of life-threatening disease activity. This technique has been incorporated in Southwest Oncology Group studies directed toward improvement of the treatment of melanoma patients with advanced disease.

The most commonly employed agent in arterial perfusion procedures is phenylalanine mustard. Presently, it is not possible to say that perfusional procedures increase survival in the management of melanoma in man.

Melanoma has traditionally been considered relatively radiotherapy-resistant when compared to many other tumors. There is no question however, that individual melanomas can be very sensitive to radiation (Hilaris *et al.*, 1963). Hence, local involvement of neoplasm with bone, biliary tree, kidney, lung, skin, brain, and meninges may respond very favorably to irradiation. Perhaps negative physician bias has played a part in the formation of clinical opinion that X-ray treatment is of limited value in the management of this malignancy. Review of this problem suggests that at least half of melanomas have substantial sensitivity to radiation and hence, if individual patient situations indicate potential benefit, there should be no hesitancy in applying this modality of therapy. Current investigations are employing prophylactic radiotherapy to the CNS because of the high incidence of metastases to this location. The aim of such treatment is to establish whether or not micrometastases may be favorably responsive; if so, control of disease in the brain may be improved in a manner similar to that in which the treatment of oat cell carcinoma of the lung has dramatically reduced CNS failure.

Chemotherapy of disseminated melanoma may be resulted in favorable palliation of disease. Unfortunately, available single-agent and combination chemotherapy are not as effective as in the case in many more sensitive neoplasms. Nevertheless, clinical research of the past decade indicates that treatment with BCNU, hydroxyurea, and imidazole carboxamide in combination may lead to partial remission in up to 40% of patients. The Southwest Oncology Group has demonstrated that such combination chemotherapy can lead to success in the palliation of advanced disease. Recently, *cis*-platinum has proved to be an efficacious drug when administered intra-arterially to the liver when extensive metastatic disease is present (Calvo *et al.*, 1979). Dramatic individual responses in this setting will undoubtedly lead to a more extensive experience in the near future if a more accurate picture of this approach should become available.

Remarkable responses have been seen to phenylalanine mustard administered intra-arterially in patients with limb lesions with in-transit metastases. As mentioned previously, this treatment has reduced the need for amputations but has not convinced many critics that benefit in survival has been achieved. Similarly, limb perfusion with phenylalanine mustard accompanied by hyperthermia may be promising, but current evaluation suggests that this modality does not affect clinical outcome dramatically. It should be emphasized that perfusion techniques are expensive and not without morbidity. In this situation it would seem reasonable to view melanoma perfusion treatment as promising in selected individual patients, but that additional experience and controlled studies are needed before a final place in the therapeutic picture is clear.

Much has been written concerning the potential use of immunotherapy in treatment of melanoma. The interest in this approach has come in part from the observation that spontaneous regression occurs in malignant melanoma in the skin and much less commonly in patients with advanced systemic disease.

Intratumoral Bacille Calmette-Guérin (BCG) injection can unquestionably cause regression of lesions (Karakousis *et al.*, 1976), but inoculation of BCG or other nonspecific immunostimulants in patients with disseminated melanomas has been disappointing in that immunotherapy alone or used with the most effective combination chemotherapy has failed to have a significant response in rates or survival. The addition of immunotherapy to chemotherapy does not, therefore, appear to increase response rates or survival times in patients with advanced disease.

VIII. CONCLUSION

Malignant melanoma represents a continuing problem in management for the clinician. Distinct improvements in available treatment choices have developed, but it is hoped that new modifications will result in programs giving a better prognosis for patients with advanced disease.

REFERENCES

Calvo, D., Patt, Y. Z., Wallace, S., Hersh, E. M., Benjamin, R. S., Pritchard, J., and Mavligit, G. M. (1979). *Am. Assoc. Clin. Oncol.* **20,** 426.

Clark, W. H., and Mihm, M. C. (1969). *Am. J. Pathol.* **55,** 39–67.

Das Gupta, T., and McNeer, G. (1964). *Cancer* **17,** 897–911.

Dellon, A. L., and Ketcham, A. S. (1973). *Arch. Surg.* (*Chicago*) **106,** 738–739.

del Regato, J. A., and Spjut, H. J. (1977). *In* "Cancer," 5th ed. pp. 200–221. Mosby, St. Louis, Missouri.

Goldsmith, H. S., Shan, J. P., and Kim, D. H. (1970). *Cancer* **26,** 606–609.

Hilaris, B. S., Robin, M., Calabrese, A. S., Phillips, R. F., and Henschke, U.K. (1963). *Cancer* **16,** 765–773.

Karakousis, C. P., Douglass, H. O., Yeracaris, P. M., and Holyoke, E. D. (1976). *Arch. Surg.* (*Chicago*) **111,** 716–718.

McBride, C. M. (1973). *Proc. Natl. Cancer Conf.* **7,** 581–585.

Nathanson, L., Sober, A., and Mihm, M. (1978). *In* ''Cancer, A Manual for Practioners,'' Am. Cancer Soc. Publ., 5th ed., p. 110. Nimrod Press, Massachusetts.

Reynolds, A. C. (1955). *J. Obstet. & Gynecol.* **6,** 205–209.

Smith, F. E., Henly, W. S., Knox, J. M., and Lane, M. (1966). *Arch. Intern. Med.* **117,** 820–823.

Stehlin, J., Giovanella, B. C., Ipolyi, P. D., Muenz, L. R., and Anderson, R. F. (1975). *Surg., Gynecol. Obstex.* **140,** 338–348.

Turnbull, A., Shah, J., and Fortner, J. (1973). *Arch. Surg.* (*Chicago*) **106,** 496–498.

14
THE SARCOMAS
Robert S. Benjamin

I.	Introduction	275
II.	Diagnosis	276
III.	Soft Tissue Sarcomas	277
	A. Classification and Incidence	277
	B. Staging and Prognosis	282
	C. Treatment	283
IV.	Sarcomas of Bone	284
	A. General	284
	B. Osteosarcoma	285
	C. Chondrosarcomas	286
	D. Ewing's Sarcoma	287
	E. Giant Cell Tumor	289
	F. Fibrous Histiocytoma	289
V.	Conclusion	290
	References	290

I. INTRODUCTION

Although sarcomas account for less than 2% of all cancers and include numerous diagnoses, they attract more attention than their relatively small numbers would indicate because they so frequently strike people in the younger age groups. Whereas the median age for patients with carcinomas lies in the seventh or eighth decades, the median age for patients with sarcomas is usually in the fourth or fifth decades. Indeed, childhood sarcomas comprise three of the top eight causes of cancer deaths in patients under the age of 15, accounting for nearly 10% of all childhood cancer deaths each year. Their occurrence in patients who are in their prime of life, coupled with the fact that their therapy involves radical surgery, frequently amputation, together with toxic chemotherapy, further increases the tragedy of these diseases.

CANCER AND CHEMOTHERAPY, VOL. II   275
Copyright © 1981 Academic Press, Inc.
All rights of reproduction in any form reserved.
ISBN 0-12-197802-8

Sarcomas are usually divided into two groups, depending on whether they arise from soft tissue or bone. In addition, there are numerous histological subtypes. Sarcomas can arise from literally any site in which the parent tissue can be found. Thus, although the soft tissues of the extremities, trunk, and retroperitoneum are the most frequent sites of soft tissue sarcomas, they can arise within the connective tissue of any organ or even in the major vessels. In addition, the three major bone sarcomas, osteosarcoma, chondrosarcoma, and Ewing's sarcoma, may all arise from soft tissues as well. The diagnosis is usually made when the patient accidentally discovers a mass in soft tissue or develops a painful area in a bone. Lesions in the soft tissues of the extremities may be quite large before they become painful, a fact that frequently delays the patient in seeking medical advice. In addition, many of the sarcomas arise in silent areas, such as the retroperitoneum, and thus are huge before causing any symptomatology.

The tumors tend to infiltrate widely in the primary area, even when they appear to be encapsulated. Thus, frequent local occurrence is the rule if a simple excision is carried out. In addition, hematogenous spread makes the lungs by far the most common site of metastases. Lymph nodes, liver, and bone are less frequently involved than with many carcinomas. Bone marrow involvement is extremely rare except in rhabdomyosarcoma and Ewing's sarcoma. Central nervous system metastases are also rare. The primary bone sarcomas metastasize to other bones as their second most frequent metastatic site.

II. DIAGNOSIS

The differential diagnosis of sarcomas includes their benign counterparts, which, in contrast to the sarcomas, are usually freely movable and of slow growth, whereas the sarcomas are attached to underlying tissue and appear to grow more rapidly. Other important differential diagnoses include sebaceous cysts, aneurysms, subcutaneous abcesses, and myositis ossificans, as well as metastatic carcinoma from an unknown primary site.

Plain X rays are often diagnostic in the case of primary bone tumors. For soft tissue sarcomas, however, plain films are less useful. Xerograms may define soft tissue masses, but these are more accurately defined by the newer techniques of ultrasound or computerized tomography (CT), especially for intra-abdominal lesions (deSantos et al., 1978). Arteriograms may aid in the diagnosis of malignancy by showing increased vascularity or abnormal tumor vessels (deSantos et al., 1977). These procedures may be helpful as well in defining the extent of primary bone tumors, particularly with regard to associated soft tissue masses. In addition, CT has been able to define skip metastases within the medullary canal of patients with osteosarcoma (deSantos et al., 1979). By defining the extent of local involvement, these tests help the surgeon to plan his initial approach to resection of the tumor.

In order to evaluate the patient for distant metastases, a plain chest film is frequently all that is required. Although many investigators prefer to obtain full lung tomograms to increase the chances of finding pulmonary metastases, others find that they rarely add to the evaluation of a patient with a truly negative plain film of the chest (Parker and Marglin, 1978). When pulmonary metastases are suspected, tomograms will find them more accurately than the plain film, and computerized tomography will define the presence of more nodules than can be seen by conventional tomography. However thoractomy may define still more nodules that were missed even by CT (Creagan *et al.*, 1978; Schaner *et al.*, 1978). In addition, the computerized tomogram may pick up lesions that are simply peripheral granulomas that may lead to a false-positive interpretation (Schaner *et al.*, 1978).

III. SOFT TISSUE SARCOMAS

A. Classification and Incidence

1. General

The soft tissue sarcomas, as defined in Table I, comprise a large variety of different tumors. Since many of the older series antedate the broad use of the diagnosis of malignant fibrous histiocytoma, it is often impossible to get an accurate picture of the distribution of diagnoses, or the natural history of the many diagnoses with which that particular tumor can be confused. The largest modern series is that of the Task Force for Soft Tissue Sarcomas of the American Joint Committee for Cancer Staging and End Results Reporting (Russell *et al.*, 1977). Their report, which is probably the most important single paper in the literature on soft tissue sarcomas, analyzed the effect of staging on prognosis in a collected series of 1215 patients from 13 institutions with a variety of diagnoses. Pathological sections were reviewed by pathologists on the task force in 600 cases, and the grade of malignancy was determined in 437 cases. Complete staging information was available in 702 cases, including 423 of those with slide review and grading, which implies that both the grade and size of the tumor, essential elements in the staging system, were known from the institutional pathologist in the remaining 279.

The distribution of all patients and those completely staged by diagnosis is shown in Table II. Note that the proportion of patients with malignant fibrous histiocytoma increases in those with slide review, probably due to the increasing frequency of reclassifying tumors previously categorized elsewhere into this

TABLE I

Soft Tissue Sarcomas

Diagnosis and variants	Synonyms
Fibrosarcoma	
Desmoid type	
Malignant fibrous histiocytoma (MHF)	Malignant fibrohistiocytoma
Pleomorphic fibrosarcoma	
Malignant histiocytoma	Reticulum cell sarcoma of soft parts
Xanthosarcoma	Malignant xanthogranuloma
	Inflammatory fibrous histiocytoma
Myxoid variant of MFH	
Malignant giant cell tumor of soft parts ⟨	Malignant giant cell tumor of tendon sheath
	Extraskeletal osteolytic osteogenic sarcoma
Dermatofibrosarcoma protuberans	
Liposarcoma	
Well-differentiated: myxoid / lipoma-like	
Mixed	
Poorly differentiated (round cell)	
Pleomorphic	
Leiomyosarcoma	Epithelioid leiomyosarcoma, malignant leiomyoblastoma
Rhabdomyosarcoma	Sarcoma botryoides
Embryonal	
Alveolar	
Mixed	
Pleomorphic	
Angiosarcoma	Malignant hemangioendothelioma
Malignant hemangiopericytoma	
Lymphangiosarcoma	
Kaposi's sarcoma	
Synovial sarcoma	Malignant synovioma
Malignant schwannoma	Neurofibrosarcoma
Primary	Triton tumor
Arising in neurofibromatosis	Neurogenic sarcoma
With rhabdomyosarcomatous change	
Alveolar soft part sarcoma	Malignant granular cell tumor, organoid
Malignant granular cell tumor	Malignant granular cell tumor, non-organoid
Clear cell sarcoma of tendon and aponeurosis	Clear cell sarcoma, malignant melanoma of soft parts
Epithelioid sarcoma	
Extraskeletal chondrosarcoma	Chondrosarcoma of soft parts
Extraskeletal Ewing's sarcoma	Ewing's sarcoma of the soft parts, small-cell sarcoma (Ewing's-like)
Extraskeletal osteosarcoma	Osteosarcoma of soft parts
Sarcomatous mesothelioma	
Unclassified sarcoma	Spindle cell sarcoma
Undifferentiated sarcoma	Malignant mesenchymoma

TABLE II

Incidence of Sarcomas

Diagnosis	All patients[a] No. (%)	Staged patients[a] No. (%)	Metastatic patients[b] No. (%)
Rhabdomyosarcoma	234 (19)	133 (19)	14 (7)
Fibrosarcoma	231 (19)	128 (18)	14 (7)
Liposarcoma	221 (18)	136 (19)	17 (8)
MFH[c]	128 (11)	96 (14)	35 (17)
Unclassified	12 (10)	67 (10)	15 (7)
Synovial sarcoma	84 (7)	42 (6)	14 (7)
Leiomyosarcoma	79 (7)	42 (6)	45 (22)
Malignant schwannoma	60 (5)	26 (4)	10 (5)
Angiosarcoma	33 (3)	17 (2)	18 (9)
Other	24 (2)	15 (2)	19 (9)
Total	1215	702	201

[a] Russell *et al.* (1977).

[b] Baker and Benjamin (1978).

[c] MFH, malignant fibrous histiocytoma.

diagnostic group. Note also, that the most frequent diagnoses in this series were rhabdomyosarcoma, fibrosarcoma, and liposarcoma, each at about 20% of the total, followed closely be malignant fibrous histiocytoma at 10–15% of the total, and unclassified sarcoma at 10%. Together, these five diagnoses comprise more than 80% of the series.

In contrast, the series of patients by Baker and Benjamin represents the findings in a series of patients referred for chemotherapy to members of the Southwest Oncology Group (Baker and Benjamin, 1978). As can be seen in Table II, leiomyosarcoma accounted for 22% of the patients in this series as compared with only 6–7% of patients in Russell's series. The second most common diagnosis was malignant fibrous histiocytoma. Third was angiosarcoma at 9%, compared with only 2–3% in Russell's series. The relatively high frequency of rhabdomyosarcoma in Russell's series compared with that of Baker does not reflect earlier presentation of that disease; rather, Baker's series excluded pediatric cases, which make up 15% of Russell's series and include the vast majority of patients with rhabdomyosarcoma. Perhaps one other reason for the higher frequency of leiomyosarcoma in the chemotherapy series is that these tumors frequently occur in primary organs such as the uterus or the gastrointestinal tract. Primary organ tumors were excluded from Russell's series. A detailed description of the pathology of these tumors is beyond the scope of this chapter and can be found in the excellent fascicles of the Armed Forces Institute of Pathology (Stout and Lattes, 1966).

2. Malignant Fibrous Histiocytoma (MFH)

The tumor that does need further discussion, however, is malignant fibrous histiocytoma, best described in the analysis of 200 cases by Weiss and Enzinger (1978) of the Armed Forces Institute of Pathology (AFIP). This tumor has varied morphological features, but is characterized by spindle (fibrous) cells and round (histiocytoid) cells arranged in a storiform pattern, other areas with a less differentiated pleomorphic appearance, and frequent giant cells. There is controversy regarding the cell of origin, with some investigators suggesting a histiocytic origin (Kauffman and Stout, 1961; Kempson and Kyriakos, 1972; Ozzello et al., 1963), whereas others suggest origin in a primitive mesenchymal cell (Fu et al., 1975). The tumors most frequently confused with MFH are pleomorphic rhabdomyosarcoma and pleomorphic liposarcoma; however, poorly differentiated fibrosarcomas and leiomyosarcomas may also be confused with it. The majority of tumors occurred on the extremities or retroperitoneum, with almost half on the lower extremity and 30% in the thigh. Typically, the tumors were deep, with peak incidence in the seventh decade; 70% of tumors occurred between the ages of 41 and 80. Two-thirds of patients were male (Weiss and Enzinger, 1978).

Forty-two percent of patients followed 2 or more years in the AFIP study developed metastases (Weiss and Enzinger, 1978). Forty-three percent of those with metastases developed a local recurrence prior to metastasis, whereas 57% developed metastasis alone or prior to local recurrence. An additional 26% of patients have shown local recurrence but no metastases at the time of their last follow-up. Only 32% had no further evidence of disease. Eighty-two percent of those with metastatic disease had metastases in the lung, as is seen with other sarcomas. In addition, lymph nodes were involved in 32% of those with metastases, liver in 15%, and bone in 11%. It should be noted, however, that lymph node metastases were present in only 12% of the patients in the entire series, and a high incidence of lymph node metastases among those with metastatic disease simply reflects biopsy and/or autopsy findings when disease was suspected (Weiss and Enzinger, 1978).

Metastases occurred in 21% of patients with tumors smaller than 2.5 cm in diameter and 57% of those with tumors larger than 10 cm in diameter (Weiss and Enzinger, 1978). However, in between these values intermediate rates of metastasis did not appear to be correlated with tumor size. In contrast, depth of invasion was a more accurate predictor of metastatic disease. Tumor confined to the subcutis showed only 9% metastasis, but a 30% local recurrence rate. Tumor in the subcutis and fascia had a similar local recurrence rate but a 27% rate of metastases. With involvement of muscle, the rate of metastases increased to 43%, and with retroperitoneal or visceral involvement the metastatic rate was 50%. Local recurrence rates in these two categories were in the 50% range.

Thirty-two percent of these patients died of their disease within 2 years of diagnosis, and an additional 14% after a longer time. In addition, 20% of survivors have evidence of recurrent disease and 15% of patients have died from other causes (Weiss and Enzinger, 1978).

Eighty patients with a myxoid variant of MFH have been described (Weiss and Enzinger, 1977). Age and sex distributions, with two-thirds of the patients being male, were similar to those with the more typical forms of MFH. The relationship of the size of tumor and depth of invasion to the recurrence or metastasis was also similar to that with standard MFH. The rate of metastases was inversely proportional to the degree of myxoid change. Only 16% of those with predominantly myxoid histology developed metastases, whereas 31% of those with predominantly cellular histology developed metastases. Those with mixed histology had an intermediate rate of metastases (24%). These tumors tended to recur locally before metastasizing. Only 27% of those that did metastasize did so prior to the development of local recurrence, as opposed to 57% of those with typical cellular MFH.

3. Rhabdomyosarcoma

Rhabdomyosarcoma is the most common soft tissue tumor of children. It is characterized by a high propensity for distant metastasis and local recurrence, as well as extraordinary sensitivity to chemotherapy with cyclosphosphamide, vincristine, and actinomycin-D, drugs that are almost inactive against the other soft tissue sarcomas. It is also somewhat more responsive to radiation than other soft tissue sarcomas. In the M.D. Anderson Hospital series, the most common initial sites were the head and neck (60%)—especially the orbit; the genitourinary tract (15%); and the extremities (14%) (Fernandez et al., 1975). Peak incidence was in children under age 5. Patients with head and neck primary tumors experienced a 90% recurrence rate within the first 18 months when not treated on a multimodality management plan involving surgery, radiation, and intensive VAC (vincristine, actinomycin-D, cyclophosphamide) chemotherapy. In contrast, 90% of patients treated on the multimodal program remained free of local recurrence, and 70% were long term survivors. The original report of this exciting series by Donaldson et al. (1973) was recently updated (Sutow et al., 1977). Only two patients have relapsed and one of these was salvaged by surgical excision of a metastasis that developed 6 years after original therapy. Prognosis depends upon clinical grouping. The group with the most favorable prognosis, Group 1, has localized disease, completely resectable, with regional nodes not involved. Group 2 has regional node involvement or incomplete excision with microscopic residual disease. Group 3 has partial excision or biopsy only. Group 4 has metastatic disease at the onset (Maurer et al., 1977). In the intergroup rhabdomyosarcoma study, patients with group 3 disease had a much poorer prognosis than patients with group 2 disease, with a 73% relapse rate as compared to 21%, and survival of 53% as compared with 91% (Hays *et al.*, 1978). Metastatic involvement most frequently involves lungs, bones, and serous membranes (Fernandez *et al.*, 1975). Bone marrow involvement occurs as well (Ruymann *et al.*, 1979), a finding that is extremely unusual in other soft tissue sarcomas.

B. Staging and Prognosis

The staging of soft tissue sarcomas is most important for prognostic purposes, more so even than diagnosis, although diagnosis is taken into account in the staging procedure (Russell *et al.*, 1977). In addition to the TNM (primary Tumor, lymph Node metastases, distant Metastases) classification used to stage other tumors, pathological grading (G) is used as well. Grading is a complex procedure and involves an expert sarcoma pathologist. Once the type of tumor has been established, histological criteria are used to determine grade; however, in some highly malignant tumors such as rhabdomyosarcoma, synovial sarcoma, and certain types of angiosarcoma, a grade 3 designation is used regardless of further histological appearance. Moreover, other factors—such as age, in fibrosarcoma, where children have better prognoses, or depth of invasion—are taken into account in assessing a grade. Three grades are used in the staging schema: grade 1 for low, grade 2, intermediate, and grade 3, high. The primary tumor is assessed as follows: T1, smaller than 5 cm; T2, 5 cm or larger; and T3, a tumor of any size that grossly invades bone, major vessel, or major nerve. Nodal involvement is assessed histologically as negative, N-0, or positive, N-1. Similarly, distant metastases are assessed as absent, M-0, or present, M-1.

Staging is determined by the grade of the tumor, the presence or absence of metastases, and tumor size. Stage 1 tumors are grade 1 tumors without regional or distant metastases. This is divided into two substages, stage 1A, with tumors smaller than 5 cm, and stage 1B with tumors larger than 5 cm. Stage 2 is identical to stage 1 except that the tumor is of grade 2 histology. Stage 3 is divided into three groups. Stages 3A and 3B are analogous to stages 1A, 1B, 2A, and 2B that involve a grade 3 tumor. Stage 3C is a tumor of any grade, but with regional lymph node metastases. Stage 4 is divided into two groups. Stage 4A involves a T3 tumor, that is, tumor of any grade that grossly invades bone, major vessel, or major nerve, with or without regional node metastases, but without distant metastases. Stage 4B involves distant metastases from any sarcoma (Russell *et al.*, 1977).

Staging is clearly of prognostic importance (Russell *et al.*, 1977). Patients with stage 1 tumors have a 75% 5-year survival rate and a 63% 10-year survival rate, as compared with 55 and 40% for stage 2, 29 and 19% for stage 3, and 7 and 3% for stage 4. Although the 5-year survival rates for fibrosarcoma, malignant fibrous histiocytoma, lipsarcoma, synovial sarcoma, and malignant schwannoma

(43 to 55%) are higher than those for angiosarcoma, rhabdomyosarcoma, leiomyosarcoma, and unclassified sarcoma (23 to 36%), survival rates within each stage are similar. Thus, for example, both patients in Russell's series with stage 1 angiosarcoma were 5-year survivors, and 1 of 2 patients with stage 2 angiosarcomas were 5-year survivors. There was only a 24% overall 5-year survivorship for patients with the diagnosis of angiosarcoma as a whole, which can be exaplained by the fact that none of 9 patients with stage 3 disease and only 1 of 4 with stage 4 disease survived 5 years (Russell *et al.*, 1977). Similarly, 8 of 14 patients with stage 1 leiomyosarcoma were 5-year survivors, despite an overall 5-year survival rate of 32% for that group. Thus, the difference in prognosis between different subgroups of sarcomas can be accounted for by the grading system, which takes into account the poor prognosis of some of these diagnoses.

C. Treatment

1. *Surgery and Radiotherapy*

The standard approach to radical resection of soft tissue sarcomas has often involved amputation. The rationale for radical surgery is the fact that although many of the soft tissue sarcomas appear to be encapsulated, enucleation of such a lesion results in local recurrence in more than 75% of patients because microscopic cells are left in the area of the so-called capsule (Clark *et al.*, 1959). Although radiation therapy can cause regression of soft tissue sarcomas, regression is rarely complete and the local recurrence rate is 66% (Lindberg, 1973). Radiation therapy is extremely useful in the adjuvant situation, however. When doses of 6000 to 6500 rads are given to patients with inadequate surgical excision, the local recurrence rate for primary lesions of the extremities is 22% (Lindberg *et al.*, 1977b). There were only 3 of 29 (10%) local recurrences for patients with stage 1 tumors as opposed to 21 of 79 (27%) for patients with stage 2 and 3 tumors in the M.D. Anderson Hospital series (Lindberg *et al.*, 1977b).

2. *Chemotherapy*

The role of adjuvant chemotherapy for adult soft tissue sarcomas is still controversial. A highly positive study has been reported from the National Cancer Institute Surgery Branch (Rosenberg *et al.*, 1978), whereas our own study had considerably less favorable results (Lindberg *et al.*, 1977a). Additional studies are confused by small patient numbers and lack of adequate staging parameters.

Adjuvant chemotherapy for adult soft tissue sarcomas would be expected to have beneficial results, however, because of the overall good results with appropriately administered chemotherapy (Benjamin *et al.*, 1977a). The Southwest Oncology Group and the M.D. Anderson Hospital have treated 1029 patients with sarcomas with Adriamycin   alone or in combination. The best results have been in the 707 patients with Adriamycin plus dimethyltriazenoimidazolecarboxamide (DTIC), where an overall response rate of 48% has been obtained. Adriamycin is clearly the backbone of sarcoma chemotherapy and has a steep dose–response curve. Similar Adriamycin combinations using lower doses of chemotherapy, longer intervals between treatments, or both, have resulted in lower response rates (Creagan *et al.*, 1976; Giuliano *et al.*, 1978; Pinedo *et al.*, 1979) whereas the highest response rate was in a study using the highest doses of chemotherapy (Rodriguez *et al.*, 1977). The addition of DTIC to Adriamycin regimens can be accomplished with little decrease in Adriamycin dose, perhaps explaining the improved results with the Adriamycin–DTIC combinations which show a slightly higher remission rate and longer remission duration and survival (Gottlieb *et al.*, 1976). When cyclophosphamide is added to such a regimen, a slightly higher response rate may be obtained (Benjamin *et al.*, 1977). However, if the Adriamycin dose is reduced to accommodate the myelosuppressive toxicity of the cyclophosphamide, the beneficial effects may be cancelled (Rosenbaum and Schoenfeld, 1977).

Approximately 15% of patients treated with aggressive combination chemotherapy will achieve complete remission. In addition, a number of patients can be rendered disease-free during chemotherapy by surgical treatment. Such patients have a prognosis equivalent to or perhaps even slightly better than that of patients who achieve complete remission from chemotherapy and substantially better than that of those who achieve only partial remission (Yap *et al.*, 1979). In addition, only a small minority of patients who achieve complete remission have remissions that will last for more than 5 years (Yap *et al.*, 1979). For this reason, efforts are being made to find new effective agents to combine with current Adriamycin-containing regimens, or to devise ways of prolonging Adriamycin therapy in an attempt to prolong complete remission (Stewart *et al.*, 1980).

IV. SARCOMAS OF BONE

A. General

The three major types of primary bone sarcomas are osteosarcoma, chondrosarcoma, and Ewing's sarcoma. Giant cell tumors of bone are occasionally malignant in location or behavior, and malignant fibrous histiocytoma of bone appears to be an increasingly diagnosed disorder. The three major types of bone sarcomas can often be differentiated radiographically. Osteosarcoma starts in the metaphysis (the area between the shaft and the end or epiphysis of a long bone), and the pattern of osteoid matrix can often be determined radiographically. In contrast, chondrosarcoma tends to arise from the epiphysis and produces a chondroid or cartilagenous matrix with a ringlike appearance which is also typical radiographically. Ewing's sarcoma more commonly involves the shaft of the bone and produces a permeative lytic lesion without sclerosis, an "onionskin" appearance of subperiosteal new bone and frequently, spiculation radiating out from the cortex. Pain is a prominent clinical manifestation of all of these tumors.

B. Osteosarcoma

1. Diagnosis

Osteosarcoma is the most common of the primary bone sarcomas. Although most osteosarcomas are of unknown etiology, Paget's disease (Price and Goldie, 1969) and irradiation (United Nations Scientific Committee of the Effects of Atomic Radiation, 1964; Soloway, 1966) are known etiologic factors in a minority of patients. The tumor is most prevalent in the 10–25 year age group and tends to concentrate near the knee (Uribe-Botero *et al.*, 1977). In the M.D. Anderson Hospital series of 243 patients, 156 (64%) had tumors in this location, with the distal femur (42%) as the primary location. Other areas of the femur were involved in 8% of patients. The predominant site of metastases is the lungs.

Two variants of osteosarcoma have a better prognosis. Parosteal osteosarcoma is characterized radiographically by a lobular lesion arising from the posterior aspect of the metaphysis of the distal femur. It does not involve the marrow cavity, and consists of well-differentiated components of bony, fibrous, and cartilagenous tissue. In fact, the pathologic diagnosis can often be confused with a benign lesion (Unni *et al.*, 1976b). Periosteal osteosarcoma is a superficial lesion arising from the periosteum and frequently involving the tibia. Radiographically, there is coarse spiculation and evidence of carlilagenous matrix; however, histologically, the varied pattern includes malignant bone, osteoid, cartilage, and a malignant stroma. The prognosis is intermediate between that of parosteal osteosarcoma and standard osteosarcoma, with 8 of 23 dead in Unni's series (Unni *et al.*, 1976a) and 3 of 13 in Spjut's (Spjut *et al.*, 1977).

Telangiectatic osteosarcoma has a particularly poor prognosis. In the Mayo Clinic study, 23 of 25 patients died of metastatic disease, another had pulmonary metastases, and the remaining survivor had developed a pneumothorax (Matsuno *et al.*, 1976). Radiographically, the lesions are permeative, lytic, or have a "blown-out" appearance. Grossly, the lesions are cystic and contain clotted blood, while histologically, the blood-filled spaces are lined with anaplastic spindle cells and benign giant cells (Matsuno *et al.*, 1976).

2. Prognosis

Five years ago it was generally accepted that osteosarcoma was a highly malignant disease with a 5-year disease-free survival rate of less than 25%. The report of Taylor *et al.* (1974) from the Mayo Clinic challenged this contention and suggested a spontaneously improving prognosis with time. They noted an increase in disease-free survival from less than 20% in 1963 to 1965 to about 40% from 1969 to 1971. The change in prognosis could not be related to a change in therapy. In contrast were reports of a 2-year disease-free survival rate of 15% unchanging with time from M.D. Anderson Hospital (Gehan et al., 1974), and of 21% without change with time from Memorial Sloan Kettering (Mike and Marcove, 1974). Several series using adjuvant chemotherapy have reported 2-year disease-free survival rate of 50% or better (Murphy et al., 1979; Cortes et al., 1979; Ettinger et al., 1979; Jaffe et al., 1978a; Sutow et al., 1978; Eilber et al., 1979; Rosen et al., 1979a). Projected survival figures are as high as 80%, but these include patients who have relapsed and can be salvaged by secondary surgical resections of metastatic foci (Rosen et al., 1979a; Jaffe et al., 1979; Rosenberg et al., 1979).

3. Treatment

The chemotherapy of osteosarcoma is similar to that for adult soft tissue sarcomas in that it is limited to a small number of active drugs. With the use of soft tissue sarcoma regimens, the best results are with a combination of Adriamycin and DTIC (Benjamin et al., 1978). In addition, high-dose methotrexate has been claimed to have even higher activity as a single agent on a weekly schedule (Jaffe et al., 1977), and there are increasing reports of the effectiveness of cis-platinum (Ochs et al., 1978; Baum et al., 1978; Rosen et al., 1979b). In addition, interferon has been used in the adjuvant situation with results similar to those of chemotherapy (Strander et al., 1979).

Because of the change in prognosis of patients with primary osteosarcoma with the addition of adjuvant chemotherapy regimens and aggressive surgical attack on metastatic deposits, new concepts in the primary surgery of osteosarcoma have been advanced. Even in cases where primary amputation is considered, there is a trend toward conservative, transmedullary amputation as opposed to disarticulation. One potential problem with this approach is that skip metastases within the intramedullary canal may be present above the site of amputation (Enneking and Kagen, 1975). Careful CT scanning of the involved bone can now identify the presence or absence of skip metastases (de Santos et al., 1979). A still more promising approach involves limb-salvage surgery (Eilber et al., 1978, 1979; Jaffe et al., 1978b, 1979; Marcove, 1978). This approach is still limited to selected cases; however, it has been possible to reconstruct involved limbs rather than amputate them because of the newer prosthetic devices and materials available to the orthopedic surgeon.

C. Chondrosarcomas

Chondrosarcomas are generally more benign than osteosarcomas and affect the older age group, the majority of patients being in their sixth or seventh decades.

Most of the lesions are in the pelvis or upper femur (Romsdahl and Ayala, 1977). Pathological grading is the primary determinant of prognosis in patients with chondrosarcoma (Evans *et al.*, 1977). None of the patients with grade 1 chondrosarcoma at M.D. Anderson Hospital showed metastases, as compared with 10% of those with grade 2 tumors and 71% with grade 3. In contrast, local recurrence was unrelated to tumor grade, but rather to the extent of the original operative procedure. Five- and ten-year survival rates were related to grade, with 90 and 83% of patients with grade 1 tumors surviving 5 and 10 years respectively. Corresponding survival figures for patients with grade 2 tumors were 81 and 64% and for those with grade 3 tumors, 43 and 29%.

Adequate surgery involves wide resection of the lesion with partial or total excision of the involved bone, or amputation, depending on the grade of lesion. Grade 3 tumors are more frequently managed by amputation (Romsdahl and Ayala, 1977).

Two variants of chondrosarcoma have been described (Dahlin, 1976). Mesenchymal chondrosarcoma is a tumor that shows low-grade malignant cartilage blending with an undifferentiated small-cell component which resembles Ewing's sarcoma. Such patients tend to develop late metastases and die, despite long survival. Dedifferentiated chondrosarcoma is a tumor composed of well-differentiated chondrosarcoma with areas of malignant spindle cells resembling fibrosarcoma. Frequently, this lesion will occur in patients with long-standing, low-grade tumors that suddenly recur or enlarge rapidly. Prognosis is uniformly poor.

Chondrosarcomas are the least responsive sarcomas to chemotherapy with Adriamycin alone or in combination (Gottlieb *et al.*, 1975); other chemotherapeutic agents have not been formally studied. The occasional good responses are seen in patients with mesenchymal chondrosarcoma or dedifferentiated chondrosarcoma.

D. Ewing's Sarcoma

1. Diagnosis

Ewing's sarcoma is a highly malignant, small-round-cell tumor of bone. The true cell of origin is unknown. With regard to its high malignancy, radiation therapy sensitivity, and VAC chemotherapy sensitivity, it is quite analogous to childhood rhabdomyosarcoma. Most commonly, it occurs during the second decade, with 90% of patients under age 30 (Dahlin *et al.*, 1961). Sixty percent of patients are males, and three-quarters of the tumors are found in the pelvis or the long tubular bones of the extremities. The tumor can produce pain, swelling, fever, leukocytosis, and anemia.

Radiographically, the lesion is characterized primarily by osteolysis, although sclerosis may occur. There is often an onionskin layering of subperiosteal new bone and spicules radiating from the cortex. The differential diagnosis includes osteosarcoma, other small-round-cell tumors, eosinophilic granuloma, and osteomyelitis. Pathologically, the differential diagnosis includes lymphoma, neuroblastoma, and metastatic round-cell rhabdomyosarcoma. A diastase-sensitive positive periodic acid–Schiff stain for glycogen aids in establishing the diagnosis; however, electron microscopy is often essential to demonstrate the presence of glycogen and the absence of intercellular reticulin fibers (lymphoma) or neural processes, junctional complexes, and neurosecretory granules (neuroblastoma) (Friedman and Hanaoka, 1971). In the case of rhabdomyosarcoma, a primary tumor is more likely to be definable, and evidence of striated muscle by light or electron microscopy establishes the diagnosis. Rhabdomyosarcomas do contain glycogen, however, and striated muscle cannot always be demonstrated. The nuclei tend to be irregular with clumped chromatin as opposed to the smooth nuclei and finely dispersed chromatin of the Ewing's cell nuclei (Ayala and Mackay, 1977).

2. Prognosis

Before the routine application of adjuvant chemotherapy to the treatment of Ewing's sarcoma, the disease had a dismal prognosis. In the Mayo Clinic series, 20 of 133 patients (15%) were 5-year survivors; however, 6 of these patients died subsequently of their disease at as late as 12 years, leaving a corrected 9% 10-year survival (Dahlin et al., 1961). On the other hand, most patients who died did so shortly after diagnosis, with 44% dead at 1 year and 71% dead at 2 years. Prognosis was best in patients with lesions of the extremities, and there were no long-term survivors with pelvic lesions. There was a suggestion that primary amputation might be more effective than radiation therapy in terms of cure.

3. Treatment

Ewing's sarcoma is quite sensitive to a number of chemotherapeutic agents that are ineffective against the majority of sarcomas. Most investigators now treat with combination chemotherapy and irradiation to the primary lesion. The most commonly used chemotherapeutic combinations include vincristine, actinomycin-D, cyclophosphamide, and Adriamycin. Utilizing this approach, Rosen and associates achieved a 76% 5-year disease-free actuarial survival (Rosen, 1977; Rosen et al., 1974). Seven of 12 who relapsed did so at metastatic sites, whereas only 5 had local recurrence. Most frequent metastatic sites were lung and bone. Because of the propensity of Ewing's sarcoma to spread within the involved bone as well as to other involved bones, radiotherapeutic practice has been to treat the entire bone involved with the tumor. The dose is usually 6000 rads. At lower doses, local recurrence was more common (Chan et al., 1979).

The M.D. Anderson Hospital series again supports the contention that the primary cause of failure is distant metastases (Chan *et al.*, 1979). With successful long-term survival from combination chemotherapy and irradiation therapy, new long-term problems are arising. Thus, of the 24 long-term survivors at M.D. Anderson, 4 developed new primary bone tumors in an irradiated area (Chan *et al.*, 1979; Strong *et al.*, 1979). With (1) the increasing ability for limb-salvage surgery, (2) the suggestive data from the Mayo Clinic that surgery may improve the prognosis in Ewing's sarcoma (Dahlin *et al.*, 1961), and (3) the fact that more effective chemotherapy, rather than irradiation, is needed to control failure due to distant metastases, we now tend to approach the treatment of Ewing's sarcoma primarily with chemotherapy and surgery, using irradiation only for patients whose primary tumor cannot be controlled without it.

E. Giant Cell Tumor

Malignant giant cell tumors will occur in the minority of patients with typical benign giant cell tumors. Histologically, high-grade osteosarcomas or fibrosarcomas may develop in an area of a previously treated tumor, the majority of which have received irradiation (Witrak *et al.*, 1979). The minority have foci of sarcoma coexisting with areas of benign giant cell tumor. Metastatic disease occasionally responds to Adriamycin combination chemotherapy. Some benign giant cell tumors are malignant by location, such as those in the sacrum or a vertebral body, and cannot be resected. Because of the high vascularity of these tumors, percutaneous vascular occlusion can often result in dramatic pain relief and stability of the bone (Wallace *et al.*, 1979).

F. Fibrous Histiocytoma

Malignant fibrous histiocytoma of bone is an increasingly common diagnosis at our institution and in the literature (Dahlin *et al.*, 1977; McCarthy *et al.*, 1979; Kahn *et al.*, 1978). The lesion is usually purely lytic in appearance and presents with pain. Histologically, it appears similar to MFH of soft tissue. In the Mayo Clinic series, one-third of patients eligible for 5-year follow-up were long-term survivors, although late deaths and metastases occurred in 5 patients (Dahlin *et al.*, 1977). McCarthy has pointed out the association with bone infarction in 4 of his 35 cases (McCarthy *et al.*, 1979). Nine of his 21 patients with 3-year, or longer, follow-up were alive and free of disease. Kahn *et al.* (1978) report 3 of 7 patients with no evidence of disease, but short follow-up. In our own experience, long-term survival in the absence of effective chemotherapy is extremely rare. In addition to Adriamycin combinations usually used for soft tissue sarcomas, we have had responses to intra-arterial *cis*-platinum. In the Mayo Clinic series, two patients were cured with radiation therapy (Dahlin *et al.*, 1977).

V. CONCLUSION

Much progress has been made in the last decade in the diagnosis and management of patients with sarcomas of soft tissue and bone. Advances in chemotherapy, primarily related to the introduction of Adriamycin, have revolutionized the treatment of soft tissue sarcomas. New approaches to radiation therapy have been utilized in place of amputation for these lesions, and limb-salvage surgery combined with adjuvant chemotherapy is becoming increasingly prevalent in the management of primary bone tumors. It is hoped that the next decade will see further refinements in these treatment approaches, together with further improved prognosis.

REFERENCES

Ayala, A. G., and Mackay, B. (1977). *In* "Management of Primary Bone and Soft Tissue Tumors," pp. 178–186. Yearbook Publ., Chicago, Illinois.

Baker, L. H., and Benjamin, R. S. (1978). *Proc. Am. Assoc. Cancer Res.* and *Am. Soc. Clin. Oncol.* **19,** 324, plus unpublished data.

Baum, E., Greenberg, L., Gaynon, P., Krivit, W., and Hammond, D. (1978). *Proc. Am. Soc. Clin. Oncol.* **19,** 385.

Benjamin, R. S., Baker, L. H., and Rodriquez, V. (1977). *In* "Management of Primary Bone and Soft Tissue Tumors," pp. 309–315. Yearbook Publ., Chicago, Illinois.

Benjamin, R. S., Baker, L. H., O'Bryan, R. M., Moon, T. E., and Gottlieb, J. A. (1978). *Cancer Treat. Rep.* **62,** 237–238.

Chan. R. C., Sutow, W. W., Lindberg, R. D., Samuels, M. L., Murray, J. A., and Johnston, D. A. (1979). *Cancer* **43,** 1001–1006.

Clark, R. L., Jr., Martin, R. G., and White, E. C. (1959). *Lancet* No. 7, 327–331.

Cortes, E. P., Holland, J. F., and Glidewell, O. (1979). *Recent Results Cancer Res.* **68,** 6816–6824.

Creagan, E. T., Hahn, R. G., Ahmann, D. L., Edmonson, J. H., Bisel, H. F., and Eagan, R. T. (1976). *Cancer Treat. Rep.* **60,** 1385–1387.

Creagan, E. T., Frytak, S., Pairolero, P., Hahn, R. G., and Muhm, J. R. (1978). *Cancer Treat. Rep.* **62,** 1404–1405.

Dahlin, D. C. (1976). Chondrosarcoma and Its "Variants" Int. Acad. Pathol. Monog. Bone and Joints, Vol. 17. Williams & Wilkins, Baltimore, Maryland.

Dahlin, D. C., Coventry, M. B., and Scanlon, P. W. (1961). *J. Bone Jt. Surg. Am. Vol.* **43,** 185–192.

Dahlin, D. C., Unni, K. K., and Matsuno, T. (1977). *Cancer* **39,** 1508–1516.

deSantos, L. A., Wallace, S., and Finkelstein, B. (1977). *In* "Management of Primary Bone and Soft Tissue Tumors," pp. 235–249. Yearbook Publ., Chicago, Illinois.

deSantos, L. A., Goldstein, H. M., Murray, J. A., and Wallace, S. (1978). *Radiology* **128,** 89–94.

deSantos, L. A., Bernardino, M. E., and Murray, J. A. (1979). *Am. J. Roentgenol. Radium Ther. Nucl. Med.* **132,** 535–540.

Donaldson, S. S., Castro, J. R., Wilbur, J. R., and Jesse, R. H. (1973). *Cancer* **31,** 26–35.

Eilber, F. R., Grant, T., and Morton, D. L. (1978). *Cancer Treat. Rep.* **62,** 213–216.

Eilber, F. R., Grant, T. T., Mirra, J., Weisenburger, T., and Morton, D. I. (1979). *Proc. Am. Assoc. Cancer Res.* **20,** 330.

Enneking, W. F., and Kagen, A. (1975). *Cancer* **36**, 2192-2205.

Ettinger, I. J., Douglass, H. O., Higby, D. J., Nime, F., Bjornsson, S., Mindell, E. R., Goorah, J., Freeman, A. I., and Moskowitz, R. M. (1979). *Proc. Am. Assoc. Cancer Res. and Am. Soc. Clin. Oncol.* **20**, 438.

Evans, H. L., Ayala, A. G., and Romsdahl, M. M. (1977). *Cancer* **40**, 818-831.

Fernandez, C. H., Sutow, W. W., Merino, O. R., and George, S. L. (1975). *Am. J. Roentgenol., Radium Ther. Nucl. Med.* **123**, 588-597.

Friedman, B., and Hanaoka, H. (1971). *J. Bone Jt. Surg. Am. Vol.* **53**, 1118-1136.

Fu, Y. S., Gabbiani, G., Kaye, G. I., and Lattes, R. (1975). *Cancer* **35**, 176-198.

Gehan, E. A., Sutow, W. W., Uribe-Botero, G., Romsdah, M., and Smith, T. L. (1963-1974). *In* "Immunotherapy of Cancer: Present Status of Trials in Man" (W. D. Terry and D. Windhorst, eds.), pp. 271-282. Raven, New York.

Giuliano, A. E., Larkin, K. L., and Eilber, F. R. (1978). *Proc. Am. Assoc. Cancer Res. and Am. Soc. Clin. Oncol.* **19**, 359.

Gottlieb, J. A., Baker, L. H., O'Bryan, R. M., Sinkovics, J. G., Hoogstraten, B., Quagliana, J. M., Rivkin, S. E., Bodey, G. P., Jr., Rodriguez, V. T., Blumenschein, G. R., Saiki, J. H., Coltman, C., Jr., Burgess, M. A., Sullivan, P., Thigpen, T., Bottomley, R., Balcerzak, S., and Moon, T. E. (1975). *Cancer Chemother. Rep.* **6**, 271-282.

Gottlieb, J. A., Benjamin, R. S., Baker, L. H., O'Bryan, R. M., Sinkovics, J. G., Hoogstraten, B., Quagliana, J. M., Rivkin, S. E., Bodey, G. P., Sr., Rodriguez, V., Blumenschein, G. R., Saiki, J. H., Coltman, C. Jr., Burgess, M. A., Sullivan, P., Thigpen, T., Bottomley, R., Balcerzak, S., and Moon, T. E. (1976). *Cancer Treat. Rep.* **60**, 199-203.

Hays, D. M., Lawrence, W., Shtow, W. W., and Teft, M. (1978). *Proc. Am. Assoc. Cancer Res. and Am. Soc. Clin. Oncol.* **19**, 415.

Jaffe, N., Frei, E., III, Traggis, D., and Watts, H. (1977). *Cancer* **39**, 45-50.

Jaffe, N., Frei, E., III, Watts, H., and Traggis, D. (1978a). *Cancer Treat. Rep.* **62**, 259-264.

Jaffe, N., Watts, H., Fellows, K. E., Vawter, G. (1978b) *Cancer Treat. Rep.* **62**, 217-223.

Jaffe, N., Traggis, D., Watts, H., and Frei, E., III (1979). *Proc. Am. Assoc. Cancer Res. and Am. Soc. Clin. Oncol.* **20**, 137.

Kahn, L. B., Webber, B., Mills, E., Anstey, L., and Heselson, N. G. (1978). *Cancer* **42**, 640-651.

Kauffman, S. L., and Stout, A. P. (1961). *Cancer* **14**, 469-482.

Kempson, R. L., and Kyriakos, M. (1972). *Cancer* **29**, 961-976.

Lindberg, R. D. (1973). *Proc. Natl. Cancer Conf. 7th, 1972,* pp. 883-888.

Lindberg, R. D., Murphy, W. K., Benjamin, R. S., Sinkovics, J. G., Martin, R. G., Romsdahl, M. N., Jesse, R. H., and Russell, W. O. (1977a). *In* "Management of Primary Bone and Soft Tissue Tumors," pp. 343-352. Yearbook Publ., Chicago, Illinois.

Lindberg, R. D., Martin, R. G., Romsdahl, M. M., and McMurtrey, M. J. (1977b). *In* "Management of Primary Bone and Soft Tissue," pp. 289-298. Yearbook Publ., Chicago, Illinois.

McCarthy, E. F., Matsuno, T., and Dorfmann, H. D. (1979). *Hum. Pathol.* **10**, 57-60.

Marcove, R. C. (1978). *Cancer Treat. Rep.* **62**, 225-231.

Matsuno, T., Unni, K. K., McLeod, R., and Kahlin, D. C. (1976). *Cancer* **38**, 2538-2547.

Maurer, H. M., Moon, T., and Donaldson, M. (1977). *In* "Management of Primary Bone and Soft Tissue Tumors," pp. 317-332. Yearbook Publ., Chicago, Illinois.

Mike, V., and Marcove, R. C. (1963-1974). *Prog. Cancer Res. Ther.* **6**, 257-269.

Murphy, W. K., Benjamin, R. S., Eyre, H. J., Thigpen, T., Groppe, C., Uribe-Botero, G., Baker, L. H., Gehan, B. A., and Gottlieb, J. A. (1979). *In* "Adjuvant Therapy of Cancer II" (S. E. Jones and S. E. Salmon, eds.), pp. 365-373. Grune & Stratton, New York.

Ochs, J. J., Freeman, A. I., Douglass, H. O., Higby, D. S., Mindell, E. R., and Sinks, L. F. (1978). *Cancer Treat. Rep.* **62**, 239-246.

Ozzello, L., Stout, A. O., and Murray, M. R. (1963). *Cancer* **16**, 331-344.

Parker, B. R., and Marglin, S. I. (1978). *Clin. Res.* **26**, 196A.

Pinedo, H. M., Vendrik, C. P. J., Bramwell, V. H., Mouridsen, H. T., Somers, R., Van Oosterom, A. T., Wagener, T., Lewis, B. J., De Pauw, M., Sylvester, R., and Bonadonna, G. (1979). *Proc. Am. Assoc. Cancer Res.* **20**, 346.

Price, C. H. G., and Goldie, W. (1969). *J. Bone Joint Surg. Br. Vol.* **51B**, 205-224.

Rodriguez, V., Bodey, G. P., and Freireich, E. J. (1977). *Proc. Am. Soc. Clin. Oncol.* **18**, 320.

Romsdahl, M. M., and Ayala, A. G. (1977). *In* "Management of Primary Bone and Soft Tissue Tumors," pp. 137-150. Yearbook Publ., Chicago, Illinois.

Rosen, G. (1977). *In* "Management of Primary Bone and Soft Tissue Tumors," pp. 187-203. Yearbook Publ., Chicago, Illinois.

Rosen, G., Wollner, N., Tan, C., Wu, S. J., Hajdu, S. I., Cham, W., D'Angio, G. J., and Murphy, M. L. (1974). *Cancer* **33**, 384-393.

Rosen, G., Marcove, R. C., Caparros, B., Nirenberg, A., Kosloff, C., and Huvos, A. G. (1979a). *Cancer* **43**, 2163-2177.

Rosen, G. Nirenberg, A., Juergens, H., and Tan, C. (1979b). *Proc. Am. Assoc. Cancer Res. and Am. Soc. Clin. Oncol.* **20**, 363.

Rosenbaum, C., and Schoenfeld, D. (1977). *Proc. Am. Soc. Clin. Oncol.* **18**, 287.

Rosenberg, S. A., Flye, M. W., Conkie, D., Seipp, C. A., Levine, A. S., and Simon, R. M. (1979). *Cancer Treat. Rep.* **63**, 753-756.

Rosenberg, S. A., Kent, H., Costa, J., Webber, B. L., Young, R., Chabner, B., Baker, A. R., Brennan, M. F., Chrétien, P. B., Cohen, M. H., De Moss, E. V., Sears, H. F., Seipp, C., and Simon, R. (1978). *Surgery* **84**, 62-69.

Russell, W. O., Cohen, J., Enzinger, F., Hajdu, S. I., Heise, H., Martin, R. G., Meissner, W., Miller, W. T., Schmitz, R. L., and Suit, H. D. (1977). *Cancer* **40**, 1562-1570.

Ruymann, F. B., Newton, W., Ragab, A. H., Donaldson, M., and Gehan, E. A. (1979). *Proc. Am. Assoc. Cancer Res.* **20**, 194.

Schaner, E. G., Chang, A. E., Doppman, J. L., Conkie, D. M., Flye, M. W., and Rosenberg, S. A. (1978). *Am. J. Roentgenol. Radium Ther. Nucl. Med.* **131**, 51-54.

Soloway, H. B. (1966), *Cancer* **19**, 1984-1988.

Spjut, H. J., Ayala, A. G., De Santos, L. A., and Murray, J. A. (1977). *In* "Management of Primary Bone and Soft Tissue Tumors," pp. 79-95. Yearbook Publ., Chicago, Illinois.

Stewart, D. J., Benjamin, R. S., Baker, L. H., Yap, B. S., and Bodey, G. P. (1980). *In* "Therapeutic Progress in Ovarian Cancer, Testicular Cancer and the Sarconias," (A. T. van Osterom, F. M. Muggia, and F. J. Cleton, eds.) pp. 453-480. Leiden University Press, The Hague

Stout, A. P., and Lattes, R. (1966). *In* "Tumors of the Soft Tissues. Atlas of Tumor Pathology," 2nd Ser., Fasc. 1, Armed Forces Inst. Pathol., Washington, D.C.

Strander, H., Adamson, U., Aparisi, T., Bronström, LÅ, Cautell, K., Einhorn, S., Hall, K., Ingimarsson, S., Nilsonne, U., and Söderberg, G. (1979). *Recent Results Cancer Res.* **68**, 40-44.

Strong, L. C., Herson, J., Osborne, B., and Sutow, W. (1979). *J. Natl. Cancer Inst.* **62**, 1401-1406.

Sutow, W. W., Fujimoto, T., Wilbur, J. R., and Okamura, J. (1977). *Proc. Am. Assoc. Cancer Res. and Am. Soc. Clin. Oncol.* **18**, 291.

Sutow, W. W., Gehan, E. A., Dyment, P. G., Vietti, T., and Maile, T. (1978). *Cancer Treat. Rep.* **62**, 265-270.

Taylor, W. F., Ivins, J. C., Dahlin, D. C., and Pritchard, D. J. (1963-1974). *Prog. Cancer Res. Ther.* **6**, 257-269.

United Nations Scientific Committee of the Effects of Atomic Radiation (1964). General Assembly/Nineteenth Session, No. 14 (A/5814), pp. 94-95. United Nations, New York.

Unni, K. K., Dahlin, D. C., and Beabout, J. W. (1976a). *Cancer* **37**, 2476-2485.

Unni, K. K., Dahlin, D. C., Beabout, J. W., and Ivins, J. C. (1976b). *Cancer* **37,** 2466–2475.

Uribe-Botero, G., Russell, W. O., Sutow, W. W., and Martin, R. G. (1977). *Am. J. Clin. Pathol.* **67,** 427–435.

Wallace, S., Granmayeh, M., De Santos, L. A., Murray, J. A., Romsdahl, M. M., **Bracken, R. B.,** and Johnson, K. (1979). *Cancer* **43,** 322–328.

Weiss, S. W., and Enzinger, F. M. (1977). *Cancer 39,* 1672–1685.

Weiss, S. W., and Enzinger, F. M. (1978). *Cancer* **41,** 2250–2266.

Witrak, G. A., Unni, K. K., Sim, F. H., Dahlin, D. C., and Beabout, J. W. (1979). *Lab Invest.* **40,** 292.

Yap, B. S., Sinkovics, J. G., Benjamin, R. S., and Bodey, G. P. (1979). *Proc. Am. Assoc. Cancer Res. and Am. Soc. Clin Oncol.* **20,** 352.

15
PEDIATRIC CANCER
Lawrence Helson

I.	Introduction	295
II.	Tumors	296
	A. Leukemias	296
	B. Non-Hodgkin's Lymphomas	298
	C. Hodgkin's Lymphoma	300
	D. Embryonal Rhabdomyosarcoma	301
	E. Wilms' Tumor	304
	F. Malignant Bone Tumors	305
	G. Brain Tumors	308
	H. Neuroblastoma	310
III.	Conclusions	315

I. INTRODUCTION

Cancer in children is rare. Although often emphasized as the second most common cause of death in children between ages 1 and 14, only 1 of 600 children will be afflicted. The most common of the cancers are childhood leukemias, followed by lymphomas and then the central nervous and peripheral nervous system tumors. Tumors of various organs, such as kidney, liver, and bone, make up a lesser proportion of the patients with childhood cancer.

The enormous emotional and financial impact of cancer in a child gives it additional importance beyond its unique biological and chemical significance. Numerous questions pertaining to heredity, carcinogenesis, and epidemiology are always raised once the diagnosis is made. Treatment methods directed at children with cancer not only have been effective, but also have served as a model for the treatment approaches to adults with solid tumors. This chapter is designed to present both specific and broad concepts of the characteristics of childhood cancer, and to provide basic ideas on treatment methods. The requirement for multidisciplinary efforts in the management of these children should be emphasized. Cancer is not one disease of one organ system, but affects the child's entire body, his or her growth and development, and psychosocial relationships with siblings, parents, and peers. The contributions of a variety of experts are often required to deliver optimal treatment and supportive care.

II. TUMORS

A. Leukemias

1. Definition

These are a group of neoplastic disorders of the cells of the blood-forming tissues. They usually occur as a malignant proliferation of poorly differentiated cells.

2. Incidence

The incidence of leukemia in the United States is approximately 1 per 10,000 population, and 50% of these are acute leukemias. Children account for 80% of these acute leukemias, whereas adults account for 90% of acute nonlymphoblastic leukemias.

3. Etiology

The causes of leukemia are unknown; however, ionizing radiation and exposure to benzene are strongly suspected as initiating agents. To date, no human viral agent such as that found in animals has been reported.

4. Classification

The leukemias may be classified according to the cell type involved—e.g., lymphocytic (actue and chronic), myelocytic (acute and chronic), or undifferentiated. More sophisticated subclassifications based upon morphology, cell-surface markers, and tinctural characteristics are in a constant state of refinement. For example, the distinctions between acute lymphocytic leukemia and lymphomas, other than Hodgkin's, may not be as clear as was previously assumed. The prognosis of children with leukemia should be considered early within the treatment planning, since there is evidence that it is possible to identify different groups of patients with variable degrees of risk and to design the intensity of chemotherapy for these patients. For example, the prognosis of children with lymphocytic leukemia may depend upon age, white count, the presence of mediastinal mass, serum immunoglobulin levels, and the rapidity of response to standard therapy. In contrast, the cells in patients with non-Hodgkin's lymphomas may be morphologically similar to leukemia cells; however, the lymphoma cell distribution—i.e., the extent of disease—appears to play a more important role in prognosis than any other factor.

5. Diagnosis

The initial workup of patients should include the following: complete physical examination, complete blood count and differential, serum immunoglobulin levels, cerebrospinal fluid cytology, chest radiographic study, and bone marrow aspiration. The latter should incorporate (1) surface markers—i.e., T-cell determinants by rosette formation with sheep red cells, and (2) immunofluorescence studies with antisera for light- and heavy-chain components for B cells and Fc and C3 receptors. Histochemical stains of cells should include periodic acid–Schiff, nonspecific esterase, acid phosphatase, chloroacetate esterase, and peroxidase. About 75% of all childhood leukemias are null-cell, 20% are T-cell, and 5% are B-cell leukemias. The latter two types frequently overlap with lymphoma patients.

6. Presenting Signs and Symptoms

At diagnosis the signs and symptoms are nonspecific: anorexia, malaise, fatigue, low-grade fever. As the bone marrow is replaced by the leukemic cells, the production of normal blood cells ceases and anemia, thrombocytopenia, and neutropenia follow. Excessive production of leukemic cells leads to organ infiltration and leukocytosis. With these developments a progression of symptoms occurs; these include marked fatigue, pallor, ecchymosis, epistaxis, gum bleeding, and bone pain. In children, adenopathy and hepatosplenomegaly are found in 50% of patients with acute lymphocytic leukemia. These are found less often in those patients with the non-lymphocytic variety. The diagnosis is confirmed by examination of the bone marrow aspirate. Normal marrow elements are usually depressed by blast cells, whose morphology is that of undifferentiated lymphoblast or myeloblast.

7. Leukemia Treatment

Most leukemia protocols include an induction phase with prednisone, and weekly treatment with vincristine and asparaginase. Cyclophosphamide or anthracyclines may be added to increase the probability of remission. Central nervous system prophylaxis is generally achieved with cranial irradiation and/or intrathecal administration of methotrexate or cytosine arabinoside, or both. Most maintenance regimens include daily 6-mercaptopurine and weekly methotrexate. Treatments extend for 2–3 years, after which the patient should be followed carefully for relapse.

It should be emphasized that the type of cell as determined by morphology and surface markers is valuable not only for classification, but also for prognosis. Subgroups of patients present and respond to therapy differently. High-risk groups such as those patients with T cells, mediastinal masses, and high white counts must be treated more aggressively and differently from patients with low-risk, null-cell types of leukemia. Although not universally agreed upon at present, standardization of leukemias and lymphomas based upon cell type will eventually permit tailored therapies and improved results with leukemias.

8. Prognosis

Statistics for all children with leukemia indicate that approximately 50% will experience long-term survival. By stratifying for cell type, improved percentages for good-risk groups will prevail, and concentration upon poor-risk patients, such as those with T-cell markers and mediastinal masses, will become the focus for more intensive effort. Therapy for patients with acute myelogenous leukemias usually includes cytosine arabinoside and anthracyclines. Research trials now involve extremely intensive cytotoxic treatment followed by compatible-bone-marrow transplantation. The role of prophylactic radiation to the head and meninges is still being actively studied, and may further improve the prognosis for children with this disease.

B. Non-Hodgkin's Lymphomas

1. Definition

The malignant lymphomas are a group of neoplastic disorders of the cells of the lymphoreticular system. They frequently occur as a tumor of the lymph nodes or spleen, and occasionally as infiltrates of organs such as the brain, bone, gonads, and gastrointestinal tract.

2. Incidence

Non-Hodgkin's lymphomas are much more common than Hodgkin's lymphomas in childhood. The former constitute a heterogeneous group of cancers arising from different cell types. The incidence in the United States for both types is about 0.5 per 10,000 population.

3. Etiology

The causes of the non-Hodgkin's lymphomas are unknown, although the Burkitt's lymphoma in Africa has been associated with Epstein-Barr virus, which is assumed to play a causative role. No evidence for this is avilable in Hodgkin's disease patients.

4. Classification

The histopathological classification can be considered to be nodular (rare in children) or diffuse, and these are subdivided into the following: lymphocytic;

well-differentiated; poorly differentiated; medullary reticulosis; and unclassifiable or Burkitt's types. There is also a clinical–diagnostic classification that is essential to staging and determination of prognosis.

5. Diagnosis

The workup of the patient includes a peripheral blood smear, determination of serum immunoglobulins, bone marrow aspiration, and determination of cell-surface markers. In general, the diffuse, well-differentiated lymphomas are B-cell types, and the remainder of the histological types are B cell, T cell, or null cell. Since the majority of patients present with a mass or lymphadenopathy, surgical biopsy is the major diagnostic gesture.

The planning of therapy is dependent upon the stage of disease and the kind of histology observed. Clinical staging should include examination of all lymph node areas, palpation, scanning, X rays, lymphangiography, and intravenous pyelography. There is little need for exploratory laparotomy or splenectomy. Patients present with either localized disease (stage I or II) or disseminated disease (stage III or IV), and may be symptomatic (B) or asymptomatic (A).

6. Treatment

Patients with localized disease and favorable histology (well-differentiated lymphocytic, mixed lymphocytic, histiocytic, and poorly differentiated lymphocytic cells) can be treated with involved field or regional radiotherapy and chemotherapy. Patients with diffuse histologies and stage III or IV disease appear to profit best from radiation therapy to critical areas, along with systemic chemotherapy. The best treatment regimens appear to be those used for leukemias, with the addition of cyclophosphamide during the induction phase. Drugs usually used are vincristine, prednisone, Adriamycin , methotrexate, and cytosine arabinoside. Radiotherapy should include adequate fields for stages I and II; for stages III and IV, radiation should be used for reduction of bulk disease. It may have a role in an emergency situation where a patient may present with a massive mediastinal tumor that is causing respiratory distress; rapid tumor lysis is then required.

7. Prognosis

Survival is related to stage and histology. With more aggressive chemotherapy and radiotherapy being applied to advanced disease in children, better survivals are being achieved. Ominous signs in any patient are testicular and central nervous system (CNS) involvement. Both meningeal and focal brain tumors can occur. These complications can be treated like leukemic involvement of the CNS—i.e., with intrathecal methotrexate, cytosine arabinoside, corticosteroids, and cranial irradiation.

C. Hodgkin's Lymphoma

1. Definition

This is a malignant lymphoma consisting of a proliferation of mononuclear or macrophage cells.

2. Incidence

Hodgkin's disease is relatively rare in children.

3. Histology

This lymphoma is more pleomorphic than the more homogeneous non-Hodgkin's lymphoma. The diagnostic cell is the Reed–Sternberg cell, which is a binucleate or multinucleate cell in a setting of abnormal mononuclear cells. The classification most commonly employed is that developed at the Rye, New York, conference in 1966.* Histopathological classification includes lymphocytic predominance (17% of patients), lymphocytic depletion (17% of patients), nodular sclerosis (40% of patients), and mixed cellularity (25% of patients).

4. Etiology

The etiology is unknown, but epidemiological studies have indicated that clusters of Hodgkin's disease have occurred in towns and in schools.

5. Classification of Hodgkins Disease

In addition to histopathological type, the extent of disease and symptoms play an important role in staging and eventual prognosis.

Stage I, disease limited to one side of the diaphragm in one or a contiguous anatomical region

Stage II, disease in more than two anatomical regions (noncontiguous) on thc same side of the diaphragm

Stage III, disease in lymph nodes on both sides of the diaphragm

Stage IV, involvement of extralymphatic organs. All patients are additionally classified A or B to indicate the absence or presence of weight loss greater than 10% of body weight, temperature over 38°C, and night sweats.

Staging laparotomy is frequently used to identify the status of the patient more accurately and when a therapeutic decision must be made. Patients who are ostensibly stage II and who have symptoms and lymphocyte-depletion histologies may benefit from such an approach, since microscopic disease in the liver and spleen and para-aortic nodes may be detected and thus change the patient's staging.

*Lukes, R. J., Craver, L. F., Hall, T. C., Rappaport, H., and Ruben, P. (1966). *Cancer Res.* **26,** 1311.

6. Diagnosis

Many patients with Hodgkin's lymphoma have cervical lymphadenopathy at diagnosis. The disease progresses from one lymphatic area to a contiguous area. About half the patients have constitutional symptoms and mediastinal lymphadenopathy. Lymphangiography is useful to detect disease in retroperitoneal nodes. Patients with more extensive disease have anemia, low serum iron, decreased iron-binding capacity, and a variety of nonspecific changes in serum copper levels, erythrocyte sedimentation rate, and alkaline phosphatase. Immunological depression, as manifested by anergy, or more subtle changes in lymphocyte activation by phytohemagglutinin (PHA) are not uncommon.

7. Treatment

The primary treatment for all localized disease is irradiation of major nodal areas using 3500–4000 rads. Chemotherapy is generally used for patients who are symptomatic or have systemic disease. The most active drugs are nitrogen mustard, cyclophosphamide, chlorambucil, vincristine, Oncovin , vinblastine, procarbazine, and prednisone. Patients are usually treated with combinations of these. One of the most popular and effective combinations is the MOPP regimen. Comprised of nitrogen mustard, Oncovin, procarbazine, and prednisone, this regimen gives a response rate of 95%. In patients with advanced disease, combinations of MOPP and radiotherapy are usually applied.

8. Prognosis

A good response is not always followed by cure, and relapse rates are causing investigators to include additional drugs in revised treatment regimens. The general tendency is to offer more vigorous therapy with the aim of attaining a higher percentage of long-term remissions and possible cures.

D. Embryonal Rhabdomyosarcoma

1. Definition

This tumor of muscle usually presents as a mass in the head and neck or pelvis regions. Sites of involvement include the orbit, nasopharynx, middle ear and sinuses, or the bladder, vagina, prostate, and paratesticular tissue. Other sites are the extremities and chest wall, but it can occur in virtually any tissue of the body.

2. Incidence

It is reported to occur from birth onward and constitutes a small percentage of childhood malignancies.

3. Classification

There are three major categories: the embryonal rhabdomyosarcoma (Fig. 1), the alveolar rhabdomyosarcoma, and the pleomorphic rhabdomyosarcoma (Fig.

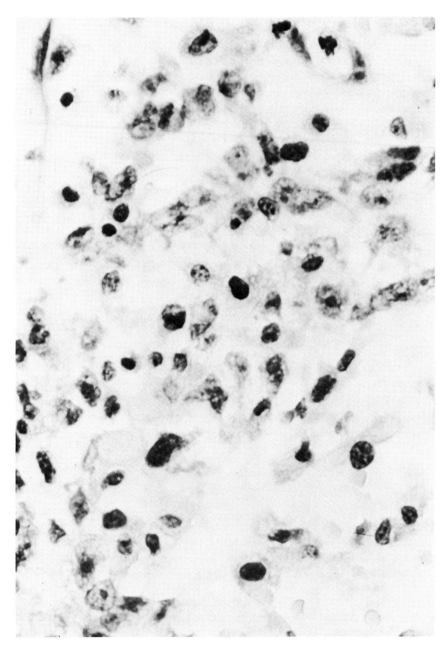

Fig. 1. Embryonal rhabdomyosarcoma. Short spindle and oval cells with pronounced nuclei and nucleoli in a myxofibrillar background (×450).

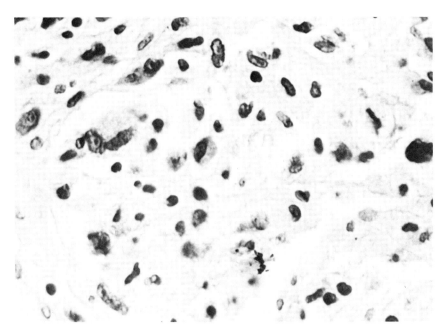

Fig. 2. Pleomorphic rhabdomyosarcoma. Oval, spindle, and giant cells in a fibrillar background (×450).

2). There are other undifferentiated sarcomas similar to the rhabdomyosarcoma but difficult to classify.

4. Diagnosis

Surgical pathology is the major method of diagnosis and includes the use of light microscopy and electron microscopy. To determine the extent of spread or matastases that are common to this tumor, radiographic and isotopic studies are essential.

5. Staging

As with all patients with a soft tissue sarcoma, the staging is essentially as follows:

Stage I, localized and grossly resected (no nodes involved)
Stage II, grossly resected with microscopic residual disease (no nodes involved)
Stage III, incomplete resection with gross residual disease
Stage IV, metastatic disease at diagnosis

6. Treatment

Surgery is used to eliminate localized diseases unless the resultant disfigurement could be avoided by radiation therapy and chemotherapy or was in an area of the body where cosmetic considerations were unimportant. In certain circumstances complete tumor removal with clear borders may eliminate the need for local radiation therapy. The use of chemotherapy has been demonstrated to be an effective adjunct. Cyclophosphamide, vincristine, actinomycin D, and Adriamycin have been the most effective drugs for this disease. The long-lasting responses have been in patients with stages I and II, whereas children with extensive disease have not fared as well.

7. Prognosis

Corresponding to the response rate, stage I and II children have long survivals, whereas more advanced stages are not as effectively controlled.

E. Wilms' Tumor

1. Incidence

Each year about 400 cases of Wilms' tumor occur in the United States. The tumor is of renal origin and may be associated with a number of congenital abnormalities in other body systems, such as aniridia and congenital hemihypertrophy.

2. Diagnosis

Wilms' tumor is virtually always discovered as an abdominal mass on routine physical examination or by the parents. The necessary workup for these patients includes a radiographic abdominal examination, an intravenous pyelogram, abdominal CAT scan and, on occasion, renal angiography. To evaluate the extent of disease, chest and bone radiographs are required. The most common site of metastasies is the lung. Upon histological examination of Wilms' tumor, one can observe an attempt at tubular formation and, not unusually, cells resembling an embryonal rhabdomyosarcoma (Fig. 3).

3. Staging

Staging of Wilms' tumor is under constant evolution and change, but in general is similar to that of the embryonal rhabdomyosarcoma.

Group I, limited to the kidney and completely resected
Group II, extends beyond the kidney but is completely resected
Group III, residual nonhematogenous tumor in abdomen
Group IV, metastases present in lung, liver, bone, or brain
Group V, bilateral renal involvement (10% of patients)

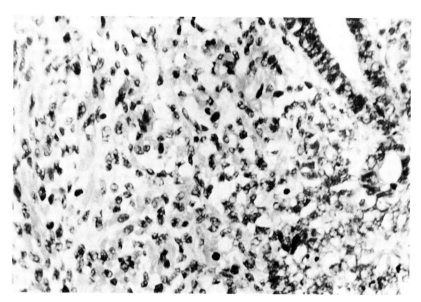

Fig. 3.   Wilms' tumor. Tubule formation and sarcomatous cells are on the same section (×450).

4. Treatment

Total resection should be attempted in all cases except where advanced disease prohibits it and chemotherapy or radiotherapy can be administered first. Definitive therapy is dependent upon the extent of disease. Radiation therapy is generally advised except for children under 1 year and in whom the tumor was completely excised. The drugs that appear to be most effective are actinomycin D, vincristine, and Adriamycin.

5. Prognosis

Approximately 85% of patients with classic Wilms' tumors with good histology and localized disease may be curable. This value diminishes with more extensive disease at diagnosis and with the presence of a sarcomatous component. Pulmonary metastases may not necessarily be an ominous sign since they may be singletons and removed surgically.

F. Malignant Bone Tumors

The most commonly encountered bone tumors of children and adolescents are osteogenic sarcoma and Ewing's sarcoma.

OSTEOGENIC SARCOMA

1. Incidence

Approximately 300 cases occur annually in the United States. It is more common in males than females. Most of the cases occur in adolescents between 13 and 14 years of age.

2. Diagnosis

The tumors usually occur in areas where bone is growing most rapidly—the proximal humerus, tibia, or distal femur. Most patients complain of pain and swelling. Radiographs of the involved regions reveal lytic and sclerotic lesions of the metaphyseal regions of the long bones with a soft tissue compound. Sometimes clacification may be present in the soft tissue in a radical or sunburst pattern. In about 40% of patients, serum alkaline phosphatase may be elevated and may be used as a measure of the degree of activity of the tumor. The final diagnosis is by biopsy and histological observation (Fig. 4), since other tumors such as lymphoma and Ewing's sarcoma can have similar presentations. The workup of the patient should include chest radiographs, because of the propensity of this cancer to metastasize to the lungs, and a bone scan or skeletal survey to detect metastatic disease on other bones.

3. Treatment

Surgical biopsy, amputation, or *en block* resection of the tumor with prosthetic replacement are practiced currently in several specialized centers. The use of chemotherapy as an adjuvant to surgery appears to have made an impact upon the natural history of the disease, with a prolongation of the time until clinically detectable metastatic growth is documented, or with an actually decrease in growth of metastases. Pulmonary metastases may be treated with surgical resection. Prolongation of life and possible cures have been obtained with this kind of aggressive approach. Currently, a variety of drug combinations including methotrexate with citrovorum rescue, vincristine, bleomycin, Adriamycin and *cis*-platinum among others is being tried in various experimental programs.

The prognosis prior to the use of chemotherapy was limited to about 20% cures following amputation. Following the use of adjuvant chemotherapy and observation of early results, it is expected that an increased percentage of cures will follows.

EWING'S SARCOMA

Most of the small-cell sarcomas of bone are Ewing's sarcoma. Although any bone in the body may be affected, this tumor tends to arise in the midshaft of the long bones and is an extremely vascular tumor.

1. Incidence

The total number of cases is small. These tumors occur mostly among teenagers, but can occur in the first and third decades as well. There is a slight predominance of male patients.

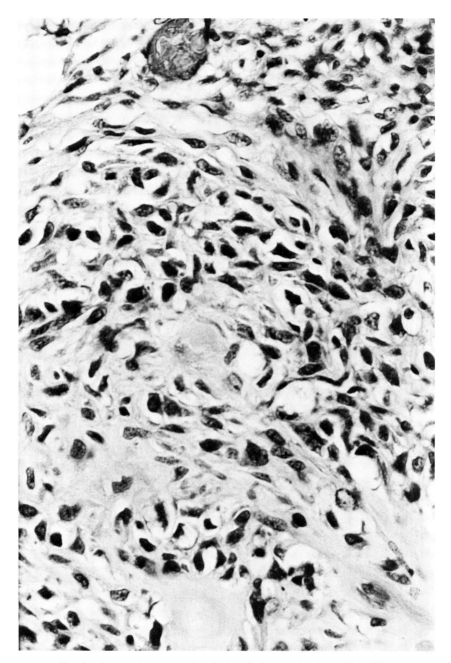

Fig. 4.   Osteogenic sarcoma. Anaplastic cells in a matrix of osteoid (×450).

2. Diagnosis

The earliest symptoms are pain and swelling. Radiographs tend to show cortical destruction and new bone formation near the periosteum, giving an "onionskin" appearance with a surrounding soft tissue mass. The lung is the most common site of spread. The diagnosis is made by biopsy since the tumor can be confused with osteomyelitis, neuroblastoma, and osteogenic sarcoma (Fig. 5).

3. Treatment

The combined use of radiation and chemotherapy is the current approach. Drugs included are vincristine, cyclophosphamide, Adriamycin, and actinomycin D. Other drugs in experimental development may have some effect on this tumor and will eventually be part of treatment programs.

4. Prognosis

Prior to the era of chemotherapy, about 5% survival was all that could be expected. With modern drugs and irradiation, expectations for cure may range as high as 60%.

G. Brain Tumors

Brain tumors are the second most common cause of death from cancer in childhood, ranking second only to leukemia. They occur with a slight predominance in males, with a peak age between 5 and 9 years. Most of the tumors are infratentorial, as opposed to those in adults, which are usually supratentorial. The most common infratentorial histological types include cerebellar astrocytoma, medulloblastoma, brain-stem glioma, and ependymoma. The supratentorial tumor types include astrocytoma, ependymoma, malignant glioma, and craniopharyngioma. There are also a number of tumors that appear to be undifferentiated and not designated in any category beyond "primitive neuroectodermal tumor."

1. Diagnosis

The diagnosis is generally based upon a few signs that may be nonspecific, but gradually direct attention to the CNS. The tumor may be localized or diffuse, interrupting neural tissue, or may be predominantly exophytic. Symptoms may be a result of increased intracranial pressure: symptoms include headache, signs of increased intracranial pressure; vomiting, usually after a night's sleep; and fatigue and lassitude. Seizures are seen in about 30% of supratentorial tumors and rarely with infratentorial tumors.

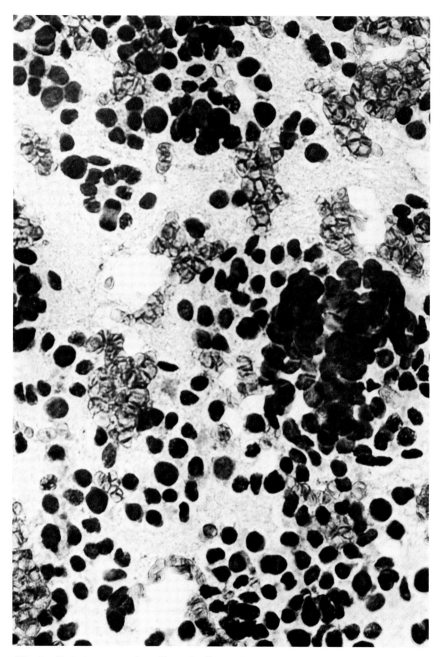

Fig. 5. Ewing's sarcoma. A small-round-cell tumor involving the bone and soft tissues (×450).

2. Signs

Visual signs such as papilledema, strabismus, diplopia, and lateral rectus palsy are important. Bulging of the fontanelle, rapidly increasing head circumference, and prominent scalp veins suggest increased intracranial pressure. Infratentorial tumors are frequently associated with ataxia. The careful neurological examination is of significant importance for future management and diagnosis of the location of the tumor. The major diagnostic technique in use today is the CAT scan. It has displaced the use of the plain skull films, radionucleotide brain scanning, electroencephalograms, and pneumoencephalography. Cerebral angiography remains an important diagnostic and localizing tool. The use of a spinal tap in the presence of a space-occupying lesion should be restricted to suspected meningeal carcinomatosis or infectious meningitis.

3. Treatment

Certain tumors are managed by surgery alone. These include meningiomas, acoustic neuromas, pituitary tumors, cystic posterior fossa astrocytomas, and optic nerve gliomas. Tumors not generally surgically resectable and requiring radiation therapy are gliomas, oligodendrogliomas, medulloblastomas, and ependymomas. Chemotherapy remains in the development stage, with some evidence of response obtained from patients failing to respond to radiotherapy. Drugs possessing antitumor activity, and which appear to cross the blood–brain barrier, include the nitrosoureas, methotrexate, and vinca alkaloids.

4. Prognosis

Many of these drugs, including corticosteroids, appear to have a beneficial effect on the symptoms caused by the tumors. However, they may not prolong life expectancy beyond that obtained from radiation and surgery. The role of surgery has been to increase the number of tumors in categories labeled "curable."

H. Neuroblastoma

The tumor of the sympathetic nervous system is the most common extracranial malignancy in infancy and childhood. Roughly 33% of neonatal cancers are neuroblastomas.

1. Incidence

About 600 cases occur each year in the United States, although there may be more, since an unknown number of infants may have undetected disease and may undergo spontaneous remission.

2. Classification

The tumors may be classified histologically as neuroblastomas or ganglioneuroblastomas. The latter are usually recognized as showing histological signs of differentiation, although the extent of disease at the time of diagnosis may be similar in both cases. Localized neuroblastomas in the neck and pelvic region are readily resected. Tumors in other areas usually involve critical surrounding structures and generally can only be partially resected. These tumors are staged as follows:

Stage I, localized tumor, totally resected
Stage II, local extension, totally resected
Stage III, tumors more extensive, lie within one body cavity, either resected or grossly resected, but with suspected residual microscopic tumor or known residual gross tumor. The distinction between these two categories, totally resected or not, may have importance in terms of prognosis.
Stage IV, tumors beyond their origin, with metastases to bones, bone marrow, liver, lymph nodes, and other regions of the body

The stage IV classification may be subject to further stratification, since some infants with presumed metastatic neuroblastoma may do well spontaneously or following treatment, whereas other infants and older patients with similar clinical presentations have a more limited prognosis. It should be emphasized that in terms of determining risk, patients at any age with bony metastases detected by skeletal survey should be distinguished from other patients with soft tissue metastases.

3. Diagnosis

The diagnosis is made by bone marrow biopsy and aspiration in patients with extensive disease. Rosette formation or clumps of neuroblastoma cells are seen (Figs. 6 and 7). In some patients a ganglioneuroblastoma may occasionally be found, characterized by a mixture of both differentiated ganglion cells and neuroblasts (Fig. 8). Biopsy of intra-abdominal or other tumor masses is the most common diagnostic procedure. Confirmation of the diagnosis may be made in the majority of cases with determination of urinary catecholamines and vanillylmandelic acid or plasma dihydroxyphenylalanine. The major presenting signs and symptoms are usually a mass (50%), leg pain or difficulty in walking (20%), neurologic signs (20%), and orbital ecchymoses with or without proptosis. A diagnostic workup should include an intravenous pyelogram, skeletal survey, radionucleotide bone scan, bone marrow biopsy and aspiration, a myelogram for any intrathoracic masses or for patients with spinal cord compression symptoms, and determination of urinary and plasma catecholamines or their metabolites.

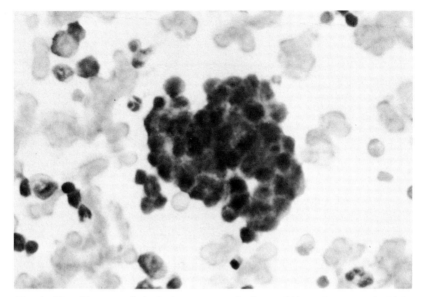

Fig. 6. Neuroblastoma cells in the bone marrow of a 2-year old boy who presented with fever and a hemoglobin of 7 gm%, with a normal white blood cell count and differential. The cytoplasm is scarce and the cells have a tendency to clump together (×250).

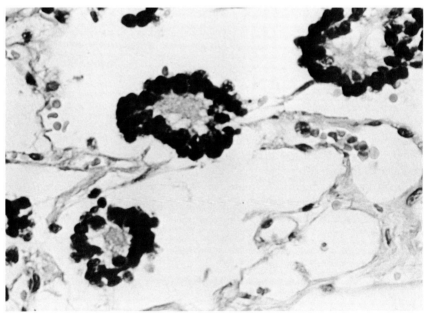

Fig. 7. As in the embryo, the neuroblasts tend to form spheres with the processes in the center. On section, these resemble rosettes. Note the fibrillar centers (×450).

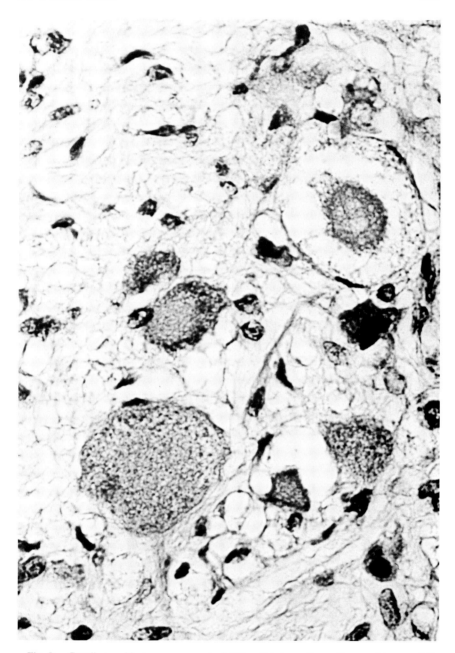

Fig. 8.   Ganglioneuroblastoma, composed of differentiated ganglion cells, neuroblasts, and fibroblasts (×450).

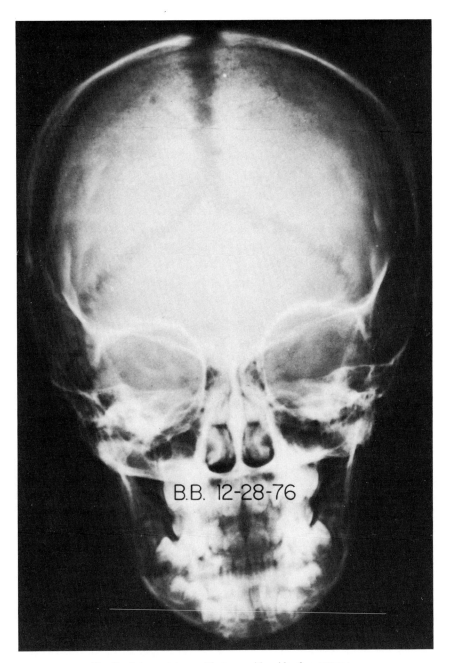

Fig. 9. Intracranial neuroblastoma with epidural metastases.

Skull X rays are valuable in demonstrating split sutures, which indicate the increased intracranial hypertension of sudden onset. Computer axial to mographic views of the head may be useful for demonstrating dilated ventricles, epidural metastases, and intracranial bone disease. Figure 9 is a typical presentation of intracranial neuroblastoma in a young child whose sutures are not closed.

4. Treatment

Surgery is curative for stage I and II patients. Stage III "resected" patients should have some systemic chemotherapy of brief duration, for 3–5 months. Stage III unresected patients should have more aggressive therapy for 5–8 months, and should be followed with a second-look laparotomy. Stage IV disease, which involves the bones, remains the most recalcitrant tumor. A series of aggressive chemotherapy programs has been studied in the last few years. A promising one appears to be a combination of gradually escalating dosages of cyclophosphamide given over a period of 5 months with the addition of other drugs, including vincristine, Adriamycin, papaverine, trifluoromethyl thymidine, cytosine arabinoside, and hydroxyurea.

The infant with stage IV nonbony involvement appears to have a better prognosis than older patients. These children may be cured if given chemotherapy, and some may spontaneously undergo remission. However, since the cure rate for infants with neuroblastoma is approximately 50%, the approach taken by some of withholding therapy from all children with such presentations without judicial use of chemotherapy is controversial.

5. Prognosis

The prognosis is good for localized disease of the neck, pelvic, and thoracic regions in general. The prognosis is poor for systemic disease in children diagnosed after the age of 2, and appears to improve with diagnosis made at an early age.

III. CONCLUSIONS

From this brief review of the characteristics of the more common tumors of childhood, it can be seen that the clinical and biological tumor patterns depend upon the site of origin, and that in comparison to what is seen in adults, a great variety of histological types may be encountered. Because of this, and since many childhood tumors are embryonal in nature, the sensitivity to various drugs and drug combinations is more specific and gratifying in child cancers than in adult cancers. It has been the experience of pediatric oncologists to have an important porportion of patients treated respond to therapy. Some responses are for long periods of time, and there appares to be a definite curability associated with children's cancer. The oncologist treating adult cancers has the opportunity to observe these responses and assuming some similarities in tumor biology may take advantage of some of the drug regimens that have been shown to be effective for children's cancer.

An additional point that should be emphasized is that the multifaceted signs, symptoms, physiological problems, and insults to the patients' physical and mental integrity associated with children's cancer require more than one physician for their care. Consequently, it is important to emphasize that the surgeon, the radiation therapist, the chemotherapist, and a variety of ancillary personnel have a role in the diagnosis and treatment of children with cancer.

There are numerous areas of research that may be of importance to the eventual goal of oncologists, which is the cure of cancer in all children. Research is needed into the mechanisms of sensitivities of tumors to drugs and radiation, and their correlation with the mechanism of tumor cell resistance. Information on the delayed effects of therapy on normal tissues, growth, development, and second cancers is of increasing importance as more prolonged clinical responses are obtained. For prophylaxis it would be important to develop a test for cancer proclivity in "normal" individuals—i.e., high-risk groups. These kinds of approaches may help us begin to develop a prophylaxis for children's cancer, earlier diagnosis, and more effective treatment.

Part III
Nutritional and
Infectious Disease
Aspects of Cancer

16
INFECTIOUS COMPLICATIONS IN THE CANCER PATIENT
Gerald P. Bodey

I.	Introduction	319
II.	Types of Infection in Cancer Patients	328
	A. Pneumonia	328
	B. Septicemia	329
	C. Skin Infection	330
	D. Organisms Causing Infection	331
III.	Diagnosis of and Therapy for Infection	343
	A. Diagnosis	343
	B. Treatment	343
IV.	Therapy for Nonbacterial Infections	353
V.	Granulocyte Transfusion	354
VI.	Prophylaxis of Infection	356
VII.	Conclusions	359
	References	359

I. INTRODUCTION

The management of infectious complications in the cancer patient remains a difficult and frustrating problem, despite impressive advances achieved during the 1970s. Unfortunately, as effective therapy is discovered for the most common infecting organism, a more resistant organism appears. For example, the introduction of carbenicillin and the new aminoglycosides led to successful therapy of most pseudomonas infections. However, this success resulted in an increase of klebsiella infections that have proved to be difficult to treat with the most antibiotic regimens (Bodey *et al.*, 1978). Many of the treatments that offer the hope of potential cure for patients with malignant diseases are associated with side effects that usually include a substantial risk of infectious complications.

CANCER AND CHEMOTHERAPY, VOL. II

Hence, the successful management of these infections becomes increasingly important as the prognosis of the underlying disease improves.

Multiple factors have been identified that predispose the cancer patient to infectious complications (Table I). The malignant process itself may be responsible for increased susceptibility to infection. Often this is a consequence of tumor growth which causes obstruction or ulceration. However, some tumors, especially hematological malignancies, may cause major defects in host defense mechanisms. Many infectious complications are a consequence of therapeutic measures. Cancer chemotherapeutic agents have multiple side effects, such as gastrointestinal ulceration and myelosuppression. A thorough understanding of these underlying factors is necessary to identify likely sources of infection and permit more effective therapy.

Some of the most difficult infections to treat are those associated with local factors. Rapidly proliferating tumor masses may outgrow their blood supply. This results in tissue hypoxia and, ultimately, tissue necrosis. It has been demonstrated in animal tumors that anaerobic organisms such as *Clostridium* spp., when injected intravenously, will migrate to areas of tissue hypoxia and establish infection (Thiele *et al.*, 1964). Indeed, this has been investigated as a possible mechanism for eradicating tumor growth. Large subcutaneous tumor masses

TABLE I

Factors Associated with Increased Susceptibility to Infection in the Cancer Patient

Local factors
   Tumor necrosis
   Obstruction to natural drainage
   Gastrointestinal ulceration
   Disruption of integument
   Prolonged catheterization
   Microbial colonization
Generalized factors
   Neutropenia
   Lymphopenia
   Impaired antibody production
   Impaired cellular immunity
   Phagocytic cell defects
   Malnutrition
Therapeutic agents
   Antitumor agents
   Adrenal corticosteroids
   Antibiotics
   Intravenous hyperalimentation
   Radiation
   Splenectomy

such as may occur in patients with breast cancer or malignant melanoma often undergo necrosis and become infected. Local control of infection becomes virtually impossible unless the tumor can be eradicated. Additionally, if these patients receive myelosuppressive chemotherapy, their infection may disseminate during periods of neutropenia.

Obstruction to natural drainage may result from tumor growth and may predispose to local infection. For example, nearly 45% of patients with bronchogenic carcinoma die of infectious complications, and 80% of these infections are pneumonias (Inagaki *et al.*, 1974). Most of these infections are caused by bronchial obstruction and atelectasis. Antibiotic therapy is often ineffective against these pneumonias even though the infecting organism is not resistant to the antibiotics used. Obstruction to urinary drainage commonly results in infection. The insertion of a catheter may relieve the obstruction, but chronic urinary tract infection is an inevitable consequence. Initially, the infecting organism is usually susceptible to multiple antibiotics, but eventually, following several courses of antibiotic therapy, superinfection with a resistant organism occurs. The best practice is to try to suppress growth of organisms in the urine with local measures but to reserve systemic antibacterial therapy until the patient develops symptoms such as fever, leukocytosis, or flank pain.

Gastrointestinal ulceration may result from a variety of factors. Perhaps the most frequent cause of these ulcerations is the use of antitumor agents that destroy the proliferating epithelial cells of the gastrointestinal mucosa. Such agents that are commonly used include methotrexate, Adriamycin , and 5-fluorouracil. Although this is a dose-related side effect, it is difficult to avoid completely since optimum antitumor response requires some degree of toxicity. Tumors of the gastrointestinal tract may undergo necrosis and ulceration, serving as a portal for infection by enteric organisms. Infection is the proximate cause of death in about 50% of patients with gastrointestinal tumors (Inagaki *et al.*, 1974). Septicemia occurs during 45% of these fatal infections. In 70% of infections, the tumor itself is the major predisposing factor. Patients with gastrointestinal tumors are among those cancer patients who have a greater susceptibility to clostridial infections. *Clostridium perfringens* may be a normal inhabitant of the gastrointestinal tract. It readily colonizes necrotic tumor tissue and thereafter invades the bloodstream.

Patients with gynecological tumors are frequently treated with pelvic irradiation. Occasionally this therapy may cause necrosis of the gastrointestinal mucosa, resulting in abscess formation or peritonitis. Infection is the cause of death in 58% of patients with genitourinary malignancies, and nearly 50% of these infections are associated with septicemia (Inagaki *et al.*, 1974).

The skin serves as a natural barrier to invasion by microorganisms that are present in the environment. These organisms may colonize the skin transiently or permanently. The cancer patient is subjected to repeated disruptions of this natural barrier. Debilitated patients who are confined to bed for prolonged periods develop decubitus ulcers which are slow to heal and may serve as a site for infection and subsequent invasion of the bloodstream. Repeated venipunctures and finger sticks for blood samples disrupt the integument and facilitate establishment of cellulitis or abscesses. Infusions of drugs may extravasate or cause phlebitis. Antitumor agents such as vincristine, Adriamycin, and nitrogen mustard cause tissue necrosis if they extravasate; this resolves slowly and may require skin grafts. The use of intravenous catheters and needles has been associated with infection. Organisms have been cultured from 5–35% of polyethylene catheters, and potential pathogens account for about 4% of contaminating organisms (Corso *et al.*, 1969). Phlebitis occurs in as many as 30% of patients, local infection in about 35%, and septicemia in 3% of patients.

Microbial colonization is a special concern because many of the organisms acquired from the hospital environment are resistant to multiple antibiotics. The administration of oral absorbable antibiotics is associated with fungal colonization of the gastrointestinal tract (Lipnik *et al.*, 1952). Both the proportion of patients colonized and the concentration of organisms in previously colonized patients increase during therapy. Colonization of the oropharynx by gram-negative bacteria during hospitalization occurs in a substantial proportion of patients, even without antibiotic administration (Glover and Jolly, 1971). Major infections have been found to occur following marked increases in the concentration of gram-negative bacilli in the oropharynx. The respiratory tracts of patients with tracheostomies are usually colonized by gram-negative bacilli which often subsequently cause tracheitis and pneumonia. The oropharynx or gastrointestinal tract of about 50% of patients with leukemia becomes colonized with *Pseudomonas aeruginosa* during hospitalization (Bodey, 1970). The frequency of subsequent pseudomonas infection is substantially higher in patients with persistent colonization. Patients may acquire potentially pathogenic organisms from the air, surfaces, bathing facilities, food, personnel, and equipment in the hospital. Even medications, intravenous fluids, and soap solutions may serve as a source of contamination. For example, an epidemic of aspergillus infections was traced to contamination of construction material in a hospital air conditioning system (Aisner *et al.*, 1976).

Generalized factors that predispose the cancer patient to infection may be a consequence of the malignant process or its therapy. Probably, the most important of these factors is neutropenia. The relation between infection and neutrophil count was studied in a group of 52 patients with acute leukemia who were followed from diagnosis until death (Bodey *et al.*, 1966a). The frequency of infection increased as the neutrophil count decreased below $1000/mm^3$. Major infections occurred 11 times more frequently when the patients' neutrophil counts were less than $100/mm^3$ than when they were greater than $100/mm^3$ (Table II). However, the frequency of infection remained constant at neutrophil

TABLE II

Relationship between Leukocyte Counts and Major Infection in Acute Leukemia

Leukocytes/mm^3	Neutrophils		Lymphocytes	
	Episodes of major infection[a]	Percentage of days with major infection	Episodes of major infection	Percentage of days with major infection
<100	43	32	25	43
101–500	19	22	26	28
501–1000	10.5	14	11	14
1001–1500	3.7	6	9	11
>1500	3.8	6	4	6

[a] Expressed as number of episodes per 1000 days without major infection.

counts greater than 1000/mm^3. Hence, a neutrophil count of 1000/mm^3 appears to be the critical level below which the risk of infection begins to increase. The risk of infection was related not only to the degree of neutropenia but also to the duration of neutropenia. About 30% of patients who maintained a neutrophil count of less than 100/mm^3 for a week acquired major infection, whereas 50% of patients who maintained a neutrophil count of less than 100/mm^3 for 3 weeks acquired major infection.

The fatality rate from major infection was related to fluctuations in the neutrophil count during the first week of infection. The rate was 80% among those patients in whom the neutrophil count at the onset of infection was less than 100/mm^3 and remained below this concentration. Among patients in whom the initial neutrophil count was less than 100/mm^3 and remained unchanged or decreased, the fatality rate was 59%. However, among those patients with the same initial neutrophil count in whom it increased to greater than 1000/mm^3, the fatality rate was only 27%.

Lymphopenia has been classically associated with advanced Hodgkin's disease. It may also result from cancer chemotherapy. The frequency of infection in patients with actue leukemia was also related to the number of circulating lymphocytes (Table II). Generally, lymphopenia is not as severe as neutropenia in patients receiving cancer chemotherapy, and patients with lymphopenia usually have normal lymph node architecture. Most patients with lymphopenia also have neutropenia, which is of greater significance. Lymphopenia may facilitate dissemination of fungal infections following colonization (Bodey, 1966).

Impaired antibody production has been described in associated with chronic lymphocytic leukemia and multiple myeloma. Gamma globulin concentrations were determined in patients with chronic lymphocytic leukemia and "lymphosarcoma'' (Ultmann *et al.*, 1959). Infections occurred in >89% of patients with gamma globulin concentrations less than 50% of normal, but in only 15% of patients with normal concentrations. The average number of days spent with infection were 145 and 57, respectively. The frequency of infection in patients with multiple myeloma and Waldenstrom's macroglobulinemia has been related to the patients' ability to respond to antigenic stimuli (Fahey *et al.*, 1963). These patients were exposed to a battery of five antigens, and the average number of antibody responses was calculated. Patients who developed infection had an average antibody response of 25%, whereas patients who did not develop infection had an average antibody response of 50%. Patients that averaged with less than 0.13 infection per month had an average antibody respone of 40%, whereas patients averaging more than 0.13 infection per month had an average antibody response of 19%.

Hodgkin's disease is a malignancy associated with impairment of cellular immunity. This impairment in host defense mechanisms occurs primarily in patients with stage III or IV disease, and is most common in patients with lymphocyte depletion and lymphocytopenia (Brown *et al.*, 1967). Impairment in cell-mediated immunity is manifested by anergy to delayed hypersensitivity skin tests, deficient mononuclear response in inflammatory exudates, and impaired homograft rejection. Patients with Hodgkin's disease are especially susceptible to infections caused by facultative intracellular parasites such as *Mycobacterium tuberculosis, Listeria monocytogenes,* and *Cryptococcus neoformans.* These organisms are resistant to bactericidal processes within normal phagocytes and multiply within these cells, causing their destruction (Simpson *et al.*, 1967). Host defense against these infections depends chiefly upon acquired cellular resistance residing in activated macrophages. Enhanced resistant to facultative intracellular parasites correlates with a greater capacity of the macrophages to ingest and inhibit multiplication of organisms. Patients with Hodgkin's disease probably have impaired macrophage function, and thus are susceptible to these infections.

The number of phagocytic cells may be normal and these cells may have a normal appearance, yet fail to function normally. Defects in neutrophil function have been identified in chronic granulomatous disease, Chediak–Higashi syndrome and Sezary's syndrome. Patients with malignant diseases may also have functional defects in phagocytic cells. For example, the bactericidal capacity of neutrophils from patients with acute leukemia has been studied (Thompson and Williams, 1974). Only 28% of the patients whose neutrophils had a normal bactericidal capacity developed infections, whereas 86% of the patients whose neutrophils had severely impaired bactericidal capacity developed infections. The number of episodes of infection per patient during the study period was 0.2 for the former group and 3.7 for the latter group.

Most patients with advanced malignancies become severely malnourished.

Often these patients are also severely immunosuppressed. Studies in malnourished children have demonstrated an increased susceptibility to infection,
and it is likely that inadequate nutrition also contributed to the increased susceptibility of cancer patients to infection. Inadequate food intake or an improper diet
may lead to vitamin deficiencies, which aggravate this problem.

Cancer chemotherapeutic agents interfere with many host defense
mechanisms. Most of these drugs cause neutropenia and lymphopenia. Some
interfere with cellular and humoral immunity at doses that do not cause
myelosuppression. The processes involved in cellular and humoral response to
antigenic stimuli are complex. Thymus-derived lymphocytes (T cells) are responsible for cell-mediated immunity, whereas bone marrow lymphocytes (B
cells) produce antibodies. Antigenic substances reach the draining lymph nodes
and are trapped in macrophages. The processed antigen is brought in contact with
lymphocytes, which proliferate, resulting in a population of effector T and B
cells. The T cells circulate through the blood and tissues, whereas the B cells
remain in the lymph node.

Antitumor agents may interfere at various stages in this response. Table III
summarizes the effects of some of these agents on both cellular and humoral
immunity (Hersh, 1974). Some drugs have a specific effect on the immune
response because of their mechanism of action. Antimetabolites affect mainly
cells in the proliferative phase, whereas alkylating agents affect cells in all
phases, but especially those in the precursor stage. Generally, antitumor agents

TABLE III

Effects of Antitumor Drugs on Host Defense Mechanisms

Chemotherapeutic agent	Antigen uptake or processing	Antigen recognition or precursor cell destruction	Blasto-genesis	Prolifer-ation	Inhibition of: 1°Ab[a]	2°Ab[b]	DHR[c]
Cyclophosphamide	x[d]	x	x	—	3+	2+	3+
Dactinomycin	x	—	x	x	±	0	±
L-Asparaginase	—	—	x	—	+	±	+
6-Mercaptopurine	—	—	x	—	2+	±	2+
Cytarabine	—	—	—	x	+	±	±
Methotrexate	—	—	—	x	2+	±	2+
Vinca alkaloids	—	—	—	x	±	0	±

[a] 1°Ab, antibody response to primary antigen.
[b] 2°Ab, antibody response to secondary antigen.
[c] DHR, delayed hypersensitivity reaction.
[d] x, interferes at this stage of immune response.

have a greater inhibitory effect upon antibody response to primary antigens than upon antibody response to antigens to which the patient has been previously exposed. Often, very toxic doses of drugs are required to inhibit the antibody response to these secondary antigens. Also, the effect on antibody production is often related to the relationship between exposure to antigen and administration of drug. Most agents are effective only if administered after the patient has been exposed to the antigen. The vinca alkaloids and dactinomycin are only weakly immunosuppressive, whereas alkylating agents are severely immunosuppressive. Continuous chemotherapy results in severe depression of antibody production and substantially greater inhibition of delayed hypersensitivity reactions than does intermittent therapy (Hersh *et al.*, 1973).

Antitumor agents also interfere with the inflammatory response, a process that can be measured by means of the skin-window technique. Initially, neutrophils migrate to the site of inflammation. They are followed by mononuclear cells. Among those agents that suppress this response are procarbazine, methotrexate, 6-mercaptopurine, dactinomycin, and cyclophosphamide. 6-Mercaptopurine is a potent anti-inflammatory agent that inhibits the mononuclear phase of the inflammatory response by reducing production and release of monocytes from the bone marrow. The administration of antitumor agents to animals increases their susceptibility to bacterial, fungal, viral, and protozoal infections.

Radiation therapy may have local or systemic effects that can increase the patient's susceptibility to infection. Rapid destruction of lymphoma of the gastrointestinal tract following irradiation has occasionally resulted in perforation and peritonitis. Necrosis of normal bowel may occur following radiotherapy of gynecological tumors, also resulting in perforation, pelvic abscess formation, or peritonitis. Radiation-induced mucositis and esophagitis often becomes superinfected by bacteria or fungi. Prophylactic craniospinal irradiation in children with acute leukemia causes a transient but significant decrease in bactericidal activity of phagocytic cells, which disappears within 2–4 weeks (Baehner *et al.*, 1973). This defect may increase susceptibility to infection, although serious infections have not been a major problem in these patients.

Adrenal corticosteroids are frequently administered to cancer patients, either as specific antitumor agents or as a supportive measure. These agents have a wide variety of effects on host defense mechanisms. They interfere with diapedesis of leukocytes, cause stabilization of lysosomal membranes, inhibit inflammation, decrease capillary permeability, decrease cellular exudation, and impair reticuloendothelial function (Robinson, 1960). Even short courses may cause substantial decreases in serum concentrations of IgG and IgA (Butler and Rossen, 1973). Recovery may be delayed for more than 4 weeks. Patients who have been on chronic adrenal corticosteroid therapy are especially susceptible to disseminated fungal infections. Patients with acute leukemia who developed disseminated candidiasis had received adrenal corticosteroids more often than leukemic patients who developed only superficial candidiasis of the gastrointestinal tract (Bodey, 1966). In experimental animal systems, adrenal corticosteroids enhance susceptibility to bacterial, fungal, viral, protozoal, and parasitic infections.

Many investigators have suggested that antibiotic therapy predisposes to superinfection, but studies in cancer patients have failed to substantiate this claim. For example, among patients with acute leukemia, those patients who developed major fungal infections did not receive more antibiotic therapy than patients who did not develop fungal infections (Bodey, 1966). Antibiotics do facilitate colonization by resistant organisms, especially if they are administered orally. In one study, the proportion of patients who became carriers of *Candida* spp. was 10% among controls but 81% among patients who received oral chloramphenicol or chlortetracycline (Lipnik *et al.*, 1952). In a study of infections caused by *Staphylococcus aureus* that were resistant to methicillin and aminoglycosides, 81% of the infected patients had received prior antibiotics compared to only 38% of a control group who were colonized by more sensitive strains of *S. aureus* (Crossley *et al.*, 1979). Hence, antibiotics may facilitate colonization by resistant bacteria or fungi. Superinfection most likely occurs for the same reasons the original infection occurred. Furthermore, the tissue damage ensuing from the original infection serves as a nidus for superinfection. For example, 70% of aspergillus infections occurred in patients with tissue damage due to other preceding or concomitant infection (Meyer *et al.*, 1973).

Intravenous hyperalimentation has been introduced in recent years as a supportive nutritional measure. This therapeutic modality facilitates establishment of infection by introducing a portal from the skin directly into the blood stream. The hypertonic nutrient solutions also may serve as a culture medium for organisms. Several reports have indicated that patients receiving intravenous hyperalimentation are susceptible to developing fungemia caused by *Candida* spp. or *Torulopsis glabrata* (Montgomerie and Edwards, 1978). Often the fungemia resolves following removal of the catheter. However, organ invasion by the fungus may occur in some patients and require antifungal therapy. It is important that catheters receive meticulous care to prevent infectious complications.

Splenectomy has become an accepted practice in the staging of patients with lymphoma. Overwhelming pneumoccocal and *Hemophilus influenzae* infections have been recognized as a potential threat in infants and children who have undergone splenectomy. Often the patients fail to respond to appropriate antibiotic therapy, and the interval between symptoms and death is less than 24 hours. The risk of such infection in adults with lymphoma who have undergone splenectomy appears to be minimal (Donaldson *et al.*, 1972). Nevertheless, a few splenectomized adults have developed overwhelming pneumococcal or *H. influenzae* septicemia. The contribution of the spleen, which prevents these infections, is not completely understood. Recently, tuftsin activity has been found to be absent in splenectomized patients. Deficiency of this phagocytosis-stimulating peptide may explain the overwhelming infection that occurs in these patients. Immunization with pneumococcal vaccine or penicillin prophylaxis should be considered in these patients.

II. TYPES OF INFECTION IN CANCER PATIENTS

The frequency of infection, the usual site of infection, and the predominant infecting organisms vary according to the patients' underlying malignant diseases. The most common types of serious infections are pneumonias and septicemias. Recurrent urinary tract infections are seldom a problem except in patients with genitourinary tumors or other malignancies causing obstruction to urinary drainage.

Occasionally, infection of other major organs may represent a serious threat. Pseudomembranous or necrotizing enterocolitis may occur in neutropenic patients (Amromin and Solomon, 1962). It may also be associated with administration of antitumor agents or antibiotics. Clinically, the patient presents with hectic fever, cramping abdominal pain, and bloody diarrhea. The lesion may be diffuse, extending from the esophagus to the rectum, and thus not amenable to therapy. However, if it is localized to a small portion of the bowel, it may be successfully resected. Central nervous system infections occur most often in patients with hematological malignancies or in patients who have undergone surgery for tumors involving the head or spine (Chernik *et al.*, 1973). Gram-negative bacilli and fungi are responsible for the majority of these infections.

A. Pneumonia

Pneumonia represents a serious threat to cancer patients because it is so difficult to treat successfully. Approximately 40% of patients with hematological malignancies acquire pulmonary infections during the course of their disease. Pneumonias are responsible for about 75% of fatal infections in patients with head and neck and lung cancers, and for about 35% to 40% of fatal infections in patients with genitourinary and gastrointestinal tumors. The pneumococcus seldom is the cause of pneumonia in cancer patients, especially if the infection is acquired in the hospital. Gram-negative baccili are responsible for most of these infections, although fungi such as *Candida* spp. and *Aspergillus* spp. are becoming an increasingly frequent cause of serious pneumonias in patients with hematological malignancies. The diagnosis of pneumonia may be overlooked in neutropenic patients who fail to develop the characteristic signs and symptoms. In an autopsy study of 50 patients with acute leukemia, 40 were found to have had major or minor pulmonary infections (Bodey, 1966). However, only 13 of 31 major infections were diagnosed premortem.

The diagnosis of pneumonia is often difficult to establish, especially in neutropenic patients, because these patients are unable to produce sputum. Frequently, pneumonia presents as a diffuse bilateral pneumonitis associated with fever and hypoxia. Usually there is nothing characteristic about the clinical presentation or the chest roentgenogram to suggest the correct diagnosis. Diffuse pneumonitis may be caused by bacteria, fungi, viruses, or protozoa. Often they are caused by multiple organisms. *Legionella pneumophila* also has been identified as a cause of pneumonitis in the compromised host. To complicate matters further, the pneumonitis may be caused by a noninfectious process. Antitumor agents such as bleomycin, busulfan, and methotrexate have been reported to cause pulmonary toxicity. Occasionally, patients with lymphangitic or hematogenous spread of tumor may present with rapidly progressing, diffuse pulmonary involvement that can be confused with an infectious process.

Often, invasive procedures are required to establish the correct diagnosis. The causative agent can be identified by transtracheal aspiration in about 30% of cases. Bronchoscopy with broncial brushings has been useful in some cases, but often the cause of pneumonitis can be identified only by a biopsy procedure. Transtracheal biopsy and needle biopsy can be attempted to avoid an open thoracotomy, but the success rate is highly variable. Often invasive procedures are unsafe because the patient is thrombocytopenic or his pulmonary function is severely compromised by his infection. A specific diagnosis can be made from only 60% of biopsy specimens (Greenman *et al.*, 1975). Open biopsy provides a specific diagnosis substantially more often than needle aspiration or needle biopsy and is generally associated with fewer complications.

B. Septicemia

Cancer patients are more susceptible to septicemia than general hospital populations. There are 2 episodes of septicemia per 100 hospital admissions in patients with solid tumors, 45 episodes in patients with leukemia, but only 1 episode in other hospitalized patients (Bodey, 1971). In most cancer institutions, gram-positive cocci cause less that 15% of episodes of septicemia. The majority of these infections are caused by *Escherichia coli, Klebsiella pneumoniae,* and *P. aeruginosa.* However, the relative distribution of organisms varies considerably in different institutions. For example, *S. aureus* infections have increased in frequency in some institutions in recent years. Epidemics of infection caused by specific organisms such as *Serratia marcescens* and *Staphylococcus epidermidis* have been observed in cancer institutions (Bodey *et al.*, 1970). In some instances, it has been possible to identify a common source for these epidemics, but in others a source has never been identified. Septicemia is especially likely to occur in patients with neutropenia since the neutrophil plays an important role in localizing infection. Among a group of 40 children with cancer who died of pneumonia, none with a neutrophil count of greater than $100/mm^3$ had septicemia, whereas 80% with a neutrophil count of less than $100/mm^3$ had septicemia in association with their pneumonia (Bodey and Hersh, 1969).

C. Skin Infection

Skin infections occasionally are a serious problem in the cancer patient. Usually, they develop at sites of intravenous infusions, but some may follow septicemia. Characteristic skin lesions can be found in some patients with pseudomonas septicemia or disseminated candidiasis, aspergillosis, phycomycosis, and varicella. The correct diagnosis often can be determined by the characteristic appearance, and the infecting organism usually can be cultured from these skin lesions. The skin of febrile patients should be carefully examined, especially the axilla, groin, and perianal areas, where lesions are likely to develop. Furthermore, patients with acute leukemia are especially susceptible to perianal infections caused by enteric organisms, which may be overlooked if these areas of the body are not examined. Frequently, these infections result in septicemia, often with multiple organisms.

D. Organisms Causing Infection

The majority of fatal infections in patients with acute leukemia, lymphoma, and solid tumors are caused by bacterial pathogens (Table IV). Nonbacterial pathogens are a common cause of fatal infection only in patients with acute leukemia, and even in these patients they account for only 26% of fatal infections (Inagaki *et al.*, 1974; Chang *et al.*, 1976; Feld *et al.*, 1974). Most bacterial infections are caused by gram-negative baccili. The relative frequency of various gram-negative bacilli depends upon the underlying malignancy. *Escherichia coli* infections are the most common type in every malignancy. Pseudomonas infections are more frequent in patients with acute leukemia than in patients with other malignancies.

Autopsy reviews are somewhat misleading because only fatal infections are included. Hence, all febrile episodes in a group of 494 patients with acute leukemia were reviewed (Bodey *et al.*, 1978). Aerobic gram-negative baccili accounted for 70% of the infections in which the infecting organism was identified. Only 6% of all infections were caused by gram-positive cocci and only 8% were caused by fungi. *Escherichia coli* and *Klebsiella spp.* were the gram-negative bacilli cultured most frequently from sites of infection, each accounting for 28% of gram-negative bacillary infections. *Pseudomonas aeruginosa* caused

TABLE IV

Causes of Death in Cancer Patients

	Acute leukemia	Lymphoma	Solid tumors
Patients studied	315	206	816
Percentage dying of infection	75	51	47
Bacterial	74	86	94
Fungal	21	13	6
Viral	3	0.3	0
Protozoal	2	0.6	0.4
Gram-negative bacillary infections	111	44	151
Percentage caused by:			
E. coli	25	34	30
K–E–S[a]	25	32	25
Pseudomonas	24	32	17

[a] Klebsiella–Enterobacter–Serratia group.

23% of these infections. The fatality rates were 16% for gram-positive coccal infections, 37% for gram-negative bacillary infections, and 86% for fungal infections.

Table V lists some of the more common organisms that cause infection in cancer patients. Some organisms such as cytomegalovirus and *Pneumocystis carinii* are infrequent causes of infection in the general cancer population, but are frequent in certain groups of patients such as children with acute leukemia or transplant recipients. Some cancer patients are more susceptible to infections caused by organisms such as *Salmonella* spp., atypical *Mycobacterium* spp., and *Cryptococcus neoformans* (Winston and Hewitt, 1979). The cancer patients with neutropenia are also susceptible to infection caused by organisms of low pathogenicity, such as *Bacillus cereus*, *Propionibacterium acnes,* and *Trichosporon cutaneum*. Both *P. acnes* and *S. epidermidis* are part of the resident skin flora and it is often difficult to ascertain whether a positive culture indicates infection or contamination. However, if these organisms are cultured on more than one occasion from a site of infection, it usually indicates that they are the causative agent. Several of these organisms will be considered in more detail because of the special problems they cause in the cancer patient.

1. Gram-Negative Bacilli

Pseudomonas aeruginosa is a frequent cause of infections in cancer patients, especially among those patients with neutropenia. In one study, 80% of cancer patients who developed pseudomonas septicemia had neutrophil counts less than

TABLE V

Organisms Causing Infections in Cancer Patients

Common	Uncommon
	Bacterial
Staphylococcus aureus	*Salmonella* spp.
Escherichia coli	*Clostridium perfringens*
Klebsiella pneumoniae	*Clostridium septicum*
Pseudomonas aeruginosa	*Listeria monocytogenes*
	Mycobacterium spp.
	Legionella pneumophila
	Fungal
Candida spp.	*Cryptococcus neoformans*
Aspergillus spp.	*Phycomycetes*
	Nocardia asteroides
	Torulopsis glabrata
	Viral
Hepatitis viruses	Cytomegalovirus
Herpes zoster-varicella	Measles virus
Herpes simplex	Papovavirus
	Protozoal and parasitic
	Pneumocystis carinii
	Toxoplasma gondii
	Strongyloides stercoralis

$100/mm^3$, and nearly 40% had neutrophil counts less than $100/mm^3$ (Whitecar *et al.*, 1970). *Pseudomonas aeruginosa* is widely disseminated in the hispital environment and is able to proliferate in moist environments. Additionally, it has been cultured from foodstuffs delivered to the hospital. A substantial number of patients become carriers of these organisms after entering the hospital, and the risk of serious pseudomonas infection is higher among carriers than noncarriers (Bodey, 1970). Pseudomonas septicemia is frequently associated with characteristic skin lesions known as ecthyma gangrenosa. These lesions have a characteristic bluish-black central area of necrosis surrounded by an erythematous halo; they usually arise in the groin, axilla, and perianal and inframammary areas. Local pseudomonas infections include orbital infections with conjunctivitis which can lead to endophthalmitis, perianal infections, necrotizing enterocolitis, meningitis, and pneumonia (Rodriguez and Bodey, 1979). Pathologically, pseudomonas infections are characterized by vasculitis of small arteries and veins that are invaded by myriads of organisms. The adjacent tissue undergoes coagulative necrosis, with surrounding hemorrhage and edema, but little inflammatory reaction. The aminoglycoside antibiotics are effective against pseudomonas infections in patients with adequate neutrophil counts, but less effective in neutropenic patients. The antipseudomonal penicillins are effective even in patients with severe neutropenia. A combination of an aminoglycoside plus an antipseudo-monal penicillin should be used for the treatment of severe infections or infec-tions in neutropenic patients. These drugs often are synergistic in their activity against *P. aeruginosa.*

The proportion of klebsiella and serratia infections has increased substantially in some cancer institutions in recent years because of better control of other types of infection. These infections usually present as septicemia, although *Klebsiella* spp. are also a common cause of pneumonia. Occasional patients develop multi-ple sites of cellulitis associated with septicemia. These organisms also may cause serious perianal infections. Infections caused by *S. marcescens* can be difficult to treat because these organisms frequently are resistant to multiple antibiotics. The usual therapy for klebsiella and serratia infections is with an aminoglycoside. Patients with serious klebsiella infections should also receive a cephalosporin. Few antibiotics other than aminoglycosides are routinely active against *S. mar-cescens.* Some strains are sensitive to carbenicillin or ticarcillin and some are sensitive to the new cephalosporin, cefamandole. Serious infections caused by susceptible strains should be treated by a combination rather than a single antibio-tic.

Salmonella infections probably do not occur more frequently in cancer pa-tients, but some cancer patients are more likely to develop serious infections when exposed to these organisms (Sinkovics and Smith, 1969). Patients with intra-abdominal tumor masses or hepatic metastases, patients receiving adrenal corticosteroids, and patients with hematological malignancies are more suscepti-ble to serious salmonella infections. *Salmonella* spp. may cause pneumonia, peritonitis, osteomyelitis, meningitis, and septicemia in these patients. Chloram-phenicol is the recommended therapy for these infections, although there has not been sufficient experience in neutropenic patients to determine its efficacy. Am-picillin may be more effective in these patients because it is a bactericidal agent, but a substantial number of *Salmonella* spp. are resistant to this antibiotic.

2. Anaerobic Organisms

Anaerobic infections occur most often in patients with gastrointestinal and genitourinary tract malignancies. Surprisingly, very few anaerobic infections occur in patients with hematological malignancies and neutropenia. Many infec-tions in these patients are thought to arise from the gastrointestinal tract since they are caused by enteric organisms. However, anaerobes comprise the largest population of organisms in the gastrointestinal tract, yet they seldom cause infection in neutropenic patients. Presumably, conditions within the local tumor mass such as tissue hypoxia and necrosis facilitate establishment of anaerobic infection, which can then disseminate via the blood stream. *Clostridium per-fringens* infections occur infrequently in cancer patients, but 90% of these infec-tions are associated with septicemia. Often the infection terminates fatally within

24 hours after onset of symptoms. Clostridial septicemia usually causes tachycardia, hypotension, oliguria, jaundice, and intravascular coagulation. Penicillin G is the drug of choice for these infections. *Bacteroides fragilis* is among the common anaerobic organisms causing infections below the diaphragm. This organism is usually resistant to penicillin G but susceptible to clindamycin, chloramphenicol, and cefoxitin. Often anaerobic organisms are found in combination with aerobic organisms in abdominal abscesses and peritonitis. Surgical drainage is necessary for successful management of most of these infections. Anaerobic organisms may cause lung abscesses, brain abscesses, sinus infections, and dental infections. Generally, the anaerobic organisms causing infection above the diaphragm are sensitive to penicillin G.

3. Other Bacterial Infections

Legionnaires' disease is a pulmonary infection caused by a bacteria, *Legionella pneumophila*, which was recognized only in 1979 (International Symposium on Legionnaires' Disease, 1979). Increasing evidence is accruing to indicate that immunocompromised patients are more susceptible to this infection. This infection may be confused with other types of pneumonitis but several findings suggest this diagnosis. These signs and symptoms include high, unremitting fever, confusion, diffuse myalgia, headache, and diarrhea. Involvement is usually unilateral with poorly marginated round opacities or diffuse patchy bronchopneumonia seen on a chest roentgenogram. The infection has occurred in epidemics and sporadically among hospitalized patients. The drug of choice appears to be erythromycin, but the compromised host may not be as responsive to therapy as other patients.

Listeria monocytogenes occasionally causes meningitis, encephalitis, septicemia, and endocarditis in cancer patients, especially in patients with lymphoma (Louria *et al.,* 1967). Whereas type 4b *L. monocytogenes* causes nearly 70% of infections in the general population of the United States, type 1 causes most infections in cancer patients. Meningitis accounts for over 60% of infections in cancer patients, and septicemia without meningitis accounts for an additional 30%. Other sites of infection, such as around pleural effusions and septic arthritis, are found rarely. The *in vitro* sensitivity of these organisms to antibiotics is variable,but they are usually sensitive to penicillin G and tetracycline. Appropriate antibiotic therapy is usually successful for cases of septicemia alone, but is less effective for cases of meningitis. *Listeria monocytogenes* infections in cancer patients may be rapidly fatal, and 20% of these patients die within 48 hours of onset of symptoms.

4. Tuberculosis

The incidence of tuberculosis has decreased substantially in the United States in recent decades. Consequently, physicians are not always alert to the possibility of mycobacteria as a cause of infection in the cancer patient. At the present time, tuberculosis occurs most often in patients with carcinoma of the head and neck and lung and in patients with lymphoma (Kaplan *et al.*, 1974). Patients with hematological malignancies are more likely to develop tuberculous pneumonia or disseminated infection. In these patients, the mortality rate approaches 50%, whereas in other cancer patients with pulmonary tuberculosis the mortality rate is less than 20%. Most of these patients should be treated with a triple-drug regimen to ensure as rapid control of the infection as possible. Most cancer patients who have a past history of tuberculosis and are receiving chemotherapy or adrenal corticosteroids should be given antituberculosis therapy to prevent reactivation when their host defense mechanisms are compromised. In some parts of the United States, an unusually high proportion of mycobacterial infections in cancer patients are caused by atypical organisms. Most of these infections are caused by *M. kansasii* and *M. fortuitum*. Frequently, they are difficult to treat because these organisms are resistant to many of the antituberculous agents, and *in vitro* susceptibility testing should be conducted routinely.

5. *Fungal Infections*

Fungal infections are increasing in frequency among cancer patients, especially among those with hematological malignancies (Bodey, 1966). These infections have been associated with a wide variety of factors, including neutropenia, impaired cellular immunity, use of intravenous catheters and intravenous hyperalimentation, and therapy with adrenal corticosteroids, antitumor agents, and antibiotics. Most fungal infections are superinfections and often arise in sites of tissue damage from previous bacterial infection. Fungal organisms can be classified into two basic groups; those that seldom cause infection except in compromised hosts, and those that usually cause limited infections in normal individuals but may cause disseminated infections in the compromised host. The former group includes *Candida* spp., *Aspergillus* spp., *Mucor* sp., and *Torulopsis glabrata*. The latter group includes *Cryptococcus neoformans, Histoplasma capsulatum, Coccidioides immitis,* and *Nocardia asteroides.*

a. Candidiasis Most fungal infections occurring in cancer patients are caused by *Candida* spp. *Candida albicans* is the most frequent infecting organism, followed by *C. tropicalis*. Other species occasionally may cause serious infection. Infection may be superficial, localized to a single organ system, or disseminated. Superficial dermatitis usually arises in the groin and perianal areas and is most prevalent in patients receiving antibiotics. It may spread extensively and cause considerable discomfort in cancer patients. Women receiving antibiotics, especially when administered orally, are subject to vaginitis. These infections respond to topical antifungal agents. Thrush, esophagitis, and gastrointestinal infection are not infrequent among patients receiving cancer chemotherapy. Gastrointestinal candidiasis is characterized by ulceration and pseudomembrane formation. Esophageal infection is diagnosed more often because it is associated with symptoms of dysphagia and retrosternal pain. Candidiasis of the lower gastrointestinal tract is diagnosed infrequently, since symptoms are often absent or mild and nonspecific. Thrush can usually be treated with topical antifungal agents. Esophageal and gastrointestinal candidiasis usually require a course of systemic therapy because of the potential for dissemination. Amphotericin B, 5-fluorocytosine, and miconazole are active agents; it has not been determined which one is most effective, although miconazole is the least toxic agent.

Disseminated candidiasis is the immediate cause of death in about 20–30% of patients with acute leukemia, but occurs much less frequently in other malignancies. Virtually every organ in the body can be involved in this infection, although the most common sites include the lungs, gastrointestinal tract, kidneys, liver, and spleen (Louria et al., 1962). Usually, there are no characteristic signs and symptoms to suggest the diagnosis. Often the only clinical features are persistent fever and gradual deterioration despite antibiotic therapy. However, some patients will have organ involvement that may suggest the diagnosis. Ocular infection manifested by white fluffy retinal exudates with vitreous haze or hemorrhage, hypopion, iritis, or conjunctivitis may result in blurred vision, pain, or scotomas (Edwards et al., 1974). Several patients have been described who developed a painful myositis in association with disseminated infection (Jarowski et al., 1978). Characteristic macronodular pinkish-purple subcutaneous skin lesions are found in about 10% of patients with disseminated candidiasis (Bodey and Luna, 1974). Rarely, cancer patients will develop cerebritis, laryngitis, or endocarditis as predominant manifestations of candidiasis. About 5% of major candida infections present as primary candida pneumonia, but usually pneumonitis is associated with disseminated infection.

The diagnosis of disseminated candidiasis is difficult to establish. Candida sp. is cultured from the blood of only about 25% of these patients, even when many blood cultures are obtained. Since Candida spp. are ubiquitous organisms, isolating them from throat, sputum, stool, and urine cultures does not establish the diagnosis. Indeed, some patients may have multiple body sites heavily colonized by Candida spp. without developing disease, whereas other patients may have extensive disease, yet Candida spp. are never isolated from any culture specimens. Some investigators have found measurements of antibody titers to be useful in establishing the diagnosis of disseminated candidiasis, whereas others have not (Filice et al., 1977; Glew et al., 1978). The major obstacle to progress in the management of this disease is the lack of a simple, reliable diagnostic procedure. Amphotericin B, 5-fluorocytosine, and miconazole all have activity against these organisms. However, therapy of disseminated candidiasis has seldom been successful unless the patient has achieved a remission of his underlying malignancy.

b. Aspergillosis and Phycomycosis Aspergillosis and phycomycosis are fungal infections that present with the same clinical and pathological features and will be considered together. Both infections occur predominantly in patients with acute leukemia. Aspergillosis is increasing in frequency, whereas phycomycosis remains an uncommon infection. Most of the aspergillus infections are caused by *A. fumigatus,* although many other species are occasionally pathogenic. Most cases of phycomycosis are caused by *Mucor* spp., but occasionally they are caused by *Rhizopus* spp. and *Absidia* spp. Pathologically, these infections are characterized by blood vessel invasion, resulting in thrombosis and infarction.

These infections may present as rhinocerebral, pulmonary, or disseminated infections. The majority of infections in cancer patients are pulmonary and may be manifested as necrotizing bronchopneumonia, hemorrhagic infarction, single or multiple abscesses, or lobar pneumonia (Young *et al.,* 1970). Some patients develop single or multiple nodular lesions which subsequently cavitate, resulting in the formation of a fungus ball. Usually, infected patients present with fever and a pulmonary infiltrate that fails to respond to antibiotic therapy. Occasional patients present with hemoptysis, pleuritic chest pain, and a pleural friction rub suggestive of acute pulmonary embolism. Neutropenic patients may have extensive pneumonitis but a normal chest roentgenogram at the onset of their infection. The organisms causing these infections are cultured infrequently from sputum specimens and, hence, the diagnosis is often established only at postmortem examination.

Rhinocerebral infection may involve the orbit, nasal cavity, paranasal sinuses, or roof of the mouth. It can lead to disfigurement due to widespread destruction of soft tissues and cartilage. Local extension into the base of the brain causes fatal meningoencephalitis. Usually, the infecting organism can be cultured from the sites of infection.

Hematogenous dissemination may lead to the infection of multiple organs. Most often the lungs, gastrointestinal tract, brain, kidneys, heart, and liver are involved (Meyer *et al.,* 1973). Organ infection can be associated with extensive infarction, leading to syndromes such as myocardial infarction, Budd–Chiari syndrome, gastrointestinal hemorrhage, and brain infarction. Disseminated infection may be associated with characteristic skin lesions, which appear as sharply demarcated areas of necrosis covered by a black eschar. Disseminated infection is seldom diagnosed clinically unless associated with these characteristic skin lesions. Many of the cases of aspergillosis and phycomycosis are diagnosed only at autopsy examination; hence, only limited experience has been obtained regarding the efficacy of antifungal therapy. The drug of choice is amphotericin B. Although 5-fluorocytosine is not active against *Aspergillus* spp. *in vitro,* some clinical evidence suggests that it may be beneficial when used in combination with amphotericin B. Therapy has not been effective unless the underlying malignancy can be treated successfully. In recent years, some patients with acute leukemia have recovered from these infections after achieving remission of their leukemia, although cavitary disease may require a long period for healing. Residual cavities with fungus balls may not resolve, and require surgical resection to prevent recurrent infection when the patient's underlying malignant disease recurs.

c. Cryptococcosis Cryptococcosis may present as primary pneumonia, meningitis, or disseminated infection (Lewis and Rabinovich, 1972). Pulmonary infection is associated with low-grade fever, pleuritic pain, and weight loss, and may follow a chronic course. Radiographic changes in the lung may indicate miliary, nodular, or cavitary lesions. Cryptococcal meningitis occurs most often in patients with lymphoma, but also may occur in patients with other hematological malignancies or solid tumors. Presenting signs and symptoms include fever, headache, vomiting, somnolence, meningismus, cranial nerve palsies, papilledema, and pathological reflexes. Occasional patients may have normal cerebrospinal fluid without any yeast cells being found on an India ink preparation. Detection of cryptococcal antigen has facilitated the diagnosis in these patients. Disseminated infection may involve the lungs, central nervous system (CNS), heart, and kidney. Bone and skin lesions may be found in occasional patients. Both amphotericin B and 5-fluorocytosine have activity against *C. neoformans,* but often cancer patients respond poorly to therapy. Cancer patients with meningitis should receive both systemic and intrathecal therapy with amphotericin B.

d. Nocardiosis Occasional cancer patients develop infections caused by *Nocardia asteroides* (Young *et al.,* 1971). Most of these patients have lymphomas. Primary pulmonary infection may be manifested as lobar pneumonia, multiple nodules, miliary abscesses, cavitary lesions, empyema, or occasionally with sinus tracts. About 30% of patients have brain abscesses that may not be recognized clinically because of minimal signs and symptoms. Disseminated infection also occurs in about 30% of infections and may involve the lungs, skin, brain, spleen, liver, kidney, and bones. Sulfadiazine is effective in many patients, although only 30% of patients with disseminated infection recover. Other drugs such as tetracycline and cycloserine may be used in combination with sulfadiazine in serious infections, and therapy should be continued for 3–6 months.

6. Viral Infections

Cancer patients are susceptible to acute viral infections that are prevalent in the community. Occasional immunosuppressed patients develop overwhelming infections that terminate fatally, but more often bacterial superinfection is likely to occur. Immunization will protect many cancer patients, but patients with hematological malignancies and patients receiving cancer chemotherapy are less likely to have an adequate antibody response (Ortbals *et al.,* 1977). The most serious viral infections in cancer patients are hepatitis, varicellazoster, herpes simplex, cytomegalic inclusion disease, and progressive multifocal leukoencephalopathy. Only hepatitis occurs frequently, although cytomegalic inclusion disease is a common complication of bone marrow transplantation. Rarely, children with cancer who contract measles develop hepatitis, encephalitis, or giant cell pneumonia, which leads to their death (Simpson and Pinkel, 1958).

a. Hepatitis Hepatitis occurs frequently among patients with hematologic malignancies who require frequent transfusions of blood products. Often it is difficult to determine whether the hepatitis is induced by a virus or by drugs. Clinically apparent infection is associated with malaise, anorexia, nausea, vomiting, abdominal pain, and jaundice. Anicteric hepatitis occurs more frequently and is detected by liver function abnormalities. Patients with impaired host defenses may be more susceptible to fulminant infection associated with acute atrophy (Good and Page, 1960). Mortality from transfusion hepatitis also may be more common in cancer patients.

It is currently believed that there are three types of viral hepatitis. Type A has an incubation period of 2–6 weeks and usually runs a mild course. Type B has an incubation period of 6 weeks to 6 months and usually is more severe. Type A hepatitis is generally transmitted orally and type B hepatitis is generally transmitted parenterally, although both viruses can be spread by either route. The hepatitis B virus antigen can be detected by several methods and has four subtype-specific determinates. The most sensitive tests for hepatitis B antigen are the radioimmunoassay and reversed passive hemagglutination. The antigen (HB_sAg) is usually detected in serum before clinically apparent illness and becomes undetectable during convalescence. Hepatitis A antibody has been detected during the acute phase of the illness. A third type of hepatitis, type C or non-A, non-B hepatitis, resembles type B infection but is not associated with HB_sAg. It is now the most common cause of post-transfusion hepatitis.

Some patients become chronic carriers of HB_sAg in their serum and may develop chronic active hepatitis. Asymptomatic HB_sAg-positive patients have caused an epidemic among personnel on an oncology ward. Leukemic children with hepatitis B have transmitted this infection to family members (Steinberg *et al.*, 1975). Cancer chemotherapy may have an adverse effect on this disease. Serial studies of HB_sAg and antibody in these patients revealed a significant decrease in antibody titers during chemotherapy with a concomitant increase in HB_sAg titer associated with evidence of hepatocellular damage. Standard immune globulin prevents or modifies the course of type A hepatitis if administered after exposure. Hyperimmune hepatitis B immune serum globulin may prevent hepatitis B infection (Prince *et al.*, 1978).

b. Herpes Virus Infections Varicella is a potentially serious infection in children with cancer, especially if they are receiving chemotherapy (Feldman *et al.*, 1975). Varicella pneumonitis occurs in about 25% of children with chickenpox

and may terminate fatally. Hepatitis, pancreatitis, and meningoencephalitis may
also complicate this infection. Bacterial superinfection of skin lesions occurs in
10% of patients. Bacterial pneumonia complicates varicella pneumonitis, and
50% of these patients develop bacteremia. The infection is highly contagious and
epidemics have been observed in pediatric cancer wards. Passive immunization
with zoster immune globulin and zoster immune plasma administered within 3
days of exposure to the virus will prevent or modify the infection.

Herpes zoster occurs in 3–15% of patients with lymphoma, myeloma, and
chronic lymphocytic leukemia, but in only 0.2–2% of the general adult population (Sokal and Firat, 1965). Infection usually represents reactivation of latent
virus which resides in the sensory cells of dorsal root ganglia, but reinfection
may also occur. If the infection remains localized, it usually presents no special
problems, although cancer patients are more likely to develop post-herpetic
neuralgia. Between 20 and 40% of cancer patients develop disseminated skin
infection, and about 35% of these develop visceral lesions. Vidarabine is an
antiviral agent that is effective in resolving the lesions of herpes zoster and
reducing pain. More experience is needed with this agent in the treatment of
visceral infection, but it is the only agent likely to be beneficial at present.

Herpes simplex lesions of the lip, oral cavity, nose, and genitalia can
cause considerable discomfort to the cancer patient. They may become extensive, and bacterial superinfection is not uncommon. Herpetic esophageal lesions
occur in 2% of cancer patients, and about 25% of these patients also develop
lesions in the larynx and trachea (Nash and Ross, 1974). Infrequently,
pneumonitis and disseminated infection occur in compromised hosts. When disseminated, infection may involve the lung, liver, gastrointestinal tract, adrenal,
pancreas, and brain. Vidarabine is effective for the treatment of herpes simplex
infections, including meningoencephalitis.

c. Cytomegalic Inclusion Disease Cytomegalic inclusion disease occurs
mainly in children with acute leukemia and recipients of bone marrow transplantation (Neiman et al., 1977). The disease may be acquired by the transfusion of
blood products obtained from infected donors. Infection is usually manifested as
a pneumonia with typical physical findings of dyspnea, cyanosis, and fine moist
rales over involved areas of the lung. A morbilliform skin rash may accompany
this infection. Diffuse reticulonodular infiltrates are found in one or both lungs
on chest roentgenogram. Although this infection may be fatal, it is often associated with a more serious bacterial or fungal pneumonia. Isolated infection of
the gastrointestinal tract may cause uncontrollable diarrhea or hemorrhage. Infection disseminates in some patients to involve other organs, including the kidneys,
liver, heart, adrenals, spleen, and pancreas. Occasional patients develop a
characteristic acute chorioretinitis. Death has resulted from myocarditis, renal
failure, and adrenal insufficiency.

Infection is recognized pathologically by identification of characteristic cells containing intranuclear or intracytoplasmic inclusions. These inclusion cells may be found in urine, sputum, gastric washings, cerebrospinal fluid, or tissue specimens. The virus may be cultured from urine, saliva, sputum, or peripheral blood cells, but viral isolation is not always indicative of disease. A fourfold rise in complement fixation antibody titers or serological conversion usually indicates the presence of disease. However, some patients are unable to mount an antibody response to infection, and other patients may show such a response without evidence of infection (Sullivan *et al.*, 1968). Hence antibody determinations are not reliable for establishing the diagnosis of cytomegalic inclusion disease. Unfortunately, there is no effective therapy for this infection.

d. Progressive Multifocal Leukoencephalopathy Progressive multifocal leukoencephalopathy appears to be caused by a papovavirus. It is an infrequent cause of CNS infection in cancer patients, especially in patients with lymphoma (Richardson, 1961). The onset of this disease is insidious, usually with progression to death in 3 to 4 months, but occasionally it lasts for as long as 2 years. The patients develop progressive mental changes including disorientation, decreased mental acuity, and abnormal emotional responses. Visual field defects and blindness are common. Other signs include aphasia or dysarthria, sensory loss, and cerebellar signs. The cerebrospinal fluid is usually normal, and electroencephalograms are always abnormal but not distinctive. Pathologically, multiple areas of demyelination are present in the cerebral hemispheres, cerebellum and brain stem. The nuclei of oligodendrocytes are enlarged, lack nuclear detail, contain intranuclear inclusions, and are densely basophilic. Hyperplastic astrocytes form bizarre cells. Electron microscopy studies have demonstrated dense collections of virus-like particles in the nuclei of some abnormal glial cells. Both the JC and SV 40 papovaviruses have been implicated in this disease, although most appear to be caused by the JC virus. Progressive multifocal leukoencephalopathy may result from reactivation of latent infection or infection in a patient who failed to acquire immunity in childhood. No therapy is currently available for this disease.

7. Protozoal Infection

Pneumocystis carinii is believed to be a protozoan that causes an interstitial pneumonia. Among cancer patients, it is responsible for as many as 45% of cases of interstitial pneumonia (Goodell *et al.*, 1970). Rarely, the organism disseminates to invade the liver, spleen, lymph nodes, and bone marrow. A substantial number of infections occur in children with leukemia who are in remission and receiving maintenance chemotherapy (Perera *et al.*, 1970). Infection may represent reactivation or recent exposure. The infection is potentially contagious and has been transmitted from patient to patient in the hospital. The characteristic clinical features of this infection are fever, nonproductive cough, dyspnea, and cyanosis. Physical findings are usually minimal or absent. The disease may develop over 1 to 2 months or may rapidly progress over a 4- to 5-day period. Chest roentgenograms reveal diffuse bilateral interstitial infiltrates which are most prominent in the hilar regions. The organism is seldom found in smears of sputum, hypopharyngeal secretions or tracheal aspirates. Needle aspiration or open lung biopsy usually is necessary to establish the diagnosis.

The earliest histological evidence of infection is the presence of cysts and trophozoites within the cytoplasm of cells attached to the alveolar walls. As the disease progresses, the alveoli become filled with an intense foamy exudate, presumably derived from the organisms. The treatment of choice is trimethoprim–sulfamethoxazole. Pentamidine isethionate also is effective therapy, but is associated with substantial toxicity. Furthermore, trimethoprim–sulfamethoxazole also can prevent infection in highly susceptible populations (Hughes *et al.*, 1977).

Toxoplasma gondii is an obligate intracellular parasite that is an infrequent but serious cause of disease in cancer patients. It occurs most often in patients with Hodgkin's disease, but also in patients with other lymphomas and leukemia (Vietzke *et al.*, 1968). The disease may represent reactivation of latent infection or newly acquired infection. The organism may be transmitted by pets, by the ingestion of improperly cooked meat products, and by blood transfusion. Infection may involve the CNS, heart, lungs, liver, kidney, lymph nodes, spleen, and bone marrow. Neurological disease is associated with confusion, seizures, and headache. Occasional patients develop focal neurological deficits, including cranial nerve palsies and paresis. The usual cerebrospinal fluid abnormalities are pleocytosis, predominantly with lymphocytes, elevated protein concentration, and normal or decreased glucose concentration. However, some patients have normal cerebrospinal fluid. There is focal necrosis of the brain with intense cellular infiltration, vascular cuffing, and endarteritis, which may lead to gelatinous softening and gliosis. Free organisms and cysts are found within the zones of necrosis. In the lungs, parasites invade alveolar cells and endothelial cells, causing intense inflammation, interstitial hemorrhage, and a homogeneous gelatinous alveolar exudate.

The diagnosis of toxoplasmosis is established by the identification of organisms in clinical specimens or by serologic tests. *Toxoplasma gondii* can be identified microscopically in the blood, sputum, cerebrospinal fluid, and tissue of infected patients. Numerous serological tests are available, including the Sabin–Feldman dye test, immunofluorescent antibody test, and IgM-fluorescent antibody. However, cancer patients often have impaired antibody production and the interpretation of serological tests may be difficult. These patients may have acute toxoplasmosis with a minimal immunofluorescent antibody titer and with no increase in antibody titer during the course of the infection. The treatment for toxoplasmosis is pyrimethamine and sulfonamides for a 4-week period. Since the regimen may cause myelosuppression and megaloblastic anemia, folinic acid may be administered without affecting the therapeutic results. The prognosis is especially poor in patients with CNS disease.

III. DIAGNOSIS OF AND THERAPY FOR INFECTION

A. Diagnosis

Fever is a common occurrence in cancer patients and its cause is often difficult to determine. The proportion of hospital days spent with fever varies from 15% for patients with metastatic cancer to 40% for patients with acute leukemia.

The proper approach to the management of fever depends upon whether or not the patient has seriously compromised host defense mechanisms, and especially whether or not he or she has neutropenia. Infection is characteristically associated with fever and leukocytosis. However, neither of these signs is a reliable indicator in this patient population. Fever may be secondary to the malignant process, transfusion of blood products, or to medications. Some antitumor agents, such as bleomycin and L-asparaginase, may cause febrile reactions. There is no characteristic pattern for fever due to infection or for fever due to other causes. Patients receiving adrenal corticosteroids may have extensive fungal infection without fever. No infectious cause is found in about 40% of febrile episodes in cancer patients.

The presence or absence of leukocytosis also may be misleading. Patients receiving myelosuppressive chemotherapy are unable to respond to infection with a leukocytosis. Leukocytosis may occur secondary to the malignant disease, especially if necrotic tumor masses are present. However, most cancer patients do not have a compromised bone marrow and will respond to infection with a leukocytosis and present with the classic signs and symptoms of infection. All patients with fever (temperature greater than 101°F) should be carefully evaluated for signs of infection, and appropriate cultures and laboratory studies should be obtained.

In patients with adequate neutrophils (more than 100/mm^3), the decision to administer antibiotics at the onset of fever should be based upon the clinical assessment of the patient. It is important to recognize those factors that may have been responsible for the infection. If infection has arisen distal to an obstruction, every effort should be made to relieve the obstruction. Intravenous catheters should be removed and cultured.

B. Treatment

The selection of antibiotics in these patients depends upon the site of infection, the events surrounding the onset of fever, and the patient's underlying malignancy. Patients who acquired their infection outside of the hospital are more likely to be infected by a gram-positive coccus or by a gram-negative bacillus susceptible to multiple antibiotics. Patients who acquired their infection in the hospital or who were recently discharged from the hospital are more likely to be infected by gram-negative bacilli. Anaerobic infection or mixed aerobic and anaerobic infection should be considered in patients with gastrointestinal or genitourinary malignancies. Usually, it is wise to administer a combination rather than a single antibiotic if the infecting organism has not been identified. Those combinations offering the broadest spectrum of coverage include an aminoglycoside plus a broad-spectrum penicillin, cephalosporin, or an anti-staphylococcal penicillin. Several randomized trials have shown an increased frequency of nephrotoxicity when the combination of gentamicin plus cephalothin is used, and this combination probably should be avoided (Wade *et al.*, 1978). Combinations of other animoglycosides and other cephalosporins may not be associated with this toxicity. If anaerobic infection exists as a possibility, clindamycin or cefoxitin should be included.

Generally, combinations of antibiotics are given in preference to a single antibiotic to provide adequate coverage against most organisms likely to cause infection. A further advantage of antibiotic combinations is potentially synergistic activity against the infecting organism. Klastersky treated patients with gentamicin plus cephalothin or with gentamicin plus ampicillin (Klastersky *et al.*, 1971). The cure rates were 58% and 67%, respectively. The antibiotic combinations selected was found to have synergistic activity *in vitro* against 44% of the infecting organisms. Eighty percent of the infections were cured when the antibiotic combination used was synergistic, but only 49% of the infections were cured when the antibiotic combination was not synergistic. Subsequently, combinations of gentamicin plus cephalothin were evaluated, gentamicin plus ampicillin and gentamicin plus carbenicillin for the treatment of infections treated in cancer patients (Klastersky *et al.*, 1971). Seventy-eight percent of the infections treated with a synergistic combination were cured, whereas only 53% of the infections treated with a nonsynergistic combination were cured ($p < .01$).

This information is important but difficult for most physicians to apply. At times, therapy must be instituted before the infecting organism is identified or the results of antibiotic sensitivity testing are known. Most clinical laboratories are not able to conduct assays for synergistic activity of antibiotic combinations. A few general rules can assist in the selection of antibiotic combinations that are likely to be synergistic. Both drugs in the regimen should be bactericidal agents, such as aminoglycosides, cephalosporins, and penicillins. Both drugs should be active against the infecting organism *in vitro*. The two drugs should have different mechanisms of action. Using these rules, the combination of an aminoglycoside plus a cephalosporin would be likely to have synergistic activity against *Klebsiella* spp., whereas the combination of an aminoglycoside plus an antipseudomonal penicillin would be likely to have synergistic activity against *P. aeruginosa.*

Several aminoglycoside antibiotics have been used for the therapy of gram-negative bacillary infections in patients with adequate neutrophil counts. Some patients received these antibiotics after failing to respond to other regimens. The majority of infections were episodes of pneumonia and septicemia. Gentamicin cured 79% of 24 infections, tobramycin cured 79% of 28 infections, and amikacin cured 74% of 43 infections (Bodey *et al.,* 1972, 1976; Valdivieso *et al.,* 1974). A prospective randomized study of amikacin and tobramycin as initial therapy for presumed infection was conducted in cancer patients (Feld *et al.,* 1977a). The most frequent infections were pneumonias, urinary tract infections, and septicemias. Tobramycin cured 57% of infections and amikacin cured 55% of infections (Table VI). All of the infections caused by gram-negative bacilli were sensitive *in vitro* to the antibiotic which the patient received. The results were similar for both antibiotics regardless of the infecting organism and the site of infection. Considering only those patients with normal renal function initially, the frequency of azotemia was 21% with tobramycin and 15% with amikacin. However, animal studies and some clinical trials have indicated that tobramycin is less nephrotoxic than other aminoglycosides. Amikacin is active against some organisms that are resistant to gentamicin. The activity of this antibiotic was evaluated in a group of cancer patients who developed infections caused by gentamicin-resistant organisms (Valdivieso and Bodey, 1977). Most of the infections were due to *P. aeruginosa* and the Klebsiella–Enterobacter–Serratia group, and were septicemias and urinary tract infections. The cure rate was 54% in this group of patients.

A prospective randomized trial of carbenicillin alone, gentamicin alone, or carbenicillin plus gentamicin was conducted in cancer patients with gram-negative bacillary infections (Klastersky *et al.,* 1973). Only a few of these patients became neutropenic during their infection. The combination regimen cured 83% of infections, whereas gentamicin cured 57% and carbenicillin cured 50% (Table VI). Considering only those infections caused by organisms that were sensitive *in vitro* to the antibiotics used, 65% responded to carbenicillin, 57% responded to gentamicin, and 91% responded to the combination. The difference in results between the combination and gentamicin was statistically significant ($p < .02$). Most infections in this study were caused by *P. aeruginosa* and *Proteus* spp. The combination was most effective against these infections, curing 87%, whereas gentamicin cured 58% and carbenicillin cured 53%.

Carbenicillin plus cephalothin was compared to carbenicillin plus cephalothin plus gentamicin as initial therapy for presumptive gram-negative bacillary infections in cancer patients, most of whom had adequate neutrophil counts (Klastersky *et al.,* 1972). Eighty percent of patients who received the two-drug regimen were cured, compared to 76% of patients who received the three-drug

TABLE VI

Studies of Antibiotic Therapy in Cancer Patients with Adequate Neutrophils

Therapy[a]	Total infections		GNB[b] infections		Pseudomonas-proteus		K-E-S[c]		Septicemia		Respiratory		References
	No.	% Cures	No.	% Cures	No.	% Cures	No.	% Cures	No.	% Cures	No.	% Cures	
Amik vs. Tobra													Feld et al., 1977a
Amik	60	55	29	69	7	57	7	71	11	64	24	33	
Tobra	51	57	18	67	5	40	8	75	6	50	32	50	
Carb vs. Gent vs. Carb + Gent													Klastersky et al., 1973
Carb	—	—	22	50	17	53	0	—	4	50	9	44	
Gent	—	—	23	57	12	58	7	71	3	33	12	58	
Carb + Gent	—	—	23	83	15	87	1	100	5	80	10	80	
Carb + Ceph vs. Carb + Ceph + Gent													Klastersky et al., 1974
Carb + Ceph	—	—	40	80	20	75	10	90	20	80	9	66	
Carb + Ceph + Gent	—	—	41	76	20	75	8	82	19	79	13	54	
Amik + Pen vs. Amik + Carb													Klastersky et al., 1977b
Amik + Pen	—	—	54	56	27	48	17	65	25	52	31	45	
Amik + Carb	—	—	63	64	22	59	17	59	27	70	19	42	

[a] Amik, amikacin; Tobra, tobramycin; Carb, carbenicillin; Gent, gentamicin; Ceph, cephalothin; Pen, penicillin G.
[b] GNB, gram-negative bacilli.
[c] K-E-S, Klebeiella-Enterobacter-Serratia group.

regimen (Table VI). The majority of patients in both groups had septicemia and the cure rates were 80% and 79%, respectively. The results in respiratory infections were less impressive, which has been true in most studies. Nephrotoxicity occurred more often with the three-drug regimen. Hence, in this group of patients, the addition of gentamicin did not improve the efficacy of carbenicillin plus cephalothin, but did increase the frequency of nephrotoxicity.

Amikacin plus penicillin G was compared to amikacin plus carbenicillin as initial therapy for presumed infection in cancer patients (Klastersky *et al.*, 1977b). Of the 250 patients entered on this study, 117 had gram-negative bacillary infections. Amikacin plus penicillin cured 56% and amikacin plus carbenicillin cured 64% (Table VI). Among patients with bacteremia, the response rates were 52% and 70%, respectively. Patients with infections caused by *E. coli* and *P. aeruginosa* had a better prognosis if treated with amikacin plus carbenicillin than if treated with amikacin plus penicillin. The cure rates for *E. coli* infections were 70% and 56%, and for pseudomonas infections were 67% and 46%, differences which were not statistically significant. Infections caused by other gram-negative bacilli responded equally well to both regimens (61% versus 57%). *In vitro* synergism of the antibiotic combination against the infecting organism was demonstrated more frequently with amikacin plus carbenicillin (64% versus 53%). When synergism was present, amikacin plus penicillin cured 70% of infections and amikacin plus carbenicillin cured 62% of infections. When synergism was absent, they cured 42% and 55% of infections, respectively.

In these studies of antibiotic regimens in patients with adequate neutrophil counts, no regimen could be considered the best. In general, a combination of antibiotics appeared to be superior to a single antibiotic, but this depended somewhat on the infecting organism and the site of infection.

The management of fever in the neutropenic patient requires a different approach from that used in patients with adequate neutrophil counts. The neutropenic patient can have extensive infection without any of the classic signs and symptoms of infection other than fever. Patients with pneumonia may have none of the clinical signs and symptoms associated with this infection, and no infiltrates are seen on chest roentgenograms. In a study of gram-negative bacillary pneumonias, in 38% of patients whose neutrophil count was less than $1000/mm^3$, the chest roentgenogram was considered to be normal at the onset of their infection (Valdivieso *et al.*, 1977). Among cancer patients who developed pneumonia, 84% of those patients whose neutrophil count was greater than $1000/mm^3$ produced purulent sputum, but only 8% of those patients whose neutrophil count was less than $100/mm^3$ produced purulent sputum (Sickles *et al.*, 1975). Likewise, among patients with urinary tract infections, pyuria was found in 97% of the former group but in only 11% of the latter group.

It is important that the physician is not misled by the absence of clinical and laboratory evidence of infection into withholding antibiotic therapy. Infection in the neutropenic patient disseminates rapidly and terminates fatally, if not treated promptly. For example, a study of pseudomonas septicemia was conducted in cancer patients before effective antibiotic therapy was available (Whitecar *et al.*, 1970). Sixteen percent of these patients had died within 12 hours after the collection of the first blood specimen from which *P. aeruginosa* was cultured, and 36% had died within 24 hours.

Antibiotic therapy must be instituted on the presumption that infection is present when he neutropenic patient becomes febrile. The majority of infections are caused by gram-negative bacilli. Pseudomonas infections are more common in neutropenic patients than in patients with adequate neutrophil counts. For many years after the introduction of the antistaphylococcal penicillins, *S. aureus* infections had become infrequent, but they have been occurring more frequently in some cancer hospitals. The neutropenic patient is also susceptible to infections caused by organisms that are usually considered to be ''nonpathogens.'' Environmental or skin contaminants, such as *Bacillus cereus* and *Propionibacterium acnes* may cause serious infections in these patients. *Staphylococcus epidermidis* is a common skin contaminant that occasionally causes serious infections in these compromised hosts. At times, it is difficult to decide whether such organisms are the causal agents of infection. Their potential pathogenicity should be recognized if they are isolated from multiple blood cultures or from sites of infection.

Broad-spectrum antibiotic therapy must be prescribed to provide adequate coverage against the wide variety of potential agents causing infection in neutropenic patients. Generally, a combination of antibiotics is necessary. Early studies suggested that not all antibiotics were effective in these patients. For example, when aminoglycosides were administered by conventional intermittent schedules, an inverse correlation was found between the patients' neutrophil counts and their response to therapy. Among patients whose neutrophil count was less than $100/mm^3$, gentamicin cured only 23% of gram-negative bacillary infections and tobramycin cured only 24% (Bodey *et al.*, 1972; Valdivieso *et al.*, 1974). However, no such correlation was observed with the antipseudomonal penicillins. Carbenicillin cured 55% of pseudomonas infections occurring in patients whose neutrophil count was greater than $1000/mm^3$, and it cured 75% of infections in patients whose neutrophil count was less than $100/mm^3$ (Bodey *et al.*, 1971a).

The poor results obtained with aminoglycosides against infections in neutropenic patients may have been due to failure to maintain adequate serum concentrations. When antibiotics are administered by intermittent schedules, there are intervals between doses when the serum concentrations may be suboptimal. Since the neutropenic patient is unable to mount an adequate inflammatory response, he is dependent upon antibiotics to control his infection. Gram-negative bacilli appear to recover rapidly from the effects of antibiotics once they are no longer present (Bodey and Pan, 1976). Hence, it is possible that these organisms may proliferate in neutropenic patients between doses of antibiotics when the concentration at the site of infection is inadequate.

Amikacin was evaluated in cancer patients, using two schedules of administration. An intermittent schedule was employed for patients with adequate neutrophil counts, and a continuous infusion schedule was employed for patients with neutropenia (Bodey *et al.*, 1976). Sixty-one percent of the 75 infections treated by the intermittent schedule and 66% of the 59 infections treated by the continuous infusion schedule were cured. This was the first study in which neutropenic patients responded as well to an aminoglycoside as patients with an adequate neutrophil count. Subsequently, a prospective randomized study was conducted in neutropenic patients in which sisomicin was administered by an intermittent or continuous schedule (Feld *et al.*, 1977b; Bodey *et al.*, 1979a). All of these patients had failed to respond to initial therapy with carbenicillin plus a cephalosporin. Forty-six percent of the 35 infections treated by the intermittent schedule were cured, whereas 61% of the 38 infections treated by the continuous infusion schedule were cured. Among patients with septicemia, the cure rates were 33% and 42%, respectively. No statistically significant differences were observed in this study, but the results were consistently better among the neutropenic patients who received the continuous infusion schedule. These and other data suggest that better results can be obtained with aminoglycosides in neutropenic patients when schedules are used that constantly maintain adequate serum concentrations of antibiotic.

A variety of antibiotic combinations has been used for the treatment of infections in neutropenic patients (Table VII). Some of these regimens have been compared in prospective randomized trials. No single regimen can be considered the most effective, although response rates have varied from 52 to 81%. Greater differences have been observed with the same regimen used by different investigators than the differences observed between different regimens used in comparative trials. For example, the combination of carbenicillin plus gentamicin produced a cure rate of 54% in one study, but a cure rate of 71% in a larger study (Rodriguez *et al.*, 1970; EORTC International Antimicrobial Therapy Project Group, 1978). Carbenicillin plus cephalothin cured 52% of infections in one study but 72% in another larger study (EORTC International Antimicrobial Therapy Project Group, 1978; Middleman *et al.*, 1972). No statistically significant differences were obtained in any of the prospective randomized trials.

The combination of carbenicillin plus gentamicin has been used most extensively as initial therapy for presumed infection in neutropenic patients. The first reported experience with this combination was in 32 cancer patients, 24 of whom had neutropenia (Rodriquez *et al.*, 1970). Most of infections were episodes of pneumonia and septicemia caused predominantly by the Klebsiella–Enterobacter—Serratia group. The cure rate in neutropenic patients was 54%. In

TABLE VII

Combination Antibiotic Regimens for Neutropenic Patients

Regimen[a]	Number	Percentage of Cures	Reference
Gent + Carb	24	54	Rodriguez et al., 1970
Tobra + Carb	80	69	Issell et al., 1979
Gent + Carb + Ceph	26	81	Bloomfield et al., 1974
Amik + Carb + Cef	39	67	Klastersky et al., 1977a
Carb + Ceph vs.	33	52	Middleman et al., 1972
Carb + Kan	28	46	Middleman et al., 1972
Carb + Ceph vs.	135	72	EORTC International Antimicrobial Therapy Project Group, 1978
Carb + Gent vs.	156	71	EORTC International Antimicrobial Therapy Project Group, 1978
Ceph + Gent	162	68	EORTC International Antimicrobial Therapy Project Group, 1978
Carb + Gent vs.	107	67	Keating et al., 1979
Carb + Amik vs.	86	69	Keating et al., 1979
Carb + Siso	89	67	Keating et al., 1979

[a] Gent, gentamicin; Tobra, tobramycin; Amik, amikacin; Siso, sisomicin; Carb, carbenicillin; Ceph, cephalothin; Cef, cefazolin; and Kan, Kanamycin.

a subsequent study, 55% of 60 cancer patients with neutropenia responded to this regimen (Schimpff et al., 1971). Sixty-seven percent of patients with pseudomonas infections responded, but only 40% of patients with infections caused by other gram-negative bacilli responded.

The combination of tobramycin plus carbenicillin was used as initial therapy during 125 documented infections, of which 84 occurred in neutropenic patients (Issell et al., 1980). Tobramycin was administered by a continuous infusion schedule. Most infections were pneumonias, septicemias, and soft tissue infections. The predominant causative agents were *K. pneumoniae* and *P. aeruginosa*. The cure rate was 69% for patients who had neutropenia at the onset of their infection. Among these patients, the cure rate was 76% for the patients whose neutrophil count increased during their infection, compared to 60% for the patients whose neutrophil count remained less than $1000/mm^3$ ($p = .005$). Among the 26 patients whose neutrophil count remained less than $100/mm^3$, the cure rate was 58%.

Two studies have reported results with three-drug combinations in neutropenic cancer patients. Gentamicin, cephalothin, and carbenicillin were used to treat 33 documented bacterial infections in 23 patients, and 82% were cured (Bloomfield and Kennedy, 1974).

Most infections were pneumonias and septicemias, and the predominant organisms were *Klebsiella* spp. and *E. coli*. The response rates were similar for patients whose neutrophil counts were less than or greater than $500/mm^3$ (88% versus 86%). Patients whose neutrophil count increased to greater than $500/mm^3$ had a response rate of 100%, whereas patients whose neutrophil count remained less than $500/mm^3$ had a response rate of 79%. The combination of carbenicillin, cefazolin, and amikacin caused a favorable response in 67% of 39 episodes of infection in neutropenic patients (Klastersky *et al.*, 1977a). Nineteen patients had gram-negative bacillary infections, and 63% responded. A response rate of 67% was obrained in patients whose neutrophil count remained less than $100/mm^3$. The neutrophil count increased in 22 patients during their infection and 73% responded, whereas the neutrophil count decreased or remained unchanged in 17 patients, and 59% responded.

A prospective randomized study of (1) carbenicillin (or ticarcillin) plus ccphalothin, (2) carbenicillin (or ticarcillin) plus gentamicin, or (3) cephalothin plus gentamicin was investigated as the initial treatment of presumed infection in neutropenic patients (EORTC International Antimicrobial Therapy Project Group, 1978). Most of the infections involved the respiratory tract, oral cavity, and soft tissues. The predominant infecting organisms were *E. coli, S. aureus, Klebsiella* spp., and *P. aeruginosa*. The overall cure rates for documented infections were 7% with carbenicillin plus cephalothin, 71% with carbenicillin plus gentamicin, and 68% with cephalothin plus gentamicin (Table VII). Patients with persistent severe neutropenia had a cure rate of only 44%, but patients whose neutrophil count increased from an initial level of less than $100/mm^3$ during their infection had a cure rate of 87%. Carbenicillin plus cephalothin was less effective than carbenicillin plus gentamicin or cephalothin plus gentamicin against *E. coli* infections (44% versus 73% versus 67%), primarily because some strains were resistant to both carbenicillin and cephalothin. Cephalothin plus gentacimin was less effective against pseudomonas infections than carbenicillin plus cephalothin or carbenicillin plus gentamicin (38% versus 50% versus 63%).

The combinations of carbenicillin plus gentamicin, sisomicin, and amikacin have been studied as initial therapy for presumed infection in cancer patients (Keating *et al.*, 1979). There were 282 documented infections in neutropenic patients. Most infections were pneumonias and septicemias, and the predominant organisms were gram-negative bacilli. There were no significant differences in overall cure rates, although relapses after therapy was discontinued occurred significantly more often with carbenicillin plus sisomicin. The response of septicemias was significantly lower with carbenicillin plus gentamicin than with carbenicillin plus sisomicin or carbenicillin plus amikacin (44% versus 75% versus 72%). The cure rates for gram-negative bacillary pneumonias were 29% for carbenicillin plus gentamicin, 35% for carbenicillin plus amikacin, and 57% for carbenicillin plus sisomicin. Patients whose initial neutrophil count was less than 100/mm^3 responded almost as frequently as patients who had a higher initial neutrophil count (63% versus 72%). Patients whose neutrophil count increased during their infection had a significantly higher response rate than those whose neutrophil count remained stable or decreased (85% versus 59%, $p = .001$). These differences were observed with all three regimens and all three regimens were equally effective in these patients.

Regardless of the combination used, about 70% of infections will respond to initial therapy. The selection of an inappropriate regimen depends upon the predominant organisms in the hospital environment and their *in vitro* susceptibilities to various antibiotics. There is no evidence at present to indicate that any particular regimen is substantially better than any other for routine use in neutropenic patients.

Once antibiotic therapy has been initiated in the neutropenic patient, a decision must be made concerning the duration of therapy if the cause of the fever remains unknown. In a study designed to resolve this problem, neutropenic patients were treated routinely with carbenicillin and cephalothin at the onset of fever (Rodriguez *et al.*, 1973). After 4 days of therapy, if the cause of fever remained undetermined, the patients were randomized either to continue or to discontinue antibiotics. Patients were randomized separately, depending upon whether they had remained febrile or had become afebrile. Among the patients who had become afebrile, infection was eventually proved to be the cause of fever in 21%. All patients who continued to receive antibiotics recovered. However, two of eight infected patients in whom antibiotic therapy had been discontinued on day 4 died of their infection, even though the infecting organism remained sensitive to either carbenicillin or cephalothin *in vitro* and although these antibiotics were promptly reinstituted when the infection was recognized. Among patients with persistent fever, infection was eventually identified in 50%. Usually, the causative agent was resistant to carbenicillin and cephalothin, and over 80% responded to the addition of gentamicin. In this group of patients, no adverse effects were observed when the initial antibiotic combination was discontinued on day 4. These data suggest that patients with fever of unknown origin which defervesces on antibiotic therapy should continue to receive this therapy for 7 to 10 days. Patients who remain febrile after 3 or 4 days should be reevaluated and treated with a different antibiotic regimen.

At least 20% of patients who fail to respond to combinations of an aminoglycoside, cephalosporin, and an antipseudomonal penicillin have a fungal infection. Since fungal infections are difficult to diagnose clinically, by the time the fungus has been identified, it may have disseminated so that antifungal therapy cannot be effective. Consequently, neutropenic patients with persistent fever that is unresponsive to antibacterial antibiotics should be considered for a therapeutic trial with an antifungal agent, if the clinical setting suggests the possibility of this diagnosis. A 5-day course of amphotericin B will cause a prompt response in about 30% of these patients. Antibiotics probably should be discontinued in patients who remain febrile after receiving this program. Although their fever most likely is not due to infection, they require close observation and frequent cultures should be obtained. The onset of infection in a cancer patient already febrile from some other cause is very difficult to recognize.

IV. THERAPY FOR NONBACTERIAL INFECTIONS

Amphotericin B remains the mainstay of therapy for most fungal infections. This antifungal antibiotic is insoluble in water and thus is administered as a colloidal material. It binds to sterols in the fungal cell membrane, resulting in loss of integrity of the cell membrane. It is active *in vitro* against *Candida* spp., *Aspergillus* spp., Phycomycetes, *H. capsulatum, C. immitis,* and *C. neoformans;* hence, it is a truly broad-spectrum antifungal agent. A major disadvantage of this agent is the high frequency of side effects (Utz *et al.,* 1964). Common reactions include headaches, chills, fever, malaise, muscle and joint pain, nausea, and vomiting. Occasional patients will experience acute hypotensive reactions. These acute reactions may be ameliorated by antipyretics, antihistamines, antiemetics, and adrenal corticosteroids. Prolonged therapy is associated with nephrotoxicity, hypokalemia, renal tubular acidosis, nephrocalcinosis, and normocytic, normochromic anemia (Bennett, 1977). During prolonged therapy, the dose of drug must usually be reduced or administered on alternate days to reduce the nephrotoxicity.

Results with amphotericin B therapy for fungal infections in compromised hosts are often suboptimal. Usually, those patients who achieve a remission of their underlying malignant disease are the only patients who benefit from this therapy, and some of these patients recover without any antifungal therapy. Perhaps some failures are due to the fact that therapy is not instituted until the fungal infection is far-advanced, because of inadequate diagnostic tests. Amphotericin B will produce dramatic results in patients with severe thrush that is unresponsive to topical agents, and in patients with candida esophagitis. Amphotericin B is being used increasingly in patients in whom the diagnosis of fungal infection is suspected but not proven. This is a difficult decision to make because of the serious toxicity of this antifungal agent.

Flucytosine (5-fluorocytosine) penetrates fungal cells where it is converted to 5-fluoruracil, which interferes with pyrimidine metabolism. It is active *in vitro* against *Candida* spp., *C. neoformans, T. glabrata,* and some *Aspergillus* spp.

(Bennett, 1977). However, up to 25% of strains of *Candida* spp. may be resistant, and some fungi develop resistance during therapy. *In vitro* synergism exists between amphotericin B and flucytosine against some fungi. Flucytosine has the advantage of being well absorbed from the gastrointestinal tract, and it penetrates into the cerebrospinal fluid. Side effects include nausea, vomiting, diarrhea, liver function abnormalities, and occasionally hepatic necrosis. Flucytosine occasionally causes myelosuppression, which may delay recovery from the myelosuppressive toxicity of antitumor agents. As with amphotericin B, recovery from major fungal infection sledom occurs unless the underlying malignancy is effectively treated. Because of the potential for emergence of resistant fungi, its use should be primarily in combination with amphotericin B against candidiasis and cryptococcosis. Some investigators have suggested that this combination is also useful for aspergillosis.

Miconazole is an antifungal agent that has been introduced for the treatment of candidiasis and coccidioidomycosis (Stevens *et al.,* 1976). This drug has the advantage over other systemic antifungal agents of having minimal toxicity. Side effects include phlebitis, pruritis, nausea and vomiting, and lipid abnormalities due to the diluent. Although some investigators have found it to be useful for the treatment of coccidioidomycosis, its role for the treatment of infections in the compromised host remains to be ascertained. However, its efficacy is likely to be dependent upon the status of the patient's underlying malignancy, as is true with the other antifungal agents. Because of its lesser toxicity, it is more likely to be used in patients suspected but not proved to have fungal infection.

Vidarabine (arabinosyl adenine) is an effective agent for the treatment of several DNA viral infections. The drug interferes with DNA synthesis. Its major toxic effects are nausea, vomiting, and myelosuppression. Vidarabine is effective for the treatment of herpes simplex and herpes zoster-varicella infections, but not for cytomegalovirus infections. In a randomized trial, untreated patients with biopsy-proven herpes encephalitis had a mortality rate of 70%, whereas patients treated with vidarabine had a mortality rate of only 28% (Whitley *et al.,* 1977). Likewise, a randomized trial of vidarabine was conducted in immunocompromised patients who developed herpes zoster infections (Whitley *et al.,* 1976). Patients who received vidarabine had more rapid clearing of virus from vesicles, more cessation of new vesicle formation, and more relief of pain than untreated controls. Hence, this drug is probably indicated for all patients except for those with very minor infections.

V. GRANULOCYTE TRANSFUSION

Extensive research has been conducted on the transfusion of leukocytes for the management of infections in neutropenic patients. A major obstacle to the routine use of granulocyte transfusions in humans has been the inability to collect adequate numbers of granulocytes from normal donors. The half-life of these cells in the blood is only about 6 hours, and the space occupied by transfused granulocytes is about 20 times the circulating blood volume. To achieve an increment of 1500 granulocytes per mm^3 of blood in the recipient requires the transfusion of 10^{11} cells, which is twice the number of granulocytes in the circulating blood volume of an average adult.

The initial solution to the problem of collecting adequate cells was the use of donors with chronic myelogenous leukemia who had high peripheral white blood counts. The response rate was related to the number of granulocytes transfused. To achieve maximum likelihood of response required the transfusion of about 10^{11} cells. In an analysis of 179 infections occurring in neutropenic patients, the response rate associated with granulocyte transfusions was 49% (Vallejos et al., 1975). Most of these infections were caused by E. coli, P. aeruginosa, K. penumoniae, and C. albicans, and they were not responding to antibiotic therapy. Responses occurred after a single transfusion, but best results were obtained with daily transfusions for several days. Fewer than 40% of patients who failed after four transfusions responded to additional transfusions.

The use of granulocyte transfusion from chronic myelogenous leukemia donors is limited by the number of available donors. Hence, a continuous blood-cell separator was developed to collect granulocytes from normal donors. The leukocytes are removed and the erythrocytes and plasma are returned to the donor. In a comparative study of gram-negative bacillary septicemia, the survival rate was 46% in patients who received granulocyte transfusions compared to 30% in patients for whom transfusions were not available (Graw et al., 1972). Among the patients who received granulocyte transfusions, survival was directly related to the number of transfusions administered. Survival after a single transfusion was 7%, compared to 100% following four transfusions.

Several randomized trials of granulocyte transfusions have been conducted in infected neutropenic patients who were failing to respond to antibiotic therapy (Table VIII). In all of these studies, the patients who received granulocyte transfusions had a higher survival rate. Survival was similar for patients whose bone marrow recovered whether they received granulocyte transfusions or not. Those patients whose bone marrow did not recover benefited significantly from granulocyte transfusions. However, it is seldom possible to predict in advance those patients in whom bone marrow recovery will occur in time to control the infection.

There can no longer be any question regarding the beneficial effects of granulocyte transfusions in infected neutropenic patients. In addition to defervesence, many patients have a substantial increment in circulating granulocytes following transfusion. By labeling the transfused granulocytes with DF^{32}P, it has been shown that they migrate to sites of infection and phagocytose

TABLE VIII

Results of Randomized Trials of Granulocyte Transfusions in Infected Neutropenic Patients

	Controls		Transfused	
	Entered	% Survival	Entered	% Survival
Herzig *et al.* (1977)	14	36	16	75
Vogler and Winton (1977)	13	15	17	59
Alavi *et al.* (1977)	19	53	14	80
Total	46	37	47	70
Marrow recovery	17	88	16	88
No marrow recovery	29	7	31	61

bacteria. Cytogenic studies have demonstrated the presence of granulocytes containing the Ph' chromosome in recipients of transfusions from donors with chronic myelogenous leukemia. Also, nuclear appendages have been demonstrated on circulating granulocytes of male recipients who received cells from female donors. Occasional recipients have developed myeloid and erythroid homografts following granulocyte transfusions from donors with chronic myelogenous leukemia.

VI. PROPHYLAXIS OF INFECTION

The high frequency of infection in cancer patients during periods of myelosuppressive treatment has led to the development of prophylactic programs. The most effective programs include the use of isolation units to protect patients against nosocomial contamination, plus antibiotic regimens to reduce the patients' endogenous microbial flora. The most popular type of isolation unit is the laminar air flow room (LAFR) in which one wall or the ceiling is comprised of high-efficiency filters. Filtered air flows across the room with a laminar distribution, providing several hundred air exchanges per hour. Additionally, a plastic curtain containing gauntlets permits personnel to perform procedures on the patient without entering the room. Bacteriostatic agents are used to clean the room initially and during patient occupancy.

Patients treated in an LAFR are exposed to a much lower level of microbial contamination in the environment than patients treated in regular hospital rooms (Bodey and Johnston, 1971). A substantial majority of samples of the air floors and settling plates from LAFR are sterile, and when organisms are recovered from these samples the concentration is considerably less than samples from regular hospital rooms. Furthermore, only about 5% of culture samples from LAFR contain potentially pathogenic organisms, whereas about 50% of the air and floor samples and 26% of settling plates from regular hospital rooms contain potentially pathogenic organisms.

While in the LAFR, the patients receive oral and topical antibiotic regimens and bathe with bacteriostatic soap preparations. These regimens cause a major reduction in the patients' endogenous microbial flora (Bodey and Rosenbaum, 1974). Over 95% of strains of bacteria and 44% of strains of fungi are no longer cultured from the stools after institution of these regimens. About 25% of patients have persistently sterile stools. About 80% of strains of bacteria, but only 5% of strains of fungi, are no longer cultured from the throat during prophylaxis. The skin, especially the groin and perianal areas, is difficult to maintain free of potentially pathogenic organisms despite the application of high concentrations of topical antibiotics. However, the bacteriostatic soap preparations reduce the skin flora by 10^3–10^5.

The first controlled study of the protected environment–prophylactic antibiotic (PEPA) program was in patients undergoing remission induction chemotherapy for acute leukemia (Bodey et al., 1971b). Control patients were selected from among patients who received the same chemotherapy and were matched with respect to those pretreatment variables that affect prognosis. The complete remission rate was 61% for the PEPA patients and 49% for the control patients, a difference that was not statistically significant. Fewer PEPA patients developed serious infections during remission induction (24% versus 42%). They had a lower fatality rate from infection (9% versus 21%) and spent significantly less time with infection than the control patients. The median duration of complete remission was 55 weeks for the PEPA patients and 26 weeks for the control patients ($p < .05$). The median duration of survival was 34 weeks for the PEPA patients and 23 weeks for the control patients ($p = .02$).

Subsequently, several randomized studies of the PEPA program have been conducted in patients undergoing remission-induction chemotherapy for acute leukemia (Table IX). Two of these studies have found significant differences in the complete remission rates, favoring the PEPA patients (Schimpff et al., 1975; Rodriguez et al., 1978). In all of these studies, the proportion of patients developing severe and fatal infections was substantially lower among the PEPA patients, and most of these differences were statistically significant. A similar study has been conducted in patients undergoing remission-induction chemotherapy for malignant lymphoma (Bodey et al., 1979b). The frequency of severe infection was also significantly lower for the PEPA patients in this study than for the control patients (7% versus 29%). Patients on the PEPA program were better able to tolerate higher doses of chemotherapy that did not increase the complete remission rate but did increase the duration of remission and survival. The PEPA program definitely reduces the risk of infection during remission-induction chemotherapy, but its long-term benefits remain to be determined.

Antibiotics have been used alone for prophylaxis of infection in cancer patients

TABLE IX

Severe Infection during Remission-Induction Therapy for Acute Leukemia

	Levine et al. (1973)		Yates et al. (1973)		Schimpff et al. (1975)		Rodriguez et al. (1978)	
	PEPA	Control	PEPA	Control	PEPA	Control	PEPA	Control
Patients entered	22	28	28	39	24	21	63	82
Patients with severe infection (%)	14	50	25	80	17	62	41	57
Patients with fatal infection (%)	0	24	5	19	17	52	13	28
Percentage of days spent with infection and								
<100 Neutrophils/mm^3	12	40	9	12	—	—	18	28
101–1000 Neutrophils/mm^3	8	10	—	—	—	—	8	15
Complete remissions (%)	45	43	33	31	54	24	71	43

with varying degrees of success. Two studies of the PEPA program included a group of patients who were randomized to receive oral nonabsorbable antibiotics in regular hospital rooms. In one of these studies, no differences existed between the control patients and the patients who received oral antibiotics (Levine et al., 1973). In the second study, the patients receiving oral antibiotic prophylaxis had fewer fatalities from infection (32% versus 52%) and fewer severe infections per patient (0.37 versus 1.0) than the control patients (Schimpff et al., 1975). Children with cancer were prospectively randomized to receive trimethoprim-sulfmethoxazole (TS) or placebo for prevention of pneumocystic pneumonia, whereas 21% of patients receiving placebo developed this infection ($p < .01$). In addition, bacterial septicemia, pneumonia, otitis media, upper respiratory infections, sinusitis, and cellulitis occurred less often in the treated group ($p < .01$). In another study, patients were randomized to receive TS or no prophylaxis during periods of neutropenia (Gurwith et al., 1979). The patients who received TS spent significantly less time with fever than the control patients. None of the patients receiving TS prophylaxis developed bacteremia, compared to 17% in the control group ($p = .001$). Soft tissue and urinary tract infections also occurred more often in the control group. These data suggest that antibiotic prophylaxis may be useful during periods of neutropenia. However, the impact of these regimens on emergence of resistant organisms remains to be ascertained.

VII. CONCLUSIONS

Infection continues to be a frequent and challenging complication in cancer patients. Considerable progress has been made in controlling some infections that had been associated with a high fatality rate in the past. Prominent among these infections that can now be treated effectively are those caused by *S. aureus* and *P. aeruginosa*. Unfortunately, these organisms have been replaced by others which are less responsive to therapy. Organisms that had been considered to be nonpathogens in the past, such as *B. cereus* and *S. marcescens,* are now causing serious infections in compromised hosts. Fungal infections are increasing in frequency. More effective diagnostic tests and therapeutic regimens must be developed to control these infections. It is not unreasonable to expect that in the future the discovery of new antimicrobial agents, the more effective use of prophylactic measures, and the increased availability of granulocyte replacement will lead to further progress in this important field of endeavor.

REFERENCES

Aisner, J., Schimpff, S. C., Bennett, J. E., Young, V. M., and Wiernik, P. H. (1976). *J. Am. Med. Assoc.* **235,** 411–412.

Alavi, J. B., Root, R. K., Djerassi, I., Evans, A. E., Gluckman, S. J., MacGregor, R. R., Guerry, D., Schreiber, A. D., Shaw, J. M., Koch, P., and Cooper, R. A. (1977). *New Engl. J. Med.* **296,** 706–711.

Amromin, G. D., and Solomon, R. D. (1962). *J. Am. Med. Assoc.* **182,** 23–29.

Baehner, R. L., Neilburger, R. G., Johnson, D. E., and Murrmann, S. M. (1973). *N. Engl. J. Med.* **289,** 1209–1213.

Bennett, J. E. (1977). *Ann. Intern. Med.* **86,** 319–322.

Bloomfield, C. D., and Kennedy, B. J. (1974). *Cancer* **34,** 431–437.

Bodey, G. P. (1966). *J. Chronic Dis.* **19,** 667–687.

Bodey, G. P. (1970). *Am. J. Med. Sci.* **260,** 82–86.

Bodey, G. P. (1971). *In* "Cancer Congress" (R. L. Clark, R. W. Cumley, J. E. McCay, and M. M. Copeland, eds.), Vol. 3, pp. 445–456. Yearbook Publ., Chicago, Illinois.

Bodey, G. P., and Hersh, E. M. (1969). *Neoplasia Childhood, Proc. Annu. Clin. Conf. 12th, 1969,* pp. 135–154.

Bodey, G. P., and Johnston, D. (1971). *Appl. Microbiol.* **22,** 828–836.

Bodey, G. P., and Luna, M. (1974). *J. Am. Med. Assoc.* **229,** 1466–1468.

Bodey, G. P., and Pan, T. (1976). *J. Antibiot.* **29,** 1092–1095.

Bodey, G. P., and Rosenbaum, B. (1974). *Medicine* **53,** 209–228.

Bodey, G. P., Buckley, M., Sathe, Y. S., and Freireich, E. J. (1966a). *Ann. Intern. Med.* **64,** 328–340.

Bodey, G. P., Powell, R. D., Jr., Hersh, E. M., Yeterian, A., and Freireich, E. J. (1966b). *Cancer* **19,** 781–793.

Bodey, G. P., Rodriguez, V., and Smith, J. P. (1970). *Cancer* **25,** 199–205.

Bodey, G. P., Whitecar, J. P., Jr., Middleman, E., and Rodriguez, V. (1971a). *J. Am. Med. Assoc.* **218,** 62–66.

Bodey, G. P., Gehan, E. A., Freireich, E. J., and Frei, E., III (1971b). *Am. J. Med. Sci.* **262,** 138–151.

Bodey, G. P., Middleman, E., Umsawasdi, T., and Rodriguez, V. (1972). *Cancer* **29,** 1697–1701.

Bodey, G. P., Rodriguez, V., Valdivieso, M., and Feld, R. (1976). *J. Infect. Dis.* **S134,** S421–S427.

Bodey, G. P., Rodriguez, V., Chang, H. Y., and Narboni, G. (1978). *Cancer* **41,** 1610–1622.

Bodey, G. P., Rodriguez, V., Cabanillas, F., and Freireich, E. J. (1979a). *Am. J. Med.* **66,** 74–81.

Bodey, G. P., Cabanillas, F., Feld, R., Keating, J., Rodriguez, V., Valdivieso, M., and McCredie, K. B. (1979b). *Curr. Ther. Res.* **25,** 814–826.

Brown, R. S., Haynes, H. A., Foley, T., Berard, C. W., and Carbone, P. P. (1967). *Ann. Intern. Med.* **67,** 291–302.

Butler, W. T., and Rossen, R. D. (1973). *J. Clin. Invest.* **52,** 2629–2640.

Chang, H. Y., Rodriguez, V., Narboni, G., Bodey, G. P., Luna, M. A., and Freireich, E. J. (1976). *Medicine (Baltimore)* **55,** 259–268.

Chernik, N. L., Armstrong, D., and Posner, J. B. (1973). *Medicine (Baltimore)* **52,** 563–581.

Corso, J. A., Agostinelli, R., and Brandriss, M. W. (1969). *J. Am. Med. Assoc.* **210,** 2075–2077.

Crossley, K., Loesch, D., Landesman, B., Mead, K., Chern, M., and Strate, R. (1979). *J. Infect. Dis.* **139,** 273–279.

Donaldson, S. S., Moore, M. R., Rosenberg, S. A., and Vosti, K. L. (1972). *N. Engl. J. Med.* **287,** 69–71.

Edwards, J. E., Jr., Foos, R. Y., Montgomerie, J. Z., and Guze, L. B. (1974). *Medicine (Baltimore)* **53,** 47–75.

EORTC International Antimicrobial Therapy Project Group (1978). *J. Infect. Dis.* **137,** 14–29.

Fahey, J. L., Scoggins, R., Utz, J. P., and Swed, C. F. (1963). *Am. J. Med.* **35,** 698–707.

Feld, R., Bodey, G. P., Rodriguez, V., and Luna, M. (1974). *Am. J. Med. Sci.* **268,** 97–106.

Feld, R., Valdivieso, M., Bodey, G. P., and Rodriguez, V. (1977a). *J. Infect. Dis.* **135,** 61–66.

Feld, R., Valdivieso, M., Bodey, G. P., and Rodriguez, V. (1977b). *Am. J. Med. Sci.* **274,** 179–188.

Feldman, S., Hughes, W. T., and Daniel, C. B. (1975). *Pediatrics* **56,** 388–397.

Filice, G., Yu, B., and Armstrong, B. (1977). *J. Infect. Dis.* **135,** 349–357.

Glew, R. H., Buckley, H. R., Rosen, H. M., Moellering, R. C., Jr., and Fischer, J. E. (1978). *Am. J. Med.* **64,** 586–591.

Glover, J. L., and Jolly, L. (1971). *Exp. Med. Surg.* **29,** 114–117.

Good, R. A., and Page, A. R. (1960). *Am. J. Med.* **29,** 804–810.

Goodell, B., Jacobs, J. B., Powell, R. D., and DeVita, V. T. (1970). *Ann. Intern. Med.* **72,** 337–340.

Graw, R. G., Jr., Herzig, G., Perry, S., and Henderson, E. S. (1972). *N. Engl. J. Med.* **287,** 367–371.

Greenman, R. L., Goodall, P. T., and King, D. (1975). *Am. J. Med.* **59,** 488–496.

Gurwith, M. J., Brunton, J. L., Lank, B. A., Harding, G. K. M., and Ronald, A. R. (1979). *Am. J. Med.* **66,** 248–256.

Hersh, E. M. (1974). *In* "Antineoplastic and Immunosuppressive Agents" (A. C. Sartorelli and D. J. Johns, eds.), pp. 577–617. Springer-Verlag, Berlin and New York.

Hersh, E. M., Gutterman, J. U., Mavligit, G., McCredie, K. B., Bodey, G. P., Freireich, E. J., Rossen, R. D., and Butler, W. T. (1973). *Transplant. Proc.* **5,** i191–1195.

Herzig, R. H., Herzig, G. P., Graw, R. G., Jr., Bull, M. I., and Ray, K. K. (1977). *New Engl. J. Med.* **296,** 701–705.

Hughes, W. T., Kuhn, S., Chaudhary, S., Feldman, S., Verzosa, M., Aur, R. J. A., Pratt, C., and George, S. L. (1977). *N. Engl. J. Med.* **297,** 1419–1426.

Inagaki, J., Rodriguez, V., and Bodey, G. P. (1974). *Cancer* **33,** 568–573.

International Symposium on Legionnaires' Disease (1979). *Ann. Intern. Med.* **90,** 489–707.

Issell, B. F., Keating, M. J., Valdivieso, M., and Bodey, G. P. (1979). *Am. J. Med. Sci.* **277,** 311–318.

Jarowski, C. I., Fialk, M. A., Murray, H. W., Gottlieb, G. J., Coleman, M., Steinberg, C. R., and Silver, R. T. (1978). *Arch. Intern. Med.* **138,** 544–546.

Kaplan, M. H., Armstrong, D., and Rosen, P. (1974). *Cancer* **33,** 850–858.

Keating, M. J., Bodey, G. P., Valdivieso, M., and Rodriguez, V. (1979). *Medicine (Baltimore)* **58,** 159–170.

Klastersky, J., Cappel, R., Swings, G., and Vandenborre, L. (1971). *Am. J. Med. Sci.* **262,** 283–290.

Klastersky, J., Cappel, R., and Daneau, D. (1972). *Antimicrob. Agents & Chemother.* **2,** 470–475.

Klastersky, J., Cappel, R., and Daneau, D. (1973). *Cancer* **31,** 331–336.

Klastersky, J., Henri, A., Hensgens, C., and Daneau, D. (1974). *J. Am. Med. Assoc.* **227,** 45–48.

Klastersky, J., Debusscher, L., Weerts-Ruhl, D., and Prévost, J. M. (1977a). *Cancer Treat. Rep.* **61,** 1433–1439.

Klastersky, J., Meunier-Carpenter, F., and Prévost, J. M. (1977b). *Am. J. Med. Sci.* **273,** 157–161.

Levine, A. S., Siegel, S. E., Schreiber, A. D., Hauser, J., Preisler, H., Goldstein, I. M., Seidler, F., Simon, R., Perry, S., Bennett, J. E., and Henderson, E. S. (1973). *N. Engl. J. Med.* **288,** 477–483.

Lewis, J. L., and Rabinovich, S. (1972). *Am. J. Med.* **53,** 315–322.

Lipnik, M. J., Kligman, A. M., and Strauss, R. (1952). *J. Invest. Dermatol.* **18,** 247–260.

Louria, D. B., Stiff, D. P., and Bennett, B. (1962). *Medicine (Baltimore)* **41,** 307–337.

Louria, D. B., Hensle, T., Armstrong, D., Collins, H. S., Blevins, A., Krugman, D., and Buse, M. (1967). *Ann. Intern. Med.* **67,** 261–281.

Meyer, R. D., Young, L. S., Armstrong, D., and Yu, B. (1973). *Am. J. Med.* **54,** 6–15.

Middleman, E. A., Watanabe, A., Kaizer, H., and Bodey, G. P. (1972). *Cancer* **30,** 573–579.

Montgomerie, J. Z., and Edwards, J. E., Jr. (1978). *J. Infect. Dis.* **137,** 197–201.

Nash, G., and Ross, J. S. (1974). *Hum. Pathol.* **5,** 339–345.

Neiman, P. E., Reeves, W., Ray, G., Flournoy, N., Lerner, K. G., Sale, G. E., and Thomas, E. D. (1977). *J. Infect. Dis.* **136,** 754–767.

Ortbals, D. W., Liebhaber, H., Presant, C. A., Van Amburg, A. L., III, and Lee, J. Y. (1977). *Ann. Intern. Med.* **87,** 552–557.

Perera, D. R., Western, K. A., Johnson, D., Johnson, W. W., Schultz, M. G., and Akers, P. V. (1970). *J. Am. Med. Assoc.* **214,** 1074–1078.

Prince, A. M., Szuness, W., Mann, M. K., Vyas, G. N., Grady, G. F., Shapiro, F. L., Suki, W. N., Friedman, E. A., Avram, M. M., and Stenzel, K. H. (1978). *J. Infect. Dis.* **137,** 131–144.

Richardson, E. P., Jr. (1961). *N. Engl. J. Med.* **265,** 815–823.

Robinson, H. J. (1960). *Antibiot. Chemother.* **7,** 199–240.

Rodriguez, V., and Bodey, G. P. (1979). *In "Pseudomonas aeruginosa:* Clinical Manifestations of Infection and Current Therapy" (R. G. Doggett, ed.), 368–407. Academic Press, New York.

Rodriguez, V., Whitecar, J. P., Jr., and Bodey, G. P. (1970). *In* "Proc. Interscience Conf. Antimicrob. Agents and Chemother., 9th" (G. L. Hobby, ed.), pp. 386–390. Am. Soc. Microbiol., Bethesda, Maryland.

Rodriguez, V., Burgess, M. A., and Bodey, G. P. (1973). *Cancer* **32,** 1007–1012.

Rodriguez, V., Bodey, G. P., Freireich, E. J., McCredie, K. B., Gutterman, J. U., Keating, M. J., Smith, T. L., and Gehan, E. A. (1978). *Medicine (Baltimore)* **57,** 253–266.

Schimpff, S. C., Satterlee, W., Young, V. M., and Serpick, A. (1971). *N. Engl. J. Med.* **284,** 1061–1065.

Schimpff, S. C., Greene, W. H., Young, V. M., Fortner, C. L., Jepsen, L., Cusack, N., Block, J. B., and Wiernik, P. H. (1975). *Ann. Intern. Med.* **82,** 351–358.

Sickles, E. A., Greene, W. H., and Wiernik, P. H. (1975). *Arch. Intern. Med.* **135,** 715–719.

Simpson, C. L., and Pinkel, D. (1958). *Pediatrics* **21,** 436–442.

Simpson, J. F., Leddy, J. P., and Hare, J. D. (1967). *Am. J. Med.* **43,** 39–49.

Sinkovics, J. G., and Smith, J. P. (1969). *Cancer* **24,** 631–636.

Sokal, J. E., and Firat, D. (1965). *Am. J. Med.* **39,** 452–463.

Steinberg, S. C., Alter, H. J., and Leventhal, B. G. (1975). *J. Pediatr.* **81,** 753–756.

Stevens, D. A., Levine, H. B., and Deresinski, S. C. (1976). *Am. J. Med.* **60,** 191–202.

Sullivan, M. P., Hanshaw, J. B., Cangir, A., and Butler, J. J. (1968). *J. Am. Med. Assoc.* **206,** 569–574.

Thiele, E. H., Arison, R. N., and Boxer, G. E. (1964). *Cancer Res.* **24,** 234–238.

Thompson, E. N., and Williams, R. (1974). *J. Clin. Pathol.* **27,** 906–910.

Ultmann, J. E., Tish, W., Osserman, E., and Gellhorn, A. (1959). *Ann. Intern. Med.* **51,** 501–516.

Utz, J. P., Bennett, J. E., Bandriss, M. W., Butler, W. T., and Hill, G. J., III (1964). *Ann. Intern. Med.* **61,** 334–354.

Valdivieso, M., and Bodey, G. P. (1977). *Am. J. Med. Sci.* **273,** 177–184.

Valdivieso, M., Horikoshi, M., Rodriguez, V., and Bodey, G. P. (1974). *Am. J. Med. Sci.* **268,** 149–156.

Valdivieso, M., Gil-Extremera, B., Zornoza, J., Rodriguez, V., and Bodey, G. P. (1977). *Medicine (Baltimore)* **56,** 241–254.

Vallejos, C., McCredie, K. B., Bodey, G. P., Hester, J. P., and Freireich, E. J. (1975). *Transfusion* **15,** 28–33.

Vietzke, W. M., Gelderman, A. H., Grimley, P. M., and Valsamis, M. P. (1968). *Cancer* **21,** 816–827.

Vogler, W. R., and Winton, E. F. (1977). *Am. J. Med.* **63,** 548–555.

Wade, J. C., Smith, C. R., Petty, B. G., Lipsky, J. J., Conrad, G., Ellner, J., and Lietman, P. S. (1978). *Lancet*, 604–606.

Whitecar, J. P., Jr., Bodey, G. P., and Luna, M. (1970). *Am. J. Med. Sci.* **260,** 216–223.

Whitley, R. J., Ch'ien, L. T., Dolin, R., Galasso, G. J., and Alford, C. A., Jr. (1976). *N. Engl. J. Med.* **294,** 1193–1199.

Whitley, R. J., Soong, S. J., Dolin, R., Galasso, G. J., Ch'ien, L. T., and Alford, C. A. (1977). *N. Engl. J. Med.* **297,** 289–294.

Winston, D. J., and Hewitt, W. L. (1979). *In* "Handbook on Hospital-Associated Infections" (D. Groschel, ed.), pp. 61–155. Dekker, New York.

Yates, J. W., and Holland, J. F. (1973). *Cancer* **32,** 1490–1498.

Young, L. S., Armstrong, D., Blevins, A., and Lieberman, P. (1971). *Am. J. Med.* **50,** 356–367.

Young, R. C., Bennett, J. E., Vogel, C. L., Carbone, P. P., and DeVita, V. T. (1970). *Medicine (Baltimore)* **49,** 147–173.

17
NUTRITION IN CANCER PATIENTS
Brian F. Issell

I.	Introduction	363
II.	Cancer–Malnutrition Associations	363
III.	Mechanisms of Cancer-Associated Malnutrition	364
IV.	Advantages of Nutritional Support	365
V.	Methods of Nutritional Support	368
VI.	Conclusion	369
	References	369

I. INTRODUCTION

Malnutrition has long been recognized as accompanying many chronic disease states, including malignancy. Much of morbidity and mortality in cancer patients may be either directly or indirectly related to their poor nutritional status. An increased susceptibility to infections is associated with malnutrition (Wittman *et al.*, 1967), and infections have been reported to be the major cause of death in cancer patients (Bodey, 1975).

II. CANCER–MALNUTRITION ASSOCIATIONS

Weight loss has been recognized as an adverse prognostic factor in different malignancies, including Hodgkin's disease, where it has been well characterized. A retrospective analysis of factors influencing the survival of patients with bronchogenic carcinoma over a 12-month period demonstrated that weight loss prior to treatment was a major prognosticator in both limited and extensive disease (Lanzotti *et al.*, 1977). It has been hypothesized that the negative impact of weight loss on survival may be mediated via the direct effect of malnutrition on host defense functions.

In a further study in non-small-cell lung cancer patients (Issell *et al.*, 1978a), the relationship of weight loss to other prognostic characteristics was analyzed. Increased survival was significantly related to pretreatment weight loss, performance status, and skin-test reactivity. A multivariate regressional analysis showed that weight loss was the most significant factor, and it predicted independently of skin-test reactivity, which was the second most important characteristic. Performance status was closely associated with weight loss. These results suggest that nutritional status may be an important prognostic characteristic in its own right rather than secondary to effects on host defense function as measured by skin-test reactivity.

III. MECHANISMS OF CANCER-ASSOCIATED MALNUTRITION

A decreased supply of nutrients (anorexia–hypophagia), ineffective gastrointestinal absorption, and an increased demand for nutrients appear to be factors contributing to malnutrition in cancer patients. These states may be due to the cancer alone or secondary to cancer therapy.

Because the successful treatment of malignancy allows a reversal of anorexia, cancer-related decreases in nutritional intake have been regarded as a distant manifestation of tumor growth. The exact nature of this is uncertain, and psychological disturbance may contribute. A decrease or perversion in taste acuity has been reported in patients with a spectrum of malignancies (DeWys, 1977), and this may contribute to food-provoked nausea, complained of by some patients, and to changes in the threshold of hunger and satiety. It is common for patients to show an aversion to a particular type of food, such as meat.

The delivery of adequate nutriments to the small intestine may not always result in nutritional repletion because of malabsorption. This may be present secondary to prior starvation (Viteri and Schneider, 1974), and thus a vicious cycle results. The growth of certain tumors in the gastrointestinal tract may also directly cause malabsorption.

Tumors are believed to be less efficient than normal tissues in utilizing energy sources, and so require increased nutriments. This has been stated to be due to anaerobic glycolysis predominating in cancer cells because of their enzymatic makeup and limited oxygen supply. An increasing recycling of lactic acid has been demonstrated in cancer patients, and has been correlated directly with the total volume of malignant tissue (Waterhouse, 1974). This has the potential for producing an energy drain on the host. In starved tumor-bearing animals, the protein and DNA metabolism of normal tissue decreases in response to starvation, but the metabolism of tumor tissue remains as before, thus creating the potential for further drain on the host (Lowry *et al.*, 1979). Other metabolic abnormalities discovered in cancer patients, including abnormal or "diabetic" glucose tolerance with increased insulin resistance, may also contribute to increased energy demands for the tumor-bearing patient (Marks and Bishop, 1959).

Surgery, radiotherapy, and chemotherapy may all either directly or indirectly nutritionally deplete cancer patients. Patients may have mechanical interruption to the continuity of their gastrointestinal tracts following surgery or radiotherapy, and nausea-promoting chemotherapy and radiotherapy may significantly decrease food intake. Also, hypermetabolism due to therapy-related infectious complications increases the nutritional demands of patients.

IV. ADVANTAGES OF NUTRITIONAL SUPPORT

The first question that must be asked is whether nutritional support may be disadvantageous in that it promotes tumor growth at the expense of the host. Animal studies related to this specific question have not shown any evidence of tumor growth out of proportion to host tissue growth (Ota *et al.*, 1977).

Several studies have been initiated that examine the effects of nutritional support in cancer patients. Some have been completed, but most are still ongoing. A positive consequence of nutritional support was suggested in a retrospective analysis of lung cancer patients receiving intravenous hyperalimentation (IVH) in addition to chemotherapy. More responses to therapy were seen in the nutritionally supported group than in a similar group of patients who did not receive intravenous hyperalimentation (Lanzotti *et al.*, 1975). A prospective randomized study in non-small-cell lung cancer patients has been reported. Toxicity advantages for the group receiving nutritional support with IVH were detected (Issell *et al.*, 1978b). The objectives of this study were to determine whether IVH given for 10 days before and during the first course of chemotherapy (1) improved the nutritional status of patients; (2) increased the response to chemotherapy; (3) reduced dose-limiting chemotherapy toxicities; and (4) increased or protected against the chemotherapy-mediated reduction of host defense functions. The study was also intended to determine if there was any evidence that tumors were fed at the expense of host tissue.

Both the nutritionally supported and unsupported groups were prognostically comparable at the start of the study, as shown in Table I. Considerably more nutritional support was given to patients who received IVH, as shown in Table II, and this resulted in a significant benefit in nutritional status for these patients after the first course of therapy. However, over subsequent courses of therapy when IVH had been withdrawn, the nutritional status of both groups became comparable, as shown in Table III.

A significant decrease in chemotherapy-induced leukopenia and neutropenia (the dose-limiting toxicity for this therapy) was noted for the group of patients

TABLE I

Patient Characteristics of Two Randomized Groups

	No. of patients receiving	
Characteristic	IVH	No IVH
Pretherapy weight loss		
< 6%	4	5
≥ 6%	9	8
Pretherapy performance status		
> 70%	6	6
≤ 70%	7	7
Pretherapy skin reaction to dermatophytin		
≥ 10 mm	4	8
<10 mm	9	5

receiving IVH over the first therapy course. However, over subsequent courses of therapy, after cessation of IVH, this advantage for the IVH group was soon lost, as shown in Table IV. A significant decrease in chemotherapy induced nausea, and vomiting was also noted for those patients receiving IVH. Although more initial responses to chemotherapy were seen for the IVH group of patients, as shown in Table V, no overall survival advantage was detected for this group. Certainly no evidence was seen suggesting that tumor growth was increased by nutritional support. An analysis of host defense parameters—including *in vivo* delayed hypersensitivity skin tests, skin window studies, *in vitro* lymphocyte blastogenesis, neutrophil chemotactic studies, and immunoglobulin concentrations—failed to show any significant differences between the two groups of patients.

The conclusions of this study were that nutritional repletion with IVH pro-

TABLE II

Total Nutritional Intake from All Sources during First Course of Chemotherapy[a]

	IVH		Non-IVH		
	Median	Range	Median	Range	p Value
Kcal	170	120–238	81	57–125	< .01
Nitrogen	270	167–320	133	102–161	< .01

[a] Average daily intake (percentage of recommended daily allowance for treatment groups, based on initial weight).

TABLE III

Relationship of Nutritional Parameters to Administration of IVH[a]

Parameter	IVH group		Non-IVH group		
	Median	Range	Median	Range	p value
First course					
Weight change (% of stated normal weight)	+7	+1 to +11	−1	−9 to + 3	< .01
Arm muscle circumference change (% of standard)	+6	−2 to +13	−4	−8 to + 1	< .01
Triceps skin-fold change (% of standard)	−2	−11 to +28	−6	−26 to +29	NS[b]
Second course					
Weight change (% of stated normal weight)	0	−7 to + 4	+1	−7 to + 7	NS
Arm muscle circumference change (% of standard)	+1	−11 to + 3	−5	−8 to 0	NS
Triceps skin-fold change (% of standard)	−8	−16 to +16	−5	−22 to +12	NS

[a] Changes over first two courses of chemotherapy: Patients were randomized to receive IVH during first course of chemoimmunotherapy only).

[b] NS, not significant.

TABLE IV

Effect of IVH on Chemotherapy-Induced Bone Marrow Toxic Effects[a]

Course number	Median lowest recorded peripheral blood cell counts × $10^3/\mu l$		
	WBCS (range)	Polymorphonuclear neutrophils (range)	Platelets (range)
First			
IVH group	2.5 (1.0–4.1)	1.6 (0.3–3.2)	259 (80–416)
Non-IVH group	1.5 (0.7–3.7)	0.4 (0.02–1.2)	185 (50–415)
	($p = .03$)	($p = .01$)	($p = $ NS)[b]
Second			
IVH group	2.3 (0.6–3.0)	1.1 (0.1–3.0)	200 (25–300)
Non-IVH group	1.9 (0.7–3.7)	0.8 (0.2–1.8)	169 (45–299)
	(NS)	(NS)	(NS)
Third			
IVH group	1.8 (0.6–4.3)	0.7 (0.2–3.0)	160 (25–270)
Non-IVH group	1.9 (0.9–4.3)	0.7 (0.2–2.8)	158 (45–305)
	(NS)	(NS)	(NS)

[a] The IVH group received only IVH during first course of chemoimmunotherapy.

[b] NS, not significant.

TABLE V

Relationship of Response to IVH Administration

Response type	No. of patients and (%)	
	IVH group	Non-IVH group
Partial	4 (31)	1 (7)
Stable disease	8 (62)	8 (62)
Progressive disease	1 (7)	4 (31)

tected against the dose-limiting chemotherapy toxicities observed for this therapy. An extrapolation from this observation is that this may allow higher dosage administration, resulting in increased response and survival in patients with tumors where higher doses of therapy lead to increased tumor response. This study also demonstrated the need for continued nutritional support in cancer patients, since benefits were rapidly lost when the support was withdrawn.

V. METHODS OF NUTRITIONAL SUPPORT

Supporting patients nutritionally on a prophylactic basis, rather than waiting for the development of malnutrition requiring nutritional repletion, would appear to be the most useful approach to cancer patient care. Methods of parenteral nutritional support are shown in Table VI. As shown above, IVH or total parenteral nutrition is an effective means of supporting and also nutritionally replenishing cancer patients. Disadvantages of this method, as it is presently most commonly employed, include the need to hospitalize patients, and the specialized technique required for the insertion and maintenance of the subclavian-vein-inserted catheter through which the concentrated nutritional solution is administered. This technique is not without the potential for life-threatening complications.

TABLE VI

Parenteral Methods of Nutritional Support

1. Total parenteral nutrition into central vein (superior vena cava) via:
   A. Subclavian vein insertion
   B. Peripheral vein insertion using silicone elastomer catheter
2. Additional parenteral nutrition via peripheral vein using:
   A. Lower tonicity solutions
   B. Intralipid Solutions
3. Home parenteral nutrition with infusion pump

TABLE VII

Enteral Methods of Nutritional Support

---

1. Small nasoenteral catheter feeding with chemically defined or meal-replacement formulations
2. Chemically defined and meal-replacement oral formulations.[a] Formulations Include Vivonex , Flexical , Ensure , Isocal.

---

[a] Main problem is palatability; also, hypertonicity with chemically defined formulations (Vivonex, Flexical).

The cost of maintaining total parenteral nutrition is also considerable. Newer methods of total parenteral nutrition under investigation are aimed at relieving some of these problems; these include using peripheral-vein-inserted silicone elastomer catheters, which are threaded into the superior vena cava, and maintaining patients at home with the aid of infusion pumps. Additional parenteral feeding into peripheral veins using Intralipid™ and solutions of lower, more tolerable concentrations has also shown promise.

Methods of enteral nutritional support are listed in Table VII. Feeding through small nasoenteral catheters with chemically defined or meal-replacement formulations has been shown to be an effective means of nutritionally supporting and repleting malnourished patients, and has been reviewed by Heymsfield *et al.* (1979).

The nutritional support of patients with oral formulations, together with good dietary counseling, may prevent much of the cancer-related malnutrition seen in the clinic. The main problem with currently available formulations is palatability. Research is needed to understand better the abnormalities of taste, satiety, and hunger in the cancer patient, so that more acceptable formulations may be developed.

VI. CONCLUSION

In conclusion, it is evident that nutritional support is an important component in the overall care of cancer patients. It is hoped that an increasing awareness of its benefits will relieve some of the mortality and morbidity seen in this patient population.

REFERENCES

Bodey, G. P. (1975). *Cancer Treat. Rev.* **2**, 89–128.
DeWys, W. D. (1977). *Cancer Res.* **37**, 2354–2358.

Heymsfield, S. B., Bethel, R. A., Ansley, J. D., Nixon, D. W., and Rudman, D. (1979). *Ann. Intern. Med.* **90**, 63–71.

Issell, B. F., Valdivieso, M., Hersh, E. M., Richman, S., Gutterman, J. U., and Bodey, G. P. (1978a). *Cancer Treat. Rep.* **62**, 1059–1063.

Issell, B. F., Valdivieso, M., Zaren, H. A., Dudrick, S. J., Freireich, E. J., Copeland, E. W., and Bodey, G. P. (1978b). *Cancer Treat. Rep.* **62**, 1139–1143.

Lanzotti, V. J., Copeland, E. W., George, S. L., Dudrick, S. J., and Samuels, M. L. (1975). *Cancer Chemother. Rep.* **59**, 437–439.

Lanzotti, V. J., Thomas, D. R., Boyle, L. E., Smith, T. L., Gehan, E. A., and Samuels, M. L. (1977). *Cancer* **39**, 303–313.

Lowry, S. F., Goodgame, J. T., Norton, J. A., and Brennan, M. F. (1979). *J. Surg. Res.* **26**, 79–86.

Marks, P. A., and Bishop, J. S. (1959). *J. Clin. Invest.* **38**, 668–672.

Ota, D. M., Copeland, E. W., Strobel, H. W., Daly, J., Gum, E. T., Guinn, E., and Dudrick, S. J. (1977). *J. Surg. Res.* **22**, 181–188.

Viteri, F. E., and Schneider, R. E. (1974). *Med. Clin. North Am.* **58**, 1487–1505.

Waterhouse, C. (1974). *Cancer* **33**, 66–71.

Wittman, W., Moodie, A. D., Hansen, J. D. L., and Brock, J. F. (1967). *Ciba Found. Study Group* **31**, 73.

INDEX

A

Acid phosphatase, in chronic lymphocytic
 leukemia, 46
Acute lymphocytic leukemia, 3–24
 bone marrow aspirate, 11
 central nervous system involvement, 18–20
 chemotherapy, 13–14
 complete remission rates, 22
 histochemical techniques, 5–6
 hypercalcemia, 11–12
 hyperuricemia, 11
 incidence, 4
 infection, 15–18
  prevention, 19
 meningeal carcinomatosis, 190–191
 platelet transfusion, 14–15
 prognostic factors, 20–22
Acute myelocytic leukemia, meningeal carcinomatosis, 190–191
Acute nonlymphocytic leukemia, 3–24
 bone marrow aspirate, 10
 central nervous system involvement, 18–20
 chemotherapy, 13–14
 chromosome abnormality, 9
 complete remission rate, 22
 erythroleukemic variant, 10–11
 histochemical techniques, 5–6
 hyperuricemia, 11
 hypokalemia, 12
 incidence, 4
 infection, 15–18
  prevention, 19
 paracoagulation syndrome, 12
 platelet transfusion, 14–15

 prognostic factors, 20–22
 as second cancer, 8–9
Adenoma, villous, 115
Adenosine deaminase, in chronic lymphocytic
 leukemia, 46
Adriamycin,
 in nonHodgkin's lymphoma, 92–94
 in small cell lung cancer, 160–163
 in soft tissue sarcoma, 284
Age, role in chronic myelocytic leukemia, 58
Alcohol, role in development, head and neck
 cancer, 127–128
Alkaline phosphatase, neutrophil, in chronic
 myelocytic leukemia, 65
ALL, See acute lymphocytic leukemia;
 leukemia, Acute
Aminoglycoside, use against infection, 17–18,
 344–353
Amphotericin B, in nonbacterial infections, 353
Anaerobic infections, 333–334
Anemia,
 chronic lymphocytic leukemia, 46, 59, 64
 pernicious, stomach carcinoma, 121
Angiography,
 brain tumor diagnosis, 180, 181
 renal cell carcinoma, 204–206
ANLL, see acute nonlymphocytic leukemia,
 leukemia, acute
Anthracycline, role in
 leukemia, 13, 34, 66
 lung cancer, small cell, 160–163
 nonHodgkin's lymphoma, 92–94
 sarcoma, soft tissue, 284
Antibiotic, use in cancer patients, 17–18, 325,
 343–353

Asbestos, role in stomach cancer, 121
Asparaginase, in leukemias, 13, 66, 297
Aspergillosis, 337–338
Aspergillus, in leukemias, 16, 35
astrocytoma,
    clinical signs, 173
    incidence, 168–170
Auer body, in acute nonlymphocytic leukemia,
    10
Autologous bone marrow transfusion, 67

B

B-cell,
    in chronic lymphocytic leukemia, 43
    monoclonal nature, 43, 45
Bacteroides fragilus, 334
barium enema, role in colorectal cancer, 117
BCNU, use in malignant melanoma, 271
Blast cell characteristic, in chronic myelocytic
    leukemia, 65–66
Bladder cancer, 231–236
    diagnosis, 233
    etiology, 231–232
    pathology, 232–233
    staging, 233–234
    treatment, 234–237
Blast crisis, chronic myelocytic leukemia, 64–65
Bleomycin,
    in head and neck cancer, 144
    in nonHodgkin's lymphoma, 92–94
Bowel, large, carcinoma. *See* Colorectal can-
    cer
Brain tumors, adult, 169–190
    clinical deterioration, 186–188
    clinical improvement, 189–190
    clinical presentation, general, 171–172
    diagnosis, 179–186
        angiography, 180, 181
        cerebral spinal fluid examination, 181
        electroencephalogram, 181, 186
        pneumoencephalography, 180
        radionuclide scanning, 180, 182
        tomography, computerized, 179–181, 183,
            185
    focal cerebral syndromes, 172–177
        acoustic neurinoma, 174
        brain stem, 173
        cerebellar, 173–174
        cerebrum, 172

corpus callosum, 173
        fourth ventricle, 173
        optic chiasma, 174
        pituitary, 175–176
        thalamus, 173
    herniation, 177–179
    histopathology, 168–170
    incidence, 169–170
    as metastases, 170
Brain tumors, pediatric, 308–310
Breast carcinoma, 99–112
    chemotherapy, 106–109
    clinical presentation, 102
    diagnosis, early, 110
    etiology, 100–101
    hormonal therapy, 106
    immunotherapy, 109
    incidence, 99–101
    metastatic disease course, 103–104
    pathology, 101
    prognostic factors, 102–103
    radiotherapy, 105–106
    surgery, 104–105
    survival, 109
Busulfan, in chronic myelocytic leukemia, 63

C

Candida, 335–336
    in leukemias, 16, 35
Carbenicillin, 17–18, 344–353
Carcinogen, chemical
    in head and neck cancer, 129
    in pancreatic cancer, 118
    in stomach cancer, 121
Carcinoembryonic antigen, in colorectal cancer,
    117
Carcinoma, *See* specific types
CCNU, in small cell lung cancer, 161
CEA. *See* carcinoembryonic antigen
Cell surface characteristic,
    in acute leukemias, 5–6
    in chronic lymphocytic leukemia, 43–44
    in nonHodgkin's lymphoma, 83, 85
Central nervous system cancer. *See* Brain
    tumors, adult; Brain tumors, pediatric; Spi-
    nal cord tumors; meningeal carcinomatosis
Cephalosporin, 17–18, 344–353
Cerebellar-foramen magnum herniation, 177–
    179

Cerebral spinal fluid,
  examination, brain tumor diagnosis, 181
  in meningeal carcinomatosis, 191, 195
Cervix cancer, 250-254
  etiology, 251
  Papanicolaou classification, 253
  prognostic factors, 251-252
  staging, 251-252
  treatment, 253
Chemotherapy,
  acute leukemias, 12-14
  bladder cancer, 236
  breast cancer, 106-109
  chronic lymphocytic leukemia, 50-51
  chronic myelocytic leukemia, 63, 66-67
  endometrium cancer, 255
  Ewing's sarcoma, 288-289
  giant cell tumor, 289
  Hodgkin's lymphoma, 81-82, 301
  head and neck cancer, 144-145
  histiocytoma, fibrous, 289
  interference with host defense, 325-327
  leukemia, pediatric, 297-298
  lung cancer,
    nonsmall cell, 154-155, 157-158
    small cell, 160-163
  melanoma, malignant, 271-272
  neuroblastoma, 315
  nonHodgkin's lymphoma, 89, 90-91, 92-94,
    299
  osteosarcoma, 286
  ovary cancer, 250
  prostate cancer, 241
  renal carcinoma, 206
  sarcoma, soft tissue, 283-284
    rhabdomyosarcoma, 304
  testis cancer, 230-231
Chlorambucil,
  in chronic lymphocytic leukemia, 50
  in chronic myelocytic leukemia, 63-65
  in Hodgkins disease, pediatric, 301
Chondrosarcoma, 286-287
Chromosome abnormality, leukemias, 9, 33, 58
Chromosome, Philadelphia, chronic myelocytic
  leukemia, 58, 60
Chronic lymphocytic leukemia, 39-55
  anemia, 46
  bone marrow involvement, 46
  cell surface characteristic, 43-44
  chemotherapy, 50

enzyme depletion, 46
genetic factors, 40
histochemistry, 45-46
hypercalcemia, 47
hyperuricemia, 47
hypogammaglobulinemia, 44, 46
infection, 45
lymphocyte morphology, 45, 47-49
lymphosarcoma cell leukemia, 47-48, 49
metastatic site, 42
prolymphocytic leukemia, 48, 49
staging system, 51, 52
thrombocytopenia, 46
Chronic myelocytic leukemia, 57-68
  chromosome abnormality, 58, 60, 65
  chronic phase, 60-63
    treatment, 63
  clonal nature, 59
  diagnosis, 59
  incidence by age, 58
  metamorphosis phase, 64-67
    laboratory findings 64-65
    treatment, 66-67
  radiation influence, 57-58
Cisplatinum,
  in bladder cancer, 236
  in head and neck cancer, 145
  in histiocytoma, fibrous, 289
  in melanoma, malignant, 271
CLL. See chronic lymphocytic leukemia
CMF, in breast carcinoma, 109
CML. See Chronic myelocytic leukemia
Colitis, chronic ulcerative, role in colorectal
  cancer, 114
Clostridium perfringens, 333-334
Colonoscope, fiberoptic, flexible, use in
  colorectal cancer, 117
Colorectal cancer, 113-117
  diagnosis, 116-117
  etiology, 114-115
  left colon presentation, 116
  right colon presentation, 115-116
Cooper regimen, in breast carcinoma, 106-107
Complement receptor,
  in chronic lymphocytic leukemia, 43
  in hairy cell leukemia, 27
Crohn's disease, role in colorectal cancer, 114
Cryptococcosis, 338
Cryptococcus, in hairy cell leukemia, 35
Cryptococcus neoformans, 331

CSF. *See* Cerebral spinal fluid.
Cyclophosphamide,
    in breast carcinoma, 106–109
    in chronic lymphocytic leukemia, 50
    in chronic myelocytic leukemia, 63, 66
    in Hodgkin's disease, pediatric, 301
    in leukemia, pediatric, 297
    in lung cancer, small cell, 160–163
    in nonHodgkin's lymphoma, 89–90
Cystectomy, 234, 236
Cytomegalic inclusion disease, 340–341
Cytosine arabinoside, leukemias, 19–20, 66

D

Daunorubicin, in chronic myelocytic leukemia,
    66
Deoxynucleotidyl transferase, terminal, in
    chronic lymphocytic leukemia, 46
DES. *See* Diethylstilbestrol
DTIC, in sarcoma, soft tissue, 284
Diet, role in
    colorectal carcinoma, 114
    pancreatic carcinoma, 118
    stomach carcinoma, 121
Diethylstibestrol, in prostate cancer, 241

E

Electroencephalogram, 181, 186
Endometrium carcinoma, 254–255
Enterobacter, in acute leukemia, 16
Epstein-Barr virus, nasopharyngeal carcinoma
    129
Erythrocyte series, abnormal, acute nonlym-
    phocytic leukemia, 4, 10
Escherichia coli, 330–331
    in leukemias, 16, 35
Ethmoid Sinus carcinoma, 135–136
Etoposide, in lung cancer, small cell, 160–163
Ewing's sarcoma, 287–289
    diagnosis, 287–288
    prognosis, 288
    treatment, 288–289

F

FAB. *See* French-American-British classifica-
    tion
Familial polyposis coli, role in colorectal cancer
    114–115

Flucytosine, 353–354
Fluoroscopy, double contrast barium, use in
    stomach cancer, 123
Fluorouracil,
    in breast cancer, 106–109
    in head and neck cancer, 144
French-American-British classification,
    acute lymphocytic leukemia, 7
    acute nonlymphocytic leukemia, 6
Fungal infection, 335–338

G

Gardner's syndrome, colorectal cancer, 115
Gastrointestinal cancer. *See* specific types
Gastroscopy, fiberoptic, in stomach cancer, 123
Genetic factor,
    breast cancer, 101
    colorectal cancer, 114–115
    melanoma, malignant, 259
Genitourinary carcinoma. *See* specific types
Giant cell tumor, 289
Glioblastoma,
    clinical signs, 173
    incidence, 168–170
Glioma, incidence, 168–170
β-glucoronidase, in chronic lymphocytic
    leukemia, 46
Glucocorticosteroid, brain tumor, 189–190
Gram negative bacilli infection, 331–333
Granulocyte, in chronic myelocytic leukemia,
    61
Granulocytopenia, absolute, acute leukemia,
    15–18
Gynecologic cancer. *See also* specific types.
    incidence, 243–245
    survival, 245
    treatment, 246

H

Hairy cell leukemia, 25–37
    chromosome abnormality, 33
    hepatomegaly, 29
    histochemical diagnostic technique, 30–31
    infection, 35
    mononuclear cell, abnormal, 29, 31–32
    morphology, 30
    pancytopenia, 31–32
    splenectomy, 33–34
    splenomegaly, 29

HCL. *See* Hairy cell leukemia; leukemia, hairy cell
Head and neck cancer, 135–146
  diagnosis, 142
  etiology, 127–129
  histopathology, 130
  hypopharynx, 140
  incidence, 127
  larynx, 141
  nasal cavity, 134–135
  nasopharynx, 137
  oral cavity, 129–134
    alveolar ridge, 132–133
    buccal mucosa, 131–132
    gingiva, retromolar, 133
    hard palate, 134
    lip, 131
    mouth, floor of, 133–134
    tongue, 134
  oropharynx, 137–139
    palatal arch, 137
    pharyngeal wall, 139
    soft palate, 137
    tongue, base, 138–139
    tonsil, 138
  paranasal sinus, 135–137
  salivary gland, 142
  staging, 142–143
  therapy, 143–145
Headache, brain tumor, 171
Hemacult test, colorectal cancer, 117
Hematuria,
  renal carcinoma, 203
  renal pelvic carcinoma, 207
Hemorrhage
  brain tumor, 186–187
  leukemias, 14–15, 35
Hepatitis, 339
Hepatomegaly,
  chronic lymphocytic leukemia, 42, 44
  hairy cell leukemia, 29
Herniation, brain tumor, 177–179
Herpes virus infection, 339–340
Histiocytoma, fibrous, 289
Hodgkin's disease, 71–82
  bone marrow biopsy, 78–79
  chemotherapy, 81–82
  clinical feature, 71–73
  diagnosis, histopathologic, 73–75
  laparotomy, staging, 79–80
  pathology, cell type

  lymphocytic depletion, 78
  lymphocytic predominance, 76, 77
  mixed cellularity, 78
  nodular sclerosis, 76–78
  pediatric, 300–301
    classification, 300
    treatment, 301
  radiotherapy, 80–81
Histochemistry,
  classification, acute leukemias, 5–6
  chronic lymphocytic leukemia, 45–46
  hairy cell leukemia, 30–32
HLA determination, acute leukemia, 15
Hormone, role in
  breast cancer, 100–101
  melanoma, malignant, 259
Hormonal therapy
  breast cancer, 106
  prostate cancer, 241
Hydrocephalus, brain tumor, 186
Hydroxyurea,
  in chronic myelocytic leukemia, 63, 66
  in head and neck cancer, 144
  in melanoma, malignant, 271
Hyperalimentation, intravenous, 365–368
Hypercalcemia,
  acute lymphocytic leukemia, 11–12
  chronic lymphocytic leukemia, 47
Hypertension, brain tumor, 187
Hyperthermia,
  head and neck cancer, 145
Hyperuricemia,
  acute leukemia, 11
  chronic lymphocytic leukemia, 47
  chronic myelocytic leukemia, 61
Hypogammaglobulinemia, chronic lymphocytic leukemia, 44, 46
Hypokalemia, acute nonlymphocytic leukemia, 12
Hyponatremia, brain tumor, 187
Hypopharyngeal carcinoma, 140
Hysterectomy, 253

I

Imidazol carboxamide, in melanoma, malignant, 271
Immunoglobulin,
  cell surface,
    chronic lymphocytic leukemia, 43–44

Immunoglobulin (*cont.*)
    hairy cell leukemia, 27–28
    hypogammaglobulinemia, chronic lymphocy-
        tic leukemia, 44, 46
Immunology,
    chronic lymphocytic leukemia, 40, 41, 43–
        44
    hairy cell leukemia, 27–28
    role in leukemic cell classification, 5–8
Immunotherapy,
    breast cancer, 109
    chronic myelocytic leukemia, 63
    melanoma, malignant, 272
Infection in cancer, 319–362
    acute leukemia, 14–15
    anaerobic organism, 333–334
    brain tumor, 188
    chronic lymphocytic leukemia, 45
    diagnosis, 343
    fungus, 335–338
    gram-negative bacilli, 331–333
    granulocyte transfusion, 354–356
    hairy cell leukemia, 35
    nutritional status, 324–325
    pneumonia, 328–329
    predisposing factors, 319–328
        chemotherapy, 325–327
        gastrointestinal ulceration, 321
        hyperalimentation, 327
        hypoxia, tissue, 320
        immunologic suppression, 323–326
        microbial colonization, 322
        neutropenia, 322–323
        obstruction, 320
        radiotherapy, 326
        splenectomy, 327
    prophylaxis, 356–358
    protozoan, 341–343
    septicemia, 329–330
    skin, 331
    superinfection, 327
    treatment
        bacterial, 343–353
        nonbacterial, 353–354
    tuberculosis, 334–335
    virus, 338–341

J

Jaundice, pancreatic cancer, 119

K

Klebsiella, 330, 333
Klebsiella pneumonia, leukemias, 16, 35

L

Laminar air flow room, 356–357
Laparotomy, staging, Hodgkin's disease, 79–80
Laryngeal carcinoma, 141
Legionella pneumophila, 334
Leukemia, acute. *See* Acute lymphocytic
    leukemia; Acute myelocytic leukemia;
    Acute nonlymphocytic leukemia
Leukemia, chronic. *See* Chronic lymphocytic
    leukemia; Chronic myelocytic leukemia
Leukemia, hairy cell. *See* Hairy cell leukemia
Leukemia, pediatric, 296–298
    diagnosis, 297
    incidence, 296
    treatment, 297–298
Leukemia, prolymphocytic, 48, 49
Leukocytosis, chronic myelocytic leukemia, 59
Leukoencephalopathy, progressive multifocal,
    341
Leukophoresis, chronic myelocytic leukemia, 63
Leukostasis,
    acute leukemia, 20
    chronic myelocytic leukemia, 62
Listeria monocytogenes, 334
Lung carcinoma, 147–165
    classification, histopathologic, 147–149
    diagnosis, 150–153
    incidence, 148
    metastatic, sites, 152
    nonsmall cell anaplastic
        extensive, 157–158
        local, 153–156
    prognostic factors, 148–150, 157, 161–163
    small cell anaplastic, 158–163
        chemotherapy, 160–163
        diagnosis, 159
        prognostic factors, 161–163
        radiotherapy, 159–160, 162
        surgery, 159
    staging, 149, 150
    survival, 150, 155, 161
Lymphangiogram, Hodgkin's disease, 74, 79
Lymphadenopathy
    benign, differential diagnosis, 70–71
    as metastatic disease, 71

Lymphocytosis, absolute, chronic lymphocytic
    leukemia, 41, 45
Lymphocyte, chronic lymphocytic leukemia
    behavior, 41–43
    cell surface characteristics, 43–44
    morphology, 45, 47–49
Lymphoma. *See also* Hodgkin's disease;
    NonHodgkin's lymphoma;lym-
    phadenopathy, benign, diagnosis, 70–71
Lymphosarcoma cell leukemia, diagnosis,
    47–48, 49
Lymphosarcoma, bone marrow involvement, 11

M

Malnutrition, cancer patients, 363–365
Mastectomy, breast cancer, 104–105
Mammography, 110
Marrow aspirate, bone
    acute leukemia, 10–11
    chronic lymphocytic leukemia, 46, 47
    chronic myelocytic leukemia, 59, 64–65
    hairy cell leukemia, 26
    Hodgkin's disease, 78–79
Maxillary sinus carcinoma, 136–137
Mediastinoscopy, lung cancer, 151, 152
Megakaryocyte series abnormality, 4, 10
Melanoma, malignant, 257–273
    clinical features, 265–268
    definition, 257
    diagnosis, 268–269
    epidemiology, 258–259
    metastatic sites, 263, 265, 266–267
    pathology, 259–265
        pigmentation, 260
        satellite lesion, 260
        staging, 260, 269
    prognostic factors, 269–270
    survival, 269–270
    treatment, 270–272
Meningeal carcinomatosis, 190–192
    cerebral spinal fluid, 191
    in leukemia, 190–191
    in solid tumors, 191–192
6-Mercaptopurine,
    chronic myelocytic leukemia, 63, 66
    leukemia, pediatric, 297
Methotrexate,
    in acute leukemia, central nervous system
        prophylaxis, 19–20

in breast cancer, 106–109
in chronic myelocytic leukemia, 66
in head and neck cancer, 144–145
in lung cancer, small cell, 160–163
Miconazole, 354
Mitomycin C, in bladder cancer, 234
Mononuclear cell, abnormal, hairy cell
    leukemia, 26, 31–32
MOPP therapy, Hodgkin's disease, 82, 301
Mucositis, 145
Myelography, diagnosis spinal cord cancer,
    195–196

N

Nasal cavity cancer, 134–135
Nasopharyngeal cancer, 137
Nausea and vomiting, brain tumors, 171
Neck cancer. *See* Head and neck cancer
Nephrectomy, 205
Neuroblastoma, 310–315
    classification, 311
    diagnosis, 311, 315
    incidence, 310
    prognosis, 315
    treatment, 315
Neutropenia, infection, 322–323
Nitrogen mustard, in Hogkin's disease, 82, 301
Nocardiosis, 338
NonHodgkin's lymphoma, 82–94
    Burkitt's type, 84, 87, 88
    chemotherapy
        combination, 90–91, 92–94
        single agent, 89
    classification, pathologic, 83–86
    clinical features, 82–83
    diffuse, 83, 85, 91–94
    histiocytic, 83, 86–87
    large cell, 83, 86–87
    nodular, 88–89, 92
    pediatric, 298–299
    staging, 89
    survival, 91, 92, 93
5'-Nucleotidase, chronic lymphocytic leukemia,
    46
Null cell, nonHodgkin's lymphoma, 85
Null cell proliferation, leukemia, 5, 43
Nutrition, cancer patient, 363–370
    malnutrition, 363–365
    nutritional support, 365–369

O

Oral cavity cancer, 129-134
Oropharyngeal cancer, 137-139
Osteosarcoma, 285-286
    chemotherapy, 286
    diagnosis, 285
    prognostic factors, 285-286
    surgery, 286
Ovary carcinoma, 245-250
    classification, histologic, 249
    clinical features, 247
    diagnosis, 248
    FIGO staging system, 248
    prognostic factors, 248
    survival, 250
    treatment, 249-250

P

Pain,
    flank, renal carcinoma, 203
    pancreatic carcinoma, 118-119
Pancreas, carcinoma, 117-121
    diagnosis, 120-121
    etiology, 118
    pathology, 118
Pancreatic oncofetal antigen, 120
Pancytopenia, hairy cell leukemia, 31-32
Papanicolaou classification, cervical cancer,
    253
Paracoagulation syndrome, acute nonlymphocy-
    tic leukemia, 12
Paranasal sinus cancer, 135-137
Parenteral nutrition, 368-369
Pediatric cancer, 295-316
    brain tumor, 308-310
    Hodgkin's disease, 300-301
    leukemia, 296-298
    neuroblastoma, 310-315
    nonHodgkin's lymphoma, 298-299
    rhabdomyosarcoma, embryonal, 301-304
    sarcoma, bone, 305-308
    Wilm's tumor, 304-305
Penectomy, 218, 221, 222
Penicillin, 344-353
Penis carcinoma, 218-222
    clinical features, 219-221
    diagnosis, 221
    incidence, geographic, 219
    pathology, 219

staging, 221
treatment, 221-222
PEPA. See Protected environment-prophylactic
    antibiotic program
Performance status, lung cancer, 149
Phagocytosis, hairy cell leukemia cell, 28
Phenylalanine mustard,
    chronic myelocytic leukemia, 63
    melanoma, malignant, 271
Philadelphia chromosome, chronic myelocytic
    leukemia, 58, 60
Phycomycosis, 337-338
Pneumoencephalography, 180
Pneumocystis carinii, 331, 341-342
    leukemia, 17, 35
Pneumonia, 328-329
    leukemia, 15, 35
Prednisone,
    in acute lymphocytic leukemia, 13
    in breast cancer, 106-109
    in chronic lymphocytic leukemia, 50
    in Hodgkin's disease, 82, 301
    in nonHodgkin's lymphoma, 89-90
Preleukemic syndrome, 7-8, 10
Procarbazine, in Hodgkin's disease, 82, 301
Prolymphocytic leukemia, 48, 49
Prostate cancer, 237-241
    diagnosis, 238, 239
    etiology, 237
    pathology, 237-238
    staging, 238
    treatment, 239-241
Prostatectomy, 239-240
Protected environment-prophylactic antibiotic
    program, 357-358
Proteus vulgaris, hairy cell leukemia, 35
Protozoan infection, 341-343
Pseudomonas aeruginosa, 330, 331-333
    acute leukemia, 16
Psychomotor activity, slow, brain tumor, 171
Pyelography, retrograde, renal pelvis car-
    cinoma, 207

R

Radiation, role in development,
    acute nonlymphocytic leukemia, 8
    breast cancer, 101
    chronic myelocytic leukemia, 57-58
Radiation morbidity, brain tumor, 187
Radiotherapy,
    acute leukemia, 20

bladder cancer, 236
brain tumor, pediatric, 310
breast cancer, 105–106
cervical cancer, 253
chronic lymphocytic leukemia, 51
chronic myelocytic leukemia, spleen, 63
head and neck cancer, 143–144
Hodgkin's disease, 80–81
    pediatric, 301
interference with host defense, 326
lung cancer
    nonsmall cell, 154–155
    small cell, 159–160, 162
melanoma, malignant, 271
nonHodgkin's lymphoma, pediatric, 299
prostate cancer, 240–241
renal carcinoma, 205–206
sarcoma,
    Ewing's, 288–289
    soft tissue, 283
testicular cancer, 227, 230
urethral carcinoma, female, 216
Wilm's tumor, 305
Radionuclide brain scan, 180, 182
Rappaport classification, nonHodgkin's lymphoma, 85
Rectal cancer, 116
Reed-Sternberg cell, Hodgkin's disease, 73, 75
Renal carcinoma, 201–206
    clinical manifestation, 203
    diagnosis, 203
    etiology, 201
    pathology, 201–202
    staging, 203–204
    treatment, 205–206
Renal pelvis carcinoma, 206–210
    diagnosis, 207, 209
    etiology, 206–207
    nephroureterectomy, 210
    pathology, 207
    staging, 209–210
Reticuloendotheliosis , leukemia. See Hairy cel leukemia; Leukemia, hairy cell
Rhabdomyosarcoma, 281–282
    embryonal, 301–304

S

Salivary gland cancer, 142
Salmonella, 331, 333
Sarcoma, 275–293
    bone, 284–290

chondrosarcoma, 286–287
Ewing's, 287–289
giant cell tumor, 289
histiocytic, fibrous, 289
osteosarcoma, 285–286, 305–308
diagnosis, 276–277
incidence, 275–276, 279
soft tissue, 277–284
    chemotherapy, 283–284
    classification, 278
    histiocytoma, fibrous, malignant, 280–281
    incidence, 279
    prognostic factors, 282–283
    radiotherapy, 283
    rhabdomyosarcoma, 281–282
    staging, 282–283
    surgery, 283
Seizure, in brain tumor, 171–172, 187–188
Septicemia, 329–330
    leukemia, 16–18, 35
Serratia marcescens, 333
    leukemia, acute, 16
Sigmoidoscopy, colorectal cancer, 117
Skin infection, 330
Splenectomy, leukemia, 33–34, 62
Sphenoidal sinus cancer, 136
Splenomegaly, leukemia, 26, 29, 41, 44
Smoking, role in development lung cancer, 147–148
Spinal cord cancer, 192–196
    classification, histopathologic, 192–194
    clinical manifestation, 194–195
    diagnosis, 195–196
    incidence, 192–194
Sputum cytology, lung cancer, 151
Staphylococcus aureus, 35
Steroid. See specific compounds
Stomach carcinoma, 121–123
    clinical presentation, 122–12
    diagnosis, 123
    etiology, 121
    pathology, 122
Sulfamethoxazole, acute leukemia, 18
Sunlight,
    lip cancer, 128–129
    melanoma, malignant, 258
Surgery,
    bladder cancer, 234, 236
    brain tumor, pediatric, 310
    breast cancer, 104–105
    cervix carcinoma, 253
    head and neck cancer, 143

Surgery (*cont.*)
  lung cancer,
    nonsmall cell, 154–155
    small cell, 159
  melanoma, malignant, 270–271
  neuroblastoma, 315
  penile carcinoma, 221, 222
  prostate cancer, 239–241
  renal carcinoma, 205
  sarcoma,
    osteosarcoma, 286
    rhabdomyosarcoma, 304
    soft tissue, 283
  testicular cancer, 230–231
  ureteral carcinoma, 210–211
  urethral carcinoma, 216, 218
  Wilm's tumor, 306
Survival,
  breast cancer, 109
  Hodgkin's disease, 76, 81
  lung cancer, 150, 155, 161
  melanoma, malignant, 269–270
  nonHodgkin's lymphoma, 91, 92, 93
  ovarian cancer, 250

T

T cell, chronic lymphocytic leukemia, 43
Temporal lobe-tentorial herniation, 177–179
Testis cancer, 222–231
  choriocarcinoma, pure, 224, 226
  clinical features, 226–227
  diagnosis, 227
  embryonal cancer, 224, 225
  etiology, 222
  nonseminoma, 224–226, 230–231
  seminoma, 223–224, 227, 230
  staging, 227
  teratoma, mature, 224, 225
  treatment, 227–231
Thiotepa, in bladder cancer, 234
Thioguanine, in chronic myelocytic leukemia,
  66
Thrombocytosis, chronic myelocytic leukemia,
  59

Thrombocytopenia, leukemia, 14–15, 46, 59, 64
TNM classification, lung cancer, 149
Tobacco, role in development
  head and neck cancer, 127–128
  lung cancer
Tomography,
  brain tumor, 179–181, 183, 185
  spinal cord tumor, 195
Toxoplasma, acute leukemia, 17
Toxoplasma gondii, 342–343
Transfusion, 14–15, 18, 354–356
Transurethral biopsy, 214, 217
Trimethoprim, in acute leukemia, 18
Tuberculosis, 334–335
Turcot's syndrome, colorectal cancer, 115

U

Ureter carcinoma, 210–211
Urethral carcinoma,
  female, 212–216
  male, 216–218

V

Vidarabine, 354
Vincristine,
  in acute lymphocytic leukemia, 13
  in breast cancer, 106–109
  in Hodgkin's disease, 82, 301
  in lung cancer, small cell, 160–161
  in nonHodgkin's lymphoma, 89–90
Viral infection, 338–341
  hairy cell leukemia, 35
Vomiting, nausea, brain tumor, 171
VP-16. *See* Etoposide

W

Weight loss, prognostic factor, 363–364
White blood cell pattern, chronic myelocytic
  leukemia, chronic phase, 61
WHO classification, lung cancer, 148
Wilm's tumor, 304–305
WPL classification, lung cancer, 146